F. Kubli N. Patel W. Schmidt O. Linderkamp (Eds.)

Perinatal Events and Brain Damage in Surviving Children

With 51 Figures and 173 Tables

Springer-Verlag Berlin Heidelberg New York
London Paris Tokyo

Prof. Dr. med. Fred Kubli †
Klinikum der Universität Heidelberg, Frauenklinik
Voßstraße 9, 6900 Heidelberg, FRG

Dr. Naren Patel
Consultant Obstetrician, The University Dundee,
Reproductive Medicine Office, Wards 37/38, Level 6,
Ninewells Hospital, Dundee DD2 1UD, UK

Prof. Dr. med. W. Schmidt
Klinikum der Universität Heidelberg, Frauenklinik
Voßstraße 9, 6900 Heidelberg, FRG

Prof. Dr. med. O. Linderkamp
Klinikum der Universität Heidelberg, Kinderklinik
Im Neuenheimer Feld, 6900 Heidelberg, FRG

ISBN-13: 978-3-642-72852-5 e-ISBN-13: 978-3-642-72850-1
DOI: 10.1007/978-3-642-72850-1

Library of Congress Cataloging-in-Publication Data
Perinatal events and brain damage in surviving children.
Based on papers presented at an international conference held in Heidelberg in 1986 under the auspices of the Committee on Perinatal Mortality and Morbidity of the International Society of Gynaecology and Obstetrics (FIGO). Includes bibliographies.
1. Birth injuries - Complications and sequelae - Congresses. 2. Fetal anoxia - Complications and sequelae - Congresses. 3. Brain damaged children - Congresses.
I. Kubli, F. (Fred) II. International Federation of Gynecology and Obstetrics. Committee on Perinatal Mortality and Morbidity. [DNLM: 1. Asphyxia, Neonatorum - complications - congresses. 2. Birth Injuries - congresses. 3. Brain Damage, Chronic - etiology - congresses. 4. Brain Damage, Chronic - in infancy & childhood - congresses. 5. Fetal Anoxia - complications - congresses. 6. Perinatology - congresses. WS 405 P445 1986]
RJ325.P46 1988 618.5 87-24331
ISBN-13: 978-3-642-72852-5

Softcover reprint of the hardcover 1st edition 1988

Typesetting, printing and binding: Appl, Wemding
2121/3145-543210

Dedication

It was with great sadness that we learnt of the untimely death of Professor Fred Kubli in Heidelberg shortly before the publication of this volume.

The proceedings recorded in this volume result from the last workshop organised by Professor Kubli as Chairman of the FIGO Standing Committee on Perinatal Mortality and Morbidity to which he gave such devoted service over many years.

His aim in bringing together various people from all over the world for this workshop was to bring awareness to obstetricians about events that occur during pregnancy and the subsequent brain damage in children and to try and reduce this.

In remembrance of his tremendous contribution to our specialty and to FIGO, this volume is dedicated to Professor Kubli.

Preface

Decision making in modern obstetrics and perinatology is controlled by a variety of different factors, but there is little doubt that in industrialized countries one of the most powerful single factors is the concern and fear of causing permanent brain damage in the unborn and newborn. The dramatic increase in the rates of abdominal deliveries in many parts of the world is certainly rooted to a substantial part in the obstetrician's concern not so much about possible perinatal death, but more so about permanent brain damage in surviving children. This trend has been accelerated by the increasing number of litigations in connection with brain damage observed in many societies. This problem itself has many aspects, but it seems evident that litigation - justified or unjustified - is one modern expression of the human and social tragedy inflicted on individuals and families by the birth of a brain-damaged child.

The medical, social, and human importance of the problem is in sharp contrast to the relative lack of scientific knowledge available. This became very clear when the National Institutes of Health published the excellent review in 1985 on "Prenatal and Perinatal Factors Associated with Brain Disorders" and its editor, J. M. Freeman, summarized the situation as follows: "Our review of the pre- and perinatal causes of mental retardation, cerebral palsy and epilepsy has revealed how little we know of the factors controlling, altering or modifying brain development - how minimal [is] our knowledge of the causes of these disabling conditions."

It was with this knowledge and against this background that an international conference was organized in Heidelberg in 1986 with special consideration of the relationship of perinatal events and brain damage in surviving children. The conference was held under the auspices of the Committee on Perinatal Mortality and Morbidity of the International Society of Gynaecology and Obstetrics (FIGO), of which one of us (F. K.) held the function of the Chairman. The aim of the conference was to more clearly separate scientifically based knowledge from myths, to determine the extent to which the enormous increase in measurable data during the perinatal period - which characterizes modern perinatal medicine - could be related both to the risk and to the event of brain damage, and thus to contribute to enabling obstetricians and neonatalogists to make more rational decisions. This book is the result of the joint effort of outstanding physiologists, epidemiologists, neurologists, obstetricians, and neonatalogists and at present undoubtedly gives the most comprehensive assessment of the known relationships between perinatal events and later brain damage. In different sections, pathophysiological mechanisms, epidemiological data, and the problems of chronic deprivation and hypoxia, of acute intrapartum asphyxia and birth trauma, and of prematurity are presented and discussed. It seems to be rather clear that isolated intelligence defects (mental retardation) are in general not due to perinatal events, but to genetic factors or early maldevelopment, whereas neurologic impairment with or without intelligence defects, notably cerebral palsy, is more likely to be related to obstetrical and neonatal conditions. Hypoxia in this context is still the most important single cause. Pathophysiological mechanisms such as loss of autoregulation and the development of hypoxic-ischemic encephalopathy are better understood. It has been shown, by prospective randomized studies as well as by hospital-based retrospective studies, that prevention of intrapartum hypoxia by modern obstetrical techniques does reduce the incidence of impaired brain function in neonates. There is ample evidence that optinization of neonatal intensive care in very premature and very low birth weight children may decrease the relative frequencies of later handicaps.

Again, however, relatively few questions can be clearly answered and many more remain unsolved. Thus, the influence of modern perinatal medicine on the incidence of cerebral palsy and other forms of brain damage remains at best controversial. Reliable epidemiologic data are widely lacking. Whereas acute and severe asphyxia are undoubtedly possible causes of cerebral palsy, their frequency and relative epidemiologic importance are felt by many to be relatively small. Moreover, the individual tolerance of the fetal or neonatal brain to hypoxia and asphyxia is widely unpredictable, and it remains unclear why some babies develop cerebral palsy after severe asphyxia and others do not. It seems clear that mild and short-lasting hypoxia does not cause brain damage, but that the relationship between pathological antepartum fetal heart rate and later impairment points to the possible role of chronic and longer lasting hypoxia. Again, however, quantitative data are widely lacking. The relative roles of maldevelopment on the one hand and of chronic or acute hypoxia on the other, including in the genesis of cerebral palsy, remains controversial but there is some evidence that multifactorial pathogenesis is not uncommon. The initial goals of the conference were only partly reached. For practical purposes, it is clear that severe peripartum asphyxia should be avoided whenever possible and if present, should be kept as short as possible since the risk of brain damage increases with severity and duration of asphyxia; a situation of substantial chronic hypoxia, as manifested for example by chronic antepartum fetal heart rate, should be kept as short as possible. Yet, data are not available which support higher cesarean section rates in order to prevent "minimal hypoxia" with respect to later brain damage. With regard to litigation, the possibility that signs of peripartum asphyxia are not a cause but rather a marker for possible pre-existing brain damage has to be paid more attention than previously.

The editors wish to express their thanks to all the authors, whose careful preparation and timely delivery of the manuscripts has made this publication possible. They are furthermore indebted to the Springer Verlag for the excellent collaboration and the careful processing of the material for publication.

It is our hope that this book will contribute to drawing the attention of those responsible for research and the support of research to the enormous need for further research on fetal and neonatal brain development and the factors interfering with it. Modern obstetrics has - in industrialized countries - successfully met the challenge of maternal mortality and, more recently and together with neonatology, has also to a large part met that of perinatal mortality. For the coming years, the major challenge for perinatal medicine will be the definition of its role with respect to the quality of life of the survivors.

F. Kubli
N. Patel
W. Schmidt
O. Linderkamp

Table of Contents

Intrauterine Deprivation - Growth Retardation and Chronic Hypoxia

Intrapartum Asphyxia and Birth Trauma

Intracranial Hemorrhage and Ischemia

Prognosis of the Very Low Birthweight and Very Preterm Infant

List of Contributors

C. AMIEL-TISON
Baudelocque Maternity Hospital, 123, Boulevard Port-Royal, 75015 Paris, France

A. AZNÁREZ
Departamento de Perinatologia, Hopital de Clinicas, Piso 16, Av. Italia S/N, Montevideo, Uruguay

R. BELITZKY
Departamento de Perinatologia, Hopital de Clinicas, Piso 16, Av. Italia S/N, Montevideo, Uruguay

J. BOUYER
INSERM Unité 170, Epidémiologie et Statistiques sur l'Environment de la Santé, Villejuif, France

M. BRAND
Abteilung Neonatologie, Klinikum der Universität, Zentrum der Kinderheilkunde, Theodor-Stern-Kai 7, 6000 Frankfurt/Main 70, FRG

G. BREART
INSERM, Unité de Recherches Epidémiologiques sur la Mère et l'Enfant, 123, Boulevard de Port-Royal, 75014 Paris, France

R. CALDEYRO-BARCIA
Departamento de Perinatologia, Hopital de Clinicas, Piso 16, Av. Italia S/N, Montevideo, Uruguay

J. L. DÍAZ ROSSELLO
Departamento de Perinatologia, Hopital de Clinicas, Piso 16, Av. Italia S/N, Montevideo, Uruguay

M. J. DIJXHOORN
University Hospital, Department of Obstetrics and Gynaecology, Oostersingel 59, 9713 EZ Groningen, The Netherlands

J. Dreyfus
Hôpital de Haguenau, France

C. M. Drillien
2 Mayfield Road, Edinburgh, EH9 2NJ, UK

P. M. Dunn
University of Bristol, Department of Child Health, Southmead Hospital, Southmead Road, Bristol, BS10 5NB, UK

J. H. Ellenberg
Biometry and Field Studies Branch, National Institute of Neurological and Communicative Disorders and Stroke, Bethesda, Maryland 20892, USA

D. Fonseca
Departamento de Perinatologia, Hopital de Clinicas, Piso 16, Av. Italia S/N, Montevideo, Uruguay

A. Fournie
INSERM U 168, Department of Obstetrics and Gynecology, Hôpital La Grave, 31052 Toulouse, France

H. Grandjean
INSERM U 168, Department of Obstetrics and Gynecology, Hôpital La Grave, 31052 Toulouse, France

A. Grant
National Perinatal Epidemiology Unit, Radcliffe Infirmary, Oxford, OX2 6HE, UK

G. Greisen
Department of Neonatology, Rigshospitalet, 2100 Copenhagen, Denmark

G. Haas
Universitäts-Kinderklinik, Abteilung Entwicklungsneurologie, Frondsbergstraße 23, 7400 Tübingen, FRG

B. Hagberg
Department of Pediatrics II, Gothenburg University, East Hospital, 41685 Gothenburg, Sweden

G. Hagberg
Department of Pediatrics II, Gothenburg University, East Hospital, 41685 Gothenburg, Sweden

E. HALBERSTADT
Abteilung Neonatologie, Klinikum der Universität, Zentrum der Kinderheilkunde, Theodor-Stern-Kai 7, 6000 Frankfurt/Main 70, FRG

P. A. HAMILTON
Department of Paediatrics, School of Medicine, The Rayne Institute, University Street, London, WC1E 6JJ, UK

K. HELMKE
Kinderklinik, Universitäts-Krankenhaus Eppendorf, Martinistraße 52, 2000 Hamburg 20, FRG

O. HJALMARSON
Department of Pediatrics II, Gothenburg University, East Hospital, 41685 Gothenburg, Sweden

E. HOCHULI
Department of Gynecology and Obstetrics, Kantonsspital Münsterlingen, 8596 Münsterlingen, Switzerland

P. HOPE
Department of Paediatrics, John Radcliffe Hospital, Headington, Oxford, UK

V. VON LOEWENICH
Abteilung Neonatologie, Klinikum der Universität, Zentrum der Kinderheilkunde, Theodor-Stern-Kai 7, 6000 Frankfurt/Main 70, FRG

C. LÓPEZ DE CAYAFFA
Departamento de Perinatologia, Hopital de Clinicas, Piso 16, Av. Italia S/N, Montevideo, Uruguay

U. LORENZ
Frauenklinik, Universitäts-Klinikum Steglitz, Hindenburgdamm 30, 1000 Berlin 45, FRG

H. C. LOU
John F. Kennedy Institute, Gl. Landevej 7, 2600 Glostrup, Denmark

H. MANZKE
Universitäts-Kinderklinik, Schwanenweg 20, 2300 Kiel, FRG

H. MENTZEL
Universitäts-Kinderklinik, Abteilung Neonatologie, Frondsbergstraße 23, 7400 Tübingen, FRG

R. L. Naeye
Department of Pathology, M. S. Hershey, Medical Center,
The Pennsylvania State University, College of Medicine,
Hershey, Pennsylvania 17033, USA

K. B. Nelson
Developmental Neurology Branch, Federal Building, Room 8C-04,
7550 Wisconsin Avenue, Bethesda, Maryland 20892, USA

K. R. Niswander
Department of Obstetrics and Gynecology, University of
California, 1621 Alhambra Blvd., Suite 2500, Sacramento,
CA 95816, USA

B. Ohrt
Universitäts-Kinderklinik, Lindwurmstraße 4, 8000 München 2,
FRG

E. Papiernik
INSERM Unité 187, Physiologie et Psychologie de
la Reproduction Humaine, Université Paris-Sud,
Hôpital Antoine Béclère, 157, rue de la Porte de Trivaux,
92141 Clamart, France

E. C. Peters
Department of Pathology, M. S. Hershey, Medical Center,
The Pennsylvania State University, College of Medicine, Hershey,
Pennsylvania 17033, USA

G. Pontonnier
INSERM U 168, Department of Obstetrics and Gynecology,
Hôpital La Grave, 31052 Toulouse, France

H. F. R. Prechtl
Department of Developmental Neurology, University of
Groningen, Oostersingel 59, 9713 EZ Groningen, The Netherlands

E. O. R. Reynolds
Department of Paediatrics, University College London, School of
Medicine, The Rayne Institute, University Street, London,
WC1E 6JJ, UK

K. P. Riegel
Universitäts-Kinderklinik, Lindwurmstraße 4, 8000 München 2,
FRG

G. ROOTH
Abteilung Geburtshilfe, Kantonsspital, 8063 Zürich, Switzerland

R. RUGGIA
Departamento de Perinatologia, Hopital de Clinicas, Piso 16, Av. Italia S/N, Montevideo, Uruguay

E. SALING
Abteilung Geburtsmedizin, Frauenklinik Neukölln, Mariendorfer Weg 28, 1000 Berlin 44, FRG

M.-F. SARRAMON
INSERM U 168, Department of Obstetrics and Gynecology, Hôpital La Grave, 31052 Toulouse, France

I. AUS DER SCHMITTEN
Universitäts-Kinderklinik, Abteilung Entwicklungsneurologie, Frondsbergstraße 23, 7400 Tübingen, FRG

F. J. SCHULTE
Kinderklinik des Universitäts-Krankenhauses Eppendorf, Martinistraße 52, 2000 Hamburg 20, FRG

Z. STEIN
G. H. Sergievsky Center, Columbia University, 630 West 168th Street, NewYork, NY 10032, USA

A. STEWART
Departments of Paediatrics and Obstetrics, University College London, School of Medicine, The Rayne Institute, University Street, London WC1R 6JJ, UK

K. STOLLHOFF
Kinderklinik, Universitäts-Krankenhaus Eppendorf, Martinistraße 52, 2000 Hamburg 20, FRG

M. SUSSER
G. Sergievsky Center, Columbia University, 630 West 168th Street, New York, NY 10032, USA

A. TWEED
Department of Anesthesia, University Hospital, P.O. Box 5339, London, Ontario N6A 5A5, Canada

N. VEELKEN
Kinderklinik, Universitäts-Krankenhaus Eppendorf, Martinistraße 52, 2000 Hamburg 20, FRG

H. T. VERSMOLD
Abteilung Neonatologie, Klinikum der Universität Großhadern, P.O. Box 701260, 8000 München 70, FRG

G. H. A. VISSER
Department of Obstetrics and Gynecology, University Hospital, Oostersingel 59, 9713 EZ Groningen, The Netherlands

F. VOGEL
Institut für Anthropologie und Humangenetik, Im Neuenheimer Feld 328, 6900 Heidelberg, FRG

H. P. VOGT
Department of Gynecology and Obstetrics, Kantonsspital Münsterlingen, 8596 Münsterlingen, Switzerland

C. B. VULLIAMY
University of Bristol, Department of Child Health, Southmead Hospital, Southmead Road, Bristol, BS10 5NB, UK

J. S. WIGGLESWORTH
Department of Paediatrics and Neonatal Medicine, Royal Postgraduate Medical School, Hammersmith Hospital, Du Cane Road, London, W12 OHS, UK

P. WINKLER
Kinderklinik, Universitäts-Krankenhaus Eppendorf, Martinistraße 52, 2000 Hamburg 20, FRG

Epidemiology

Definitions, Risks, and Indices

M. SUSSER and Z. STEIN

Certain words, often used loosely in everyday language, have acquired a more precise meaning in epidemiology. As a contribution to this exchange between obstetricians, pediatricians, pathologists, and epidemiologists, we begin by defining some of these terms; next, we describe some concepts of risk basic to epidemiologic judgments; lastly, we introduce the terminology we have found useful in approaching neurodevelopmental disability. A fuller source for all this discussion, and one that includes the key references, is Susser et al. (1985).

Definitions

First, we need to distinguish *incidence* from *prevalence. Incidence* describes the frequency with which disorders arise in a population during a defined period of time. This is straightforward, when the origin of the disorder (i.e., the time when it arises) is a well-marked event, as for instance, a case of influenza or measles. The time period needs to be specified; most often it will be defined as one calendar year. The incidence rate is then the number of cases divided by the population multiplied by 1000.

If there is uncertainty as to when the disorder arises, however, incidence is less straightforward, and this is a problem that besets us with neurodevelopmental disorders, for instance, cerebral palsy (CP). Did the disorder arise at birth, or earlier? As this question will probably arise many times in this volume, there is no need to belabor it here, save to illustrate the ambiguities that the uncertainty creates in the use of the term incidence.

Prevalence describes the amount of disorder existing in a population at a particular time, regardless of time of onset. It is clear that the prevalence of CP at birth could be measured without making any assumptions about the time at which the disorder set in. On the one hand, if the prevalence at birth is to yield a complete picture of that condition in the population, all cases would need to be apparent at birth and diagnosed at that stage. In practice, all cases cannot be diagnosed at birth: in some infants, the manifestations only appear some time after birth. On the other hand, if prevalence is assessed only at, say, 3 years of age, then some severely affected children will not have survived to enter the count; at the same time, in some children CP is diagnosed in infancy, but later in childhood (3 years) the criteria for the diagnosis are no longer met. Therefore prevalence poses problems of both under- and over-ascertainment.

Whether the chosen measure of disease frequency is incidence or prevalence, care is needed in the description of the data, its collection, and its interpretation.

A relationship, of course, exists between the incidence and the prevalence of a disorder: prevalence is a function of the incidence and the duration of the disorder. When either incidence or duration is known, inferences about the other can be drawn from prevalence studies. Again, however, one must be cautious because this relationship does not hold if either incidence or duration has changed over the period between the usual age of incident cases and the age of the subjects contributing to prevalence. In CP we have reason to believe that incidence (at birth) and duration (survival of affected cases) have indeed changed over the short term. Thus Hagberg et al. (1984), in interpreting time trends in the prevalence of CP in early childhood in south-western Sweden over the years 1959–1978, invoke changes in both incidence and mortality to explain the observed fluctuations in prevalence. These interpretations must remain tentative, pending further studies.

Risks

Relative Risk and Odds Ratios: Establishing Associations

Relative Risk (RR) is the ratio of the frequency of a disorder in a group that experiences a risk factor to the frequency of the disorder in a comparable group without the risk factor.

$RR = Ie/Iu$, where Ie is the incidence rate in the "exposed" group that experiences the factor, and Iu is the incidence rate in the "unexposed" group that does not. In studies of cause, this ratio is the most useful index of the strength of the relationship of a factor to a particular outcome. The value of the ratio can be adjusted as needed to control the unwanted effects of related factors that occur together with the factor under study.

RR estimates use different equations and assumptions depending on the study design. Looking forward, cohort studies compare frequencies of a given outcome among exposed and unexposed cohorts. They define their study populations from a common point of entry to observation, whether the recruitment is at birth, or attendance at prenatal clinic, or admission to hospital, etc. Those exposed to a given or suspected factor are compared in terms of the frequency of the specified outcome with those unexposed. Looking backward, case-control studies compare the frequencies of a history of a given risk factor among persons affected by a disorder and among persons unaffected (controls). They define their study populations in terms of persons known to have, or to be free from, the disease or outcome of interest.

The schema of Table 1 encompasses risk estimates for both cohort and case-control studies. In cohort studies, in which we begin with the knowledge of who is exposed and discover who becomes affected, the ratio of those affected among the

Table 1. Risk estimates for cohort and case-control studies

Exposure	Disorder		All
	Affected	Not affected	
+	a	b	$a+b$
−	c	d	$c+d$
All	$a+c$	$b+d$	$a+b+c+d$

exposed $(a/a+b)$ is compared to the ratio among those unexposed $(c/c+d)$. $RR=(a/a+b)/(c/c+d)$. In case-control studies the frequency of exposure in the population, $(a+b)$ and $(c+d)$, is not known. We begin with cases, persons who have the disorder $(a+c)$, and controls who do not $(b+d)$, and discover the frequency of exposure (obtained retrospectively) among each group. Because $a+b$ and $c+d$ are not known, the RR, $(a/a+b)/(c/c+d)$, cannot be estimated directly. Fortunately, a simple approximation of the RR, the *odds ratio*, ad/bc (also known as the cross products ratio), gives a robust estimate under most conditions (but not all). This expression can be derived intuitively from the RR, as follows: $(a/a+b)/(c/c+d)=a(c+d)/c(a+b)$.

The derivation to the odds ratio requires the assumption that the disease is rare among both the exposed and the unexposed. Then $a(c+d)$ is approximately equal to ad (because c is so rare) and $c(a+b)$ is approximately equal to cb (because a is rare). Thus $a(c+d)/c(a+b)$ becomes ad/cb.

Thus ad/cb, the odds ratio, may be estimated directly from the terms present in case-control studies. The odds ratio is a stable and extremely useful statistic for case-control studies. Odds ratios are the cornerstone for such studies, which comprise the great majority of epidemiological studies today. With a rare disease, a sufficient number of cases to test a hypothesis can often not be obtained from cohort studies without cohort studies of enormous size observed over many years. In case-control studies, the researcher can usually select a series of well-described cases of a disease, however rare, that are sufficient in number to test a hypothesis. Thus a range of investigations that would otherwise be quite impractical becomes possible.

A relevant example is the relationship of CP to neonatal asphyxia. Because CP is rare, in a cohort study; literally tens of thousands of deliveries would need to be evaluated for asphyxia and followed through the period of risk for the appearance of CP in order to generate a sufficient number of neonates to study this association in detail. To study the same question in a case-control study, a sufficient number of incident or prevalent cases and of suitable controls could be much more readily assembled, provided only that the exposure to asphyxia could be adequately described retrospectively.

As with incidence and prevalence, the complexities of design and analysis in both cohort and case-control studies need attention. Multivariate statistics have added to the range and precision and to the sophistication of interpretation of such studies. Their ultimate statistical base remains, as in Table 1, a risk estimate. With categorical disorders like CP these are risk ratios. - RR or odds ratios. (With continuous variables, other statistics come into play).

Attributable Risks

Attributable risk (AR) is the amount or proportion of a disorder in a given population that can be attributed to that factor. This risk estimate provides a means of expressing the public health significance of association. In other words, AR describes the presumed amount or proportion of a disorder that would not occur if the factor were to be removed. A risk factor is not necessarily a cause or determinant, however. It indicates only that a raised frequency of the condition under study is associated with the factor. AR is useful as an index of the quantitative importance of a given risk factor in the occurrence of a disorder. AR, in the first place, is a means of retrospective attribution of risk; that is, AR is a means of apportioning to a given "causal" factor an amount or proportion of cases of a disorder that has already occurred. In the second place, AR is a means of prediction; that is, AR is a means of estimating the excess risk of the disorder that would be produced by the factor. In ordinary circumstances, AR estimates can be made only for cohort studies and not for case-control studies.

Essential to estimates of AR, besides a group which experiences - or is exposed to - the factor, is an unexposed comparison group. Without comparison, the best that can be done is to state the proportion of a particular disorder ascribed to a given causal factor within a collection of cases of that disorder. Since this type of statement is often to be found in papers, and indeed by necessity in this review, we shall term this value "proportional morbidity by factor" (PMF).

However representative cases may be of the incidence of a disorder in the population from which the cases are drawn, the PMF does not take account of frequency of the factor among unaffected persons in that population. Hence the PMF is inherently likely to produce an overestimate, because the value does not offset for the frequency with which the factor occurs without contributing to the occurrence of cases. Moreover, the PMF does not indicate the presence of an association between factor and outcome; any so-called cause can only be presumed to have an association with the outcome, since the factor may be as frequent in the unexamined population at large as it is among cases. Despite its weakness, the PMF may be the only statement that can be made from available data. The PMF can be useful in flagging strong associations, especially with exposures known to be rare in the general population, or with rare diseases occurring in special contexts such as industry.

Two common ways of stating attributable risk differ somewhat in concept and in arithmetic. The "excess risk"[1] (ER) describes the amount of a disorder that a given factor is presumed to cause, over and above the amount that would occur in its absence. That is, ER is the simple arithmetical difference by which incidence of the disorder in the exposed group exceeds that in the unexposed group. Another formulation has been described as the "attributable fraction" (AF)[2]. This estimate indicates the fraction or proportion of cases that can be attributed to the factor. That is, to obtain AF, the difference in *frequency* between exposed and unexposed

[1] Also called the "rate difference" or "risk difference" or "simple difference." "Rate" and "risk," while not themselves synonymous, are often used indiscriminately in this and other contexts.

[2] Called "etiological fraction" by Miettinen (1974).

groups is converted into a proportion of *frequency* in the exposed. Thus, removal of the factor in question can be expected to reduce the number of cases either by an *absolute* amount as indicated by the excess risk, or by a *proportion* as indicated by the AF.

Terminology for AR has not been standard and there is much confusion in the literature: as one example, sometimes AR has been used to describe both ER and AF, or only one or the other. Another difficulty is that available formulae use incidence as the measure of frequency, a natural step if one is trying to convey the magnitude of benefits to the public health that would accrue from prevention. We have already pointed to some complexities of incidence in assessing neurodevelopmental disorders. The formulae we present will respect the convention that the frequency measure is *incidence,* but the data presented in the analysis in the paper that follows may often use point prevalence or age-specific prevalence. In our view, these measures reflect the ultimate public health significance of each problem as well or better than incidence, although they incorporate duration and survival and are thus at one remove from the immediate impact of a causal factor upon the occurrence of a disorder.

In the usage chosen here, the ER and the AF must be qualified to distinguish three different values: (a) estimates that pertain to cases exposed to the factor; (b) estimates that pertain to all cases in the study population, both exposed and unexposed; (c) estimates that pertain to all cases in the population at large. With all these estimates an unexposed comparison group is essential to provide a reference standard for the frequency of the disorder that would occur in the absence of the factor; the differences between them reside in the choice of the group of cases within which the presumed effects of the risk factor are apportioned.

In the first instance, all cases are derived from the exposed cohort, and risk is apportioned solely among those cases; a subscript to indicate the restriction to exposed cases is convenient, as in ER_e and AF_e. ER_e is obtained by subtracting the incidence of the disorder among unexposed individuals from the corresponding rate among the exposed, on the assumption that all causes of the disorder other than the risk factor under study are equal in the two groups. ($Ie-Iu$, where Ie is the incidence rate among the exposed and Iu the incidence rate among the unexposed.) This arithmetical difference between the incidence in the two groups is sometimes expressed as the percentage by which frequency in the exposed group exceeds that in the unexposed, with the unexposed group taking the value of 100%. As a percentage excess, ER_e becomes $Ie-Iu/Iu \times 100$. Note that an equivalent expression can be obtained from the relative risk, namely $RR-1$.

In the AF, the excess of cases becomes the numerator of the fraction; the denominator of the fraction is the incidence rate of the disorder among the exposed (now, the frequency among the exposed takes the value of 100%). AF_e is described by the expression $Ie-Iu/Ie$. This expression can be written equivalently as $RR-1/RR$ where RR is the relative risk in the exposed versus the unexposed population; hence an estimate can be made if relative risk alone is known.

In the second instance, estimates go beyond exposed cases to apportion the risks pertaining to all cases in the *population under study* (ps), both the exposed and unexposed. The incidence of cases in the study population (I_{ps}) is, of course, the combined incidence in the exposed and unexposed cohorts under comparison.

Thus $I_{ps} = P_e I_e + P_u I_u$ where P_e is the proportion of the population exposed to the risk factor, and P_u the proportion unexposed. It is convenient to indicate the extension of the estimate by a subscript, as in ER_{ps} and AF_{ps}.

$$ER_{ps} = I_{ps} - I_{psu}$$

$$AF_{ps} = \frac{I_{ps} - I_{psu}}{I_{ps}}$$

The crucial difference from ER_e and AF_e is that ER_{ps} and AF_{ps} take into account the frequency of exposure to the factor in the population studied; since not all cases are likely to be exposed to a single factor, the estimates are to that extent reduced. These estimates are, of course, restricted by the character of the study population, which will be unrepresentative of the population at large because, deliberately or otherwise, the cohorts are selected for entry to a study by a variety of criteria.

In the third instance, when estimates are extrapolated from the study samples to the population at large, estimates must take account of the frequency of the causal factor in that population. To indicate AR in the population at large, in our usage the ER will be designated ER_{pl}[3] and the AF will be designated AF_{pl}.[4] The equations do not differ in principle for estimates for the study population or the population at large, although additional data are needed to extrapolate from the one to the other. Thus $ER_{pl} = I_{pl} - I_{pu}$, where I_{pl} is the frequency of the disorder in the population and I_{pu} the frequency in the segment of the population unexposed to the factor, i.e., $AF_{pl} = I_{pl} - I_{plu}/I_{pl}$. An equivalent expression is

$$AF_{pl} = \frac{P_e(RR-1)}{1+P_e(RR-1)}$$

hence an estimate can be made if only RR and P_e are known. As will be noted below, this is of importance for case-control studies.

If a cohort study contains exposed and unexposed individuals in proportions similar to those of the general population, the AF_{ps} calculated from the cohort study may be usable as an estimate of AF_{pl} in the population at large. If that is not the case, and many cohort studies are especially selected and not representative, the restrictions on AF_{ps} calculated from the study should be kept in mind.

For populations, AR may diverge quite markedly from RR. For the same factor in the same disorder, AR may diverge from RR because the estimate AR depends both upon RR and on the proportion of the given risk factor among other risk factors for the disorder in the population under study. For the same factor in different disorders, ARs may diverge from each other even when the RRs are the same because, unlike RR, ARs depend also upon the frequency in the population of the disorder under study.

A further caution is in order. We noted the implication of the term "attributable" in that elimination of the factor would reduce the incidence of the disease by the amount or fraction indicated by the AR estimate. We also noted that a risk factor is not necessarily causal. ARs are usually calculated from data generated from

[3] Also termed "population attributable risk".

[4] Well-named "Levin's attributable risk", and sometimes "population attributable risk per cent".

observational studies rather than from preventive intervention studies. It cannot, therefore, simply be assumed that all differences in disease incidence between the exposed and unexposed are in fact causally related to the factor under study. Other uncontrolled or unmeasured factors may be involved and not accounted for.

In addition, several factors may overlap in their effects to produce less than their sum, while others may interact to produce more than their sum. For this reason, some authors have developed AR estimates which are adjusted for potential confounding variables. The usual AR estimates calculated for single factors in cohort studies are perhaps best interpreted as upper limits of the amount or proportion of disease that could be prevented by eliminating the factor.

Under the circumstances of ordinary case-control studies, as noted, *attributable risk* cannot be derived since outcome rates are not observed. Under special circumstances - studies in which either all incident cases of the given disorder in a population are included, or studies in which the frequency of the factors under study is known - a reasonable estimate can be derived by extrapolation.[5]

Using CP again as our example, the fraction of cases attributable to perinatal mishaps could vary in different populations or at different times. They could vary with obstetrical policies and practices if such practices were to affect the incidence. Carefully collected population-based data, as we exemplified by the papers already mentioned from Sweden (Hagberg et al. 1984) and others (see review by Paneth and Kiely 1984), are needed to assess the public health significance of these changes.

Indices

Besides the complexities of measures and risks, there is yet another set of problems attached to epidemiological studies of neurodevelopmental disorders, and these relate to case definition. To be counted, cases must be distinguished from non-cases, but the lines of demarcation in many developmental disorders are blurred by confused definition. Thus, recognized disorder is in part a social attribute. With mental retardation, for example, recognition is a consequence of failures to perform the social roles demanded of individuals at each stage of life. The order of society determines how taxing these roles shall be. What is expected in particular social roles, therefore, varies with time and among societies, and among the classes of a single society. In particular, we emphasize the distinctions between "impairment", "disability", and "handicap", a classification of Stein and Susser that has since been adopted by the World Health Organization.

A handicapping condition encompasses organic, functional, and social components. The organic component, which we term "impairment", can be any persist-

[5] Levin's attributable risk (AF_{pl}) can be estimated from a case-control study where the proportion of controls exposed is a good estimate of the proportion exposed in the entire population (P_e). Then $AF_{pl} = E_{ca} - E_{co}/1 - E_{co}$, where E_{ca} and E_{co} are the proportions of cases and controls exposed, respectively.

ing physical or psychological defect which stems from molecular, cellular, physiological, or structural disorder. The functional component, which we term "disability", refers to persisting physical or psychological dysfunction; it stems from the limitations imposed both by the impairment, and by the individual's psychological reaction to it. The social component, which we term "handicap", refers to persisting social dysfunction, a social role that stems not from the individual but from the social expectations of others and the individual's interaction with society.[6] Handicap describes the manner and degree in which the expected performance of social roles is altered in the presence of primary impairment and functional disability.

Organic, psychological, and social criteria yield different frequencies and make different contributions to our understanding of a given condition. To take mental retardation as an example, components of the disorder measured by each criterion do not have a one-to-one relationship with each other, and they are made apparent by different circumstances. Impairments that can be recognized at birth and for which a one-to-one relationship with functional disability and social handicap can be predicted, as in Down's syndrome, are not common. CP is an impairment recognized by the signs of brain damage. Not all cases of CP suffer the functional disability of intellectual deficit, nor are all assigned the special social role of the handicapped person. Hydrocephalus is an anatomical deformity that may or may not be accompanied by cerebral impairment, or functional disability, or social handicap. Phenylketonuria is an inherited impairment of metabolism that does not always lead to functional disability and, when it does, treatment may avert or reduce the disability or handicap.

Conversely, recognized functional disability cannot always be related to definitive organic lesions. In a large proportion of cases of mental retardation even with severe intellectual deficits, a specific clinical diagnosis cannot be made. In these cases, the presence of organic impairment is merely assumed.[7] Severe mental retardation of unspecified diagnosis thus describes a residual class of cases that is heterogeneous in terms of organic impairment. Yet it is a homogeneous class in terms of functional disability and social handicap.

In mild mental retardation, on the other hand, the intellectual deficit and functional disability of the "cultural-familial" syndrome is not preceded by detectable organic impairment, and is not always accompanied by the social role of mental handicap. Sometimes the social role of mental handicap is assigned to individuals who have neither impairment of the brain nor intellectual disability. Their social roles are inadvertently acquired by their admission to "treatment" because of a combination of behavior disorders and lack of social support. Thus, even in the recent past, a proportion of the inmates of many institutions for mental deficiency have often had neither detectable clinical lesions nor IQ scores below the normal range.

---

[6] The dynamic analogues of these components of static and persisting disorders are disease (physiological or psychic pathology), illness (the subjective perception of physiological or psychic dysfunction), and sickness (the social role that accompanies the recognition of sickness by others).

[7] In uncontrolled studies of severe mental retardation, brain lesions have been found in 90% or more at autopsy.

Postcript

In this paper, we purposely chose to point to the complexities and limitations, as well as to the strengths, of the epidemiologists' craft in the joint enterprise of assessing the risks perinatal factors pose for neurological development. An interdisciplinary attack on a difficult problem calls for mutual understanding and demystification.

References

Freeman JM (ed) (1985) Prenatal and perinatal factors associated with brain disorders. USDHHS, April

Hagberg B, Hagberg G, Olow I (1984) The changing panorama of cerebral palsy in Sweden. IV. Epidemiological trends 1959-1978. Acta Pediatr Scand 73: 433-440

Miettinen OS (1974) Proportion of disease caused or prevented by a given exposure, trait or intervention. Am J Epidemiol 99: 325-332

Paneth N, Kiely JL (1984) The frequency of cerebral palsy: review of population studies in industrialized nations since 1950. In: Stanley F, Alberman E (eds) Epidemiology of cerebral palsies. Spastics International Medical Publications, London, pp 46-56

Susser M et al. (1985) Quantitative estimates of prenatal and perinatal risk factors for perinatal mortality, cerebral palsy, mental retardation and epilepsy. In: Freeman JM (ed) Prenatal and perinatal factors associated with brain disorders. USDHHS, pp 359-439

The Quantification of Risk Factors in Major Neurodevelopmental Disorders

M. SUSSER

My task is to review those risks that are subject to quantification for three major groups of neurodevelopmental disorders, namely, mental retardation, epilepsy, and cerebral palsy. The material is in large part taken from a chapter in the book *Prenatal and Perinatal Factors Associated With Brain Disorders* (Freeman 1985). The work for that chapter was shared with my Sergievsky Center colleagues, Hauser, Kiely, Paneth, and Stein. Since the publication of the book, two papers by Nelson and Ellenberg (1985 a, b) have appeared on the subject of risk factors in cerebral palsy in the National Collaborative Perinatal Project (NCPP). I have also drawn freely on this large body of new material.

We pointed out in the preceding paper that many measurement problems attend the effort to quantify risks. It may be wise here to re-emphasize some of these as they relate to inference about the causal role of the factors under review. Some large assumptions underly the application of the attributable risk idea which we use so freely in our presentation. First, a risk factor is not necessarily a part of a direct causal sequence leading from the factor to the outcome; quite often it will be a surrogate or index of some other underlying factor, or even of a group of heterogeneous factors, and its removal may not prevent the occurrence of the condition to which it relates. For many factors to be discussed the available evidence and the level of analysis are not enough to establish that they occur within a causal sequence. A risk factor indicates no more than that a raised risk for a given condition occurs in association with the factor. By itself, a raised risk associated with a particular factor does not confer on the factor a place in a causal sequence.

Secondly, risk factors are almost invariably multiple. For the most part, in the available data on neurodevelopmental impairment, they have been analyzed only one factor at a time. The result, in most cases, is to assign a maximum effect to the factor. The main reason for this is that the factors may overlap one another or occur in sequence; no account is taken of this often substantial overlap. In an analysis of one factor alone, the whole of the association will be consigned to that factor alone. It follows - as we shall see - that the sum of all single factors added together without adjustment can be more than 100%. If these problems are kept in mind, then attributable fractions, as described in the preceding paper, can give a useful idea of the size of a particular problem attached to a given indicator of risk, if not of the causal sequence that leads to it.

Even when analysis is multivariate, in an effort to deal with the problems of overlap, severe difficulties of interpretation persist. In multivariate analyses of the relationship of risk factors to outcomes, the construction of the analysis and the sequence in which variables are entered can have profound effects on the apparent contribution of any given factor or set of factors. In interpreting results of these kinds, it is essential to keep in mind what the possible causal models can be which could account for the results. This is often a difficult and complicated task. It does not readily yield to simple interpretation (Susser 1973).

Mental Retardation

Surprisingly, few studies of mental retardation in the population at large have examined its relation to prenatal and perinatal factors. In any such analysis, it is wise first to put aside cases that arise before the risk period of interest, namely, those of known chromosomal or genetic origins and, secondly, also to put aside mild mental retardation (MMR). With MMR, perinatal factors are overwhelmed by the frequency of the sociocultural or cultural/familial syndrome, which in many developed countries may comprise some 70% of the population ascertained with MMR (excepting, in recent years, in Sweden and, possibly, in Japan). Thus, MMR with detectable central nervous system signs that can reasonably be attributed to prenatal and perinatal impairment of the brain are by far the minority of cases, have a different origin and course from the sociocultural syndrome, and generally need to be analyzed separately.

Mental retardation, like all neurological handicaps, is measured differently according to the level of organization involved, whether impairment, disability, or handicap. The central concern here is with impairment, because we have in mind in this discussion a particular causal chain:

```
Prenatal/perinatal insult→impairment→disability→handicap
                          (brain      (cognitive (failure in
                          disorder)   deficit)   social role)
```

Thus we hypothesize that brain impairment owed to perinatal insult underlies the cognitive deficits and role failure that characterize mental retardation syndromes. The ascertainment of cases of mental retardation does not precisely meet the needs of the hypothesis, for it is generally psychometric (IQ, by definition) which yields indices of dysfunction and disability; or if not psychometric, ascertainment is social (school failure, job failure, social deviance) which yields indices of handicap. Thus the frequencies given by most population surveys are not direct measures of impairment; to get an estimated rate of impairment we need detailed clinical data on neurological state, which is seldom available in surveys. For the purposes of the hypotheses under test, then, surveys without these data are of limited use, and a first requirement for usefulness is for adequate diagnostic information. A second requirement is, of course, that information is provided on prenatal and perinatal risk factors. A third requirement is that the survey relates to a definable population. Data that meet these three requirements are quite rare.

Two Swedish surveys by the team of Hagberg, Gustavson and their colleagues proved useful in meeting the diagnostic and population requirements (Gustavson

Table 1. PMF in serious mental retardation in Sweden

Assigned Cause	PMF Uppsala (N=122) (%)	PMF Vasterbotten (N=161) (%)
Chromosomal	36	36
Single locus gene	7	16 (Intermarriage high)
Malformations:		
Recognized	2	8
Unclassifiable	18	-
Prenatal infection	2	0
"Fetal deprivation of supply"	8	8
Unknown, presumed prenatal	14	23
Perinatal (intrapartum and early neonatal)	10	8
Postnatal (any factor)	3	1

et al. 1976, 1977a, b; Hagberg 1978; Hagberg et al. 1981a). In these surveys, serious mental retardation is defined by an IQ level below 50, i.e., a functional psychometric criterion. Details of "presumed causes" are given, and at this level of severity, neuropathological studies allow us to assume that some kind of impairment is present in virtually all cases. Unfortunately, no reference or comparison group was examined, so that we cannot obtain either relative risks or attributable fractions and must make do with proportional morbidity by factor (PMF). Table 1 summarizes the data from these two studies. In this table we see that prenatal factors comprise 24% and 31%, respectively; together with perinatal factors, they comprise 34% and 39%, respectively. An important clue in these data is that among all cases assigned to prenatal and perinatal causes, 70% have frank signs of central nervous system damage. This high percentage, which is confined to the presumed prenatal/perinatal cases, suggests that both serious mental retardation, and the neurological signs, are the common consequence of overt cerebral abnormality or, in our interpretation, that they reflect cerebral palsy complicated by mental retardation. A second important result is that if the causal assignments of the Swedish surveys are correct - and one must emphasize that these rest on clinical judgment and not on epidemiological assessments of relative risks derived from the use of comparison groups - then it seems also that much the larger part of the damage arose prenatally and not perinatally.

The only risk factor that we can usefully examine in relation to mental retardation, in studies that meet the requirements we lay out above, is asphyxia, or various indices of asphyxia. In the 1958 British birth cohort, Peters, Golding and Lawrence (1984) used "respiratory delay" as an index of asphyxia. While the index did relate to newborn deaths and cerebral palsy, it did not relate to mental retardation (nor did it relate to epilepsy). Another attempt to relate asphyxia to mental retardation was made by Broman (1979) using the 54,000 births from 1959

Table 2. Neonatal respiratory difficulty among retarded children at 7 years, compared with children of average IQ (white children)

	%	RR (CL)	AF_{ps}
MR with CNS genetic abnormalities			
SMR	10.4	7.4 (3.6, 15.2)	8.2
MMR	14.3	10.2 (4.0, 25.6)	11.4
MR without CNS genetic abnormalities			
SMR	4.0	2.9 (0.4, 20)	2.5
MMR	3.6	2.6 (1.2, 5.8)	2.1

to 1966 of the NCPP. Broman used ten indicators including Apgar score, apnea, resuscitation, meconium, and fetal heart rate. Nine of the ten indicators had no association with mental retardation when they were screened in a discriminant function analysis. From this one might justifiably conclude that no association exists between asphyxia and mental retardation. The only indicator that did relate was "respiratory difficulty" recorded by pediatricians in the nursery. For what it is worth, we shall examine the results for this variable. The examination turns out, after all, to shed a little light on the problem.

In line with the perinatal hypothesis, we need to explore whether this one indicator of asphysia relates to detectable neurological impairment combined with mental retardation, or to mental retardation regardless of frank neurological deficit. We are able to extract some indication, if an imperfect one, of the risks for the separate conditions.

Table 2 separates the presence or absence of central nervous system abnormalities imperfectly since they are grouped together with genetic and chromosome abnormalities. What it shows is that when a detectable central nervous system lesion is present, then this single indicator of respiratory difficulty has a high relative risk and a high attributable fraction. When no detectable central nervous system lesion is present, then the relative risk and the attributable fraction are much reduced and are not statistically significant. Surprisingly, severe mental retardation (SMR) and MMR look much the same. The findings for black children are much the same as they are for whites.

If we can assume that this sign of respiratory difficulty as observed by pediatricians indicates an abnormal perinatal state, then the results, again, suggest that the association of mental retardation with prenatal/perinatal factors is, in the main, a reflection of clinically detectable central nervous system abnormality. Thus we incline to interpret the available data as showing that when or if mental retardation is associated with asphyxia or related indicators, then the mental retardation is an expression of frank brain abnormality.

The corollary of this interpretation is equally, or more, important. We find no good evidence, nor even any suggestive evidence, that prenatal and perinatal factors cause mental retardation in the absence of detectable central nervous system lesions. In another result of the NCPP, very severe asphyxia occurred in 120 births and two-thirds of the neonates survived. Among the survivors, the risk of cerebral palsy was very high and mental retardation was frequently associated with cerebral palsy. However, among those survivors without cerebral palsy, no single case was mentally retarded.

Epilepsy

With epilepsy we face a problem similar to that with mental retardation, in that large proportions of cases also have frank neurological abnormalities or cerebral palsy. In cerebral palsy, the relative risk for epilepsy is between 30 and 60; if cases of epilepsy with cerebral palsy are not separated from those without cerebral palsy, we cannot know if the associated risk factors reflect the cerebral palsy, or the epilepsy, or both. So, again, we must try and separate epilepsy with frank central nervous system signs from epilepsy without such signs. This we can sometimes do, sometimes not. Furthermore, while we are able to calculate several relative risks for epilepsy from the available data, we cannot calculate attributable fractions.

Maternal Complications

In four studies, all maternal complications were combined and treated as a group. Two of these studies were cohort studies and two case-control studies (Ross et al. 1980; Nelson and Ellenberg 1984; Lilienfeld and Pasamanick 1954; Henderson et al. 1964) (Table 3). In these four studies the relative risks of maternal complications for epilepsy were not significant except in one subgroup in one study, namely, among the white children in the early case-control study by Lilienfeld and Pasamanick (1954). Maternal complications carried a raised risk for epilepsy in these white children whether or not the epilepsy was accompanied by an associated defect. A reasonable interpretation of the data from these four studies taken together, however, is that no effect has been demonstrated. With regard to the single inconsistent result there is reason to think that selection of controls for the subgroup of white children led to an underestimate of the frequency of maternal com-

Table 3. Risk ratios for epilepsy - maternal complications

Nelson and Ellenberg (1984)	Not significant	
Ross et al. (1980)	Not significant	
Lilienfeld and Pasamanick (1954)		
No associated defect	White	1.62 (1.04–2.53)
	Nonwhite	1.14 (0.68–1.92)
Associated defect	White	1.73 (1.0–3.0)
	Nonwhite	n for estimates too small
Henderson et al. (1964)	Black	1.1

Table 4. Risk ratios for epilepsy - maternal bleeding

Nelson and Ellenberg (1984)	Not significant
Ross et al. (1980)	$p<.05$
Lilienfeld and Pasamanick (1954)	12.4 (6.6-95.8)
Henderson et al. (1964)	3.6 (1.0-12.7)

plications among them. Cases in white children were drawn from a public clinic population, a distinctly poor and disadvantaged group; controls were selected from birth records contiguous to that of the case and were more likely to reflect the general population.

It is possible to calculate the relative risks for one specific complication, *maternal bleeding,* in the same four studies (Table 4). The strongest study in terms of size, detail, and prospectively collected data, that is, the NCPP, yields no association of maternal bleeding with epilepsy. A report on the British national cohort of 1958 makes the statement that maternal bleeding is statistically significant in epilepsy, but provides no backup of data or analysis for the statement. However, in the two case-control studies the odds ratios are distinctly high. Unfortunately, we cannot say whether a high relative risk would persist if cases of epilepsy with cerebral palsy were separated from those without cerebral palsy. In the NCPP, while maternal bleeding did not relate to epilepsy, the relative risks for cerebral palsy with various kinds of maternal bleeding ranged from 1.6 to 3.9.

Low Birthweight

By the nature of the phenomenon, low birthweight reflects some prenatal problem of pregnancy, either in mother or in child. A neurodevelopmental impairment related to birthweight does not have the same constraint on its time of origin. The impairment may arise either prenatally as a result of the prenatal problem that causes the low birthweight (Freud's hypothesis, 1897), or it may arise postnatally in an infant vulnerable because it is premature and of low birthweight (Little's hypothesis, 1862). The available data suggest that in the absence of neurological defect, low birthweight carries no raised risk for epilepsy (Nelson and Ellenberg 1984; Ross et al. 1980; Van den Berg and Yerushalmy 1969; Lilienfeld and Pasamanick 1954; Henderson et al. 1964).

In five available studies - three cohort and two case-control (Table 5) - the risk ratio was raised only when cerebral palsy or associated defects were not excluded; even then, in two of the studies the raised risk ratio was a modest one. In the one study (Lilienfeld and Pasamanick 1954) that provides the necessary data, at least in one subgroup, for cases with and without associated defects, the odds are 5.19 with added defects, and 0.84 without.

If infants with low birthweight in consequence of retarded growth alone are considered [that is, small for gestational age (SGA) infants] then in the two available studies for which the calculations can be made there seems to be a modest increase in risk with intrauterine growth retardation in one study (Nelson and Ellenberg 1984) which excluded cases with associated cerebral palsy (the NCPP), and

Table 5. Risk ratios for epilepsy - low birthweight and SGA

	Birthweight < 2500 g (no maternal complications)	SGA
Nelson and Ellenberg (1984) (excludes cerebral palsy)	Not significant	1.7 (1.1-2.6)
Ross et al. (1980)	Not significant	
Van den Berg and Yerushalmy (1969)	1.6 (0.6 -4.5)	3.0 (2.2-4.0)
Lilienfeld and Pasamanick (1954)		
White: with neuro. defect	5.19 (1.95-13.8)	
without neuro. defect	0.84 (0.23- 2.54)	
Non-white: with neuro. defect	?	
without neuro. defect	0.93 (0.28- 3.14)	
Henderson et al. (1964)	1.7 (1.5 - 1.8)	

Table 6. Risk ratios for epilepsy - eclampsia and long labor

	Eclampsia	Duration labor > 20 h
Nelson and Ellenberg (1984)	Not significant	Not significant
Lilienfeld and Pasamanick (1954) (without associated defects)		
White	2.26 (1.9-2.7)	
Nonwhite	1.5 (1.2-1.8)	
Henderson et al. (1964)	0.9	1.0 (all complications)

a higher risk in the California cohort of Van den Berg and Yerushalmy (1969), in which cerebral palsy was not commented on. In summary, the birthweight data do not suggest that either the antecedents of low birthweight or the perinatal vulnerability of the small infant contribute much to the risk of epilepsy in the absence of frank neurological damage.

Parturition

Factors close to and around parturition again seem to contribute little to the risk for epilepsy (Table 6). Eclampsia carries a risk for epilepsy in only one (Lilienfeld and Pasamanick 1954) of three studies, and in that study the problem of the comparison group has already been mentioned. Duration of labor, in two studies (Nelson and Ellenberg 1984; Henderson et al. 1964), carries no added risk for epilepsy.

Abnormal Neonatal State

There is no doubt that an abnormal neurological state detected in the newborn infant carries a high relative risk for epilepsy (Table 7). Unfortunately, once again,

Table 7. Risk ratios for epilepsy - abnormal neonatal state (seizures; cyanosis; asphyxia)

Holden et al. (1982)	
Seizures	16.6 (11.3-24.3)
Lilienfeld and Pasamanick (1954)	
White	3.5 (1.9- 6.4)
Nonwhite	4.6 (2.4- 8.8)
Henderson et al. (1964)	9.3 (1.2-73.9)

the three studies that permit the necessary quantification (Lilienfeld and Pasamanick 1954; Henderson et al. 1964; Holden et al. 1982) do not permit cases of epilepsy with cerebral palsy to be distinguished from cases of epilepsy alone. Certainly, there is good reason to think that in many infants, the abnormal neonatal state (for instance, those who had seizures or other frank neurological signs in the newborn period) indicated neurological impairment.

To summarize with regard to epilepsy, then, we are inclined to conclude, as for mental retardation, that, in the absence of cerebral palsy or frank neurological abnormality, the prenatal and perinatal factors so far studied contributed in only a small way, if at all, to the risk of the condition. In the presence of frank neurological damage, however, some prenatal and perinatal factors relate strongly to epilepsy; these may contribute substantially to epilepsy as a secondary manifestation of the primary neurological impairment.

Cerebral Palsy

Our review of mental retardation and epilepsy leads us to expect that prenatal and perinatal factors will contribute substantially to cerebral palsy. Data from Nelson and Ellenberg (1985a, b) have added much to the data base for quantifiable risks. [We draw especially on Nelson and Ellenberg (1985a). The authors provide both the relative risk and the prevalence of the risk factor so that an attributable fraction (AF_{ps}) can be calculated.] The analyses in these papers treat each risk factor one by one, as yet taking no account of the overlap and redundancy between the factors. We can take advantage of the way the data are presented to examine these single of factors grouped at successive stages of pregnancy.

Maternal Factors Independent of Reproduction

Several new factors relating to the mother's attributes have been brought to light in these NCPP data. Each of these now awaits thorough testing and exploration in terms of causal role and pathogenesis. Table 8 shows a selection of the factors studied. In each case the relative risks are fairly high, but because the prevalence of the risk factor is low, the attributable fractions are all around 2%, which is modest.

Table 8. Cerebral palsy: nonreproductive maternal factors. (Data from Nelson and Ellenberg 1985)

Factor	Relative risk		AF_{ps} (%)
	All infants	> 2500 g	
Mental retardation	6.5	10.3	2
Active seizures	3.5	4.5	2
Hyperthyroidism	4.9	4.7	2
Heart disease (asymptomatic)	3.1	3.0^{ns}	2
Prior hospitalization	1.6	1.2^{ns}	7.5

ns Not significant

Table 9. Cerebral palsy: reproductive history. (Data from Nelson and Ellenberg 1985a)

Factor	Relative risk		AF_{ps} (%)
	All infants	> 2500 g	
Long menstrual cycle	1.9	2.4	3
Previous birthweight < 2000 g	2.7	0.5	6
Previous child			
Motor deficit	3.8	2.7^{ns}	3
Sensory deficit	2.8	1.6^{ns}	2
Mental retardation	2.7	2.8	2

ns Not significant

Reproductive History

The NCPP data suggest that a woman's own hormonal state may be a factor in cerebral palsy. Not only long menstrual cycles, but also the administration of estrogens and progesterone were associated with cerebral palsy. The recurrent theme of all the remaining four variables in Table 9 could be an underlying deficiency in an individual woman's reproductive performance. Thus Bakketeig (1977) demonstrated the relationship between the outcome of one pregnancy and the next in terms of birthweight and also of mortality. The same pathogenetic process could underly the risk these factors carry for subsequent cerebral palsy, as well as for the recurrence risk indicated by the sensory or mental deficit in a previous child and the apparent association of neurological impairment in one child with cerebral palsy in the next. One must bear in mind here that we have no notion from this univariate analysis of the extent to which all these risks may be additive. All might overlap, and on multivariate analysis all of them might be absorbed by a factor like previous low birthweight or, indeed, by low birthweight in the index or study pregnancy.

Prenatal Risk Factors

Prenatal risk factors as a group emerge in greater numbers than do risk factors from the earlier stages. This plethora may be real, or it may arise merely because more prenatal factors were recorded. The risk factors that operate in late pregnancy, shown in the first four rows of Table 10, yield no great surprises: toxemia-related factors are predominant in the risk for cerebral palsy. The main surprise is that the relative risks and attributable fractions are so modest. However, the association of hormones administered during pregnancy already referred to is new and interesting. The problem presented by these medical interventions is to disentangle the risks of the treatments themselves from the risks of the conditions that were being treated.

The findings of the last two rows in Table 10, relating to incompetent cervix and prenatal visits, are included more as a warning about possible problems of circularity and confounding than for any substantive role they may have. Without further analysis, it is difficult to interpret either of these two factors. In the United States, at any rate, the discovery of an incompetent cervix generally did not follow from a routine or systematic procedure, but was likely to be stimulated by the existence of some previous problem like miscarriage or preterm delivery. Subjective bias governed by a preconceived hypothesis cannot be ruled out. In the matter of prenatal visits, it is not possible to determine from the data presented whether fewer prenatal visits are the cause of the preterm delivery or whether, by an inevitable process of selection, they are the result of the reduced opportunity for prenatal visits entailed by a preterm delivery.

With regard to the prenatal stage, we are fortunate to find consistency of risk on replication for at least two factors, namely, toxemia and bleeding. Thus, Hagberg et al. (1976) in Sweden showed relations of toxemia and bleeding to cerebral palsy which are comparable to those found in the NCPP in the United States (Table 11).

Table 10. Cerebral palsy: prenatal factors. (Data from Nelson and Ellenberg 1985a)

Factor	Relative risk		AF_{ps} (%)
	All infants	> 2500 g	
Late pregnancy			
Severe proteinuria	3.9	5.1	3
Severe hypertension	2.1	2.2^{ns}	3
Bleeding	1.8	1.6	10
Polyhydramnios	2.5	3.2	2
Hormones			
Estrogen	3.3	1.1^{ns}	2
Progesterone	2.7	2.0^{ns}	2
Thyroid	2.3	2.3^{ns}	3
Incompetent cervix	5.9	–	1
Prenatal visits ≤ 6	1.7	1.0	18

ns Not significant

Table 11. Relations of toxemia and hemorrhage to cerebral palsy, western Sweden (Data from Hagberg et al. 1976)

Condition	Relative risk	AF_{pl} %
Bleeding during pregnancy	8	6.7
Toxemia	5	1.6

Table 12. Cerebral palsy: labor and delivery factors. (Data from Nelson and El-lenberg 1985a)

Factor	Relative risk		AF_{ps} (%)
	All infants	>2500 g	
Bleeding at admission	2.3	1.0	6
Placental bleeding	3.9	2.4	8
Membrane rupture > 24 h	2.7	0.8	8
Chorionitis	2.8	1.0	4
Breech presentation	4.6	3.9	9
Fetal heart rate < 60 beats per min	4.5	2.9	4

Parturition

When one examines factors that operate more closely in time to the outcome of interest, it is a general rule that one can expect to account for more of the risk in a given condition. This occurs as expected with factors in labor and delivery (Table 12). It is evident that each factor at labor and delivery accounts for a fairly substantial attributable fraction. One must bear in mind, again, that there is likely to be much overlap and many complex relationships among these variables. They cannot be simply summed.

Factors at Birth

When we come to factors observed more closely and, also, more directly in the infant, we begin to see even more substantial relative risks and attributable fractions in relation to cerebral palsy (Table 13). The strong associations of cerebral palsy with birthweight and with asphyxia (as measured by Apgar score) are both to be expected from all that has gone before. A new and important addition, however, is the association with congenital malformations (excluding the central nervous system).

The analysis of low birthweight can be carried a little further by differentiating preterm deliveries from fetal growth retardation. For this analysis, we used an NCPP report of an earlier vintage (Ellenberg and Nelson 1979). From Table 14, we see that the predominant contribution to cerebral palsy is made by preterm deliver, which, taken on its own, has a high relative risk and an attributable frac-

Table 13. Cerebral palsy: factors at birth. (Data from Nelson and Ellenberg 1985a)

Factor	Relative risk		AF_{ps} (%)
	All infants	> 2500 g	
Birthweight			
≤2500 g	4.9	-	26
≤2000 g	13.7	-	20
Apgar score 0-3			
1 min	6.4	5.2	21
5 min	20.8	20.0	15
Malformation, non-CNS	3.8	3.9	16

Table 14. Relative risks and attributable fractions for cerebral palsy by birthweight/gestational age (NCPP)

Birthweight (g)	Gestational age (weeks)	Terms commonly used for each to refer to this group	Relative risk	AF_{ps} (%)
<1501	Any gestational age	Very low birthweight	24.4	9 } 23
1501-2500	≤36	Low birthweight and appropriate for gestational age; preterm	6.2	14 } 23
1501-2500	≥37	Low birthweight and small for gestational age; full term	1.8	3
>2500	≤36	Large for gestational age; preterm	1.4	4
>2500	≥37	Normal and high birthweight; full term	1.0	(70)

tion of 23%. An SGA infant at term has a modest increase in relative risk of 1.8 and accounts for an attributable fraction of only 3%, less than do preterm infants of birthweight greater than 2500 g.

Asphyxia and Newborn State

Table 15 shows substantial relative risks for severe asphyxia in cerebral palsy and a considerable attributable fraction for all levels of asphyxia for any Apgar score less than 6. We cannot neglect to point out, at the risk of repetitiveness, the great overlap between asphyxia and birthweight. Asphyxia is predominantly a manifestation of low birthweight infants. We do not know whether asphyxia in low birthweight infants is an antecedent or a consequence of the brain impairment. It might reflect antecedent prenatal insult which causes both low birthweight and asphyxia:

Table 15. Relationship of birth asphyxia to cerebral palsy in the NCPP

Apgar score at 5 min	Relative risk	AF_{ps} (%)
0-3 (severe asphyxia)	21.0	15
4-6 (moderate asphyxia)	5.0	10
Total 0-6	10.0	25

$$\text{Prenatal insult} \begin{array}{l} \nearrow \text{low birthweight} \\ \searrow \text{brain impairment} \rightarrow \text{asphyxia} \end{array}$$

Alternatively, asphyxia might be the antecedent of brain impairment:

Prenatal insult→low birthweight→asphyxia→brain impairment

Some other indicators of the abnormal state of the newborn infant also have strong relative risks and attributable fractions (Table 16). The observation of newborn seizures in particular carries a very high risk. Presumably the risk with lowered hematocrit points to the presence of intraventricular hemorrhage.

Obstetrical Efficiency

A final point remains to be made about the contribution of obstetric practice to the risk of cerebral palsy. During the period when the births for the NCPP were collected (1959-1966), a total of 50 children who had both severe mental retardation and cerebral palsy were observed. Of the 50, 41 had a birthweight of more than 2500 g; all had asphyxia, but there was also a very high frequency of abnormal labors, including such difficulties as arrested progress of labor, and the application of midforceps. There is persuasive evidence in these 50 cases, comprising about one in 1000 births, that they were caused by obstetric difficulties. These births occurred about 30 years ago, from 1959 to 1964. There is no good contemporary evidence for attributing a causal role to obstetric practice as a risk factor in cerebral palsy. However, this is not to say that such a risk would not be discovered if populations of sufficient size were to be examined in a rigorous fashion.

Table 16. Cerebral palsy: newborn state. (Data from Nelson and Ellenberg 1985 a)

Factor	Relative risk		AF_{ps} (%)
	All infants	>2500 g	
Seizures	53.6	63.3	14
Activity depressed	14.6	13.6	21
Respiratory problem	9.2	7.7	11
Hematocrit < 40%	10.9	6.2	20

A Canadian study (MacManus et al. 1977) found that among all cerebral palsy cases, 29% had had "inappropriate care." Unfortunately, this result is not interpretable, because the frequency of such care among normal births is unknown. In a study of the whole Oxford region in Britain, Niswander et al. (1984) did make appropriate comparisons and, in addition, they made assessments of the quality of care provided in a standardized manner and blind to the outcome. In this study, it turned out that obstetric care for cerebral palsy was in several respects better than average. For example, prenatal care carried an odds ratio of 0.7, and poor care during labor carried a risk ratio of 0.2. Care for fetal distress was slightly worse than average with an odds ratio of 1.2.

Conclusions

The marked overlap among risks attached to the many variables examined has been re-emphasized in the previous discussion and is evident in the tables. The partial selection of variables arrayed in the tables from the NCPP data of Nelson and Ellenberg (1985), if simply summed, account for an attributable fraction of at least 180%, that is, almost twice as much cerebral palsy as exists in the population. Table 17 shows our best estimates from all the available literature for each type of variable, again disregarding redundancy among them. To comprehend this redundancy and gain a true understanding of the causal processes will involve a repetitive two-stage procedure. The first is to gather data in appropriate form and with the protection of adequate research design. Some reservoirs of the necessary data, as in the NCPP, are already available. The analysis of such data calls for two kinds of skills. The first of these is the *quantitative skill* required for the deployment of suitable multivariate techniques with which to demonstrate the numerical relationships and the redundancies among multiple variables. The second is the *logical skill* with which to construct, explore, and, when possible, eliminate the multitude of causal models that can plausibly represent multiple variables (Susser 1973; Susser and Stein 1982). In the nature of the research process, the repetition of these two stages must follow in order to test the plausible hypotheses that are not eliminated from consideration.

At this time, it is possible to draw the following conclusions from our review of those available data that can be quantified:

Table 17. Risk for various factors in cerebral palsy

Factor	PMF (%)	RR	AF_{ps} (%)
Prenatal etiology	30	3.5	20
Prematurity (short gestation)	35	9	25
Fetal growth retardation	10	2.3	6
Perinatal asphyxia	40	10	25
Other perinatal causes (e.g., trauma)	5	?	3-5

1. Prenatal and perinatal factors have a circumscribed, but as yet ill-specified, role in neurodevelopmental impairment.
2. In mental retardation and epilepsy, when uncomplicated by frank neurological impairment, prenatal/perinatal factors do not contribute in a major way, if at all.
3. In cerebral palsy, prenatal/perinatal factors have a distinct and powerful role, but as yet the many factors involved cannot be clearly separated from each other, nor placed in their appropriate positions in the causal chain. A unique risk value cannot be given to any one factor because, between the overlapping factors, the overlap with other factors cannot be assigned with regard either to the amount of variance explained or their time order.

References

Bakketeig L (1977) The risk of repeated preterm or low birth weight delivery. In: Reid DM, Stanley FJ (eds) The epidemiology of prematurity. Urban and Schwartzenberg, Baltimore, pp 231-241

Broman SH (1979) Perinatal anoxia and cognitive development in early childhood. In: Field TM (ed) Infants born at risk. S.P. Medical and Scientific Books, Jamaica New York, pp 29-52

Ellenberg J, Nelson K (1979) Birth weight and gestational age in children with cerebral palsy or seizure disorders. Am J Dis Child 133: 1044-1048

Freeman JM (ed) (1985) Prenatal and perinatal factors associated with brain disorders. US DHHS, April 1985

Freud S (1897) Infantile Cerebrallähmung. Hölder, Wien, tr. (1967), University of Miami Press, p 137

Gustavson KH, Hagberg B, Hagberg G et al. (1976) Severe mental retardation in a Swedish county. II. Etiologic and pathogenetic aspects of children born 1959-1970. Neuropaediatrie 8: 293-304

Gustavson KH, Hagberg B, Hagberg G et al. (1977a) Severe mental retardation in a Swedish county. I. Epidemiology, gestational age, birth weight and associated CNS handicaps in children born 1959-1970. Acta Paediatr Scand 66: 373-379

Gustavson KH, Holmgren G, Jonsell R et al. (1977b) Severe mental retardation in children in a northern Swedish county. J Ment Defic Res 21: 161-177

Hagberg B (1978) Severe mental retardation in Swedish children born 1959-1970: epidemiological panorama and causative factors. Ciba Found Symp 59; 29-51

Hagberg G, Hagberg B, Olow I (1976) The changing panorama of cerebral palsy in Sweden 1954-1970. III. The importance of foetal deprivation of supply. Acta Paediatr Scand 65: 403-408

Hagberg B, Hagberg G, Lewerth A et al. (1981a) Mild mental retardation in Swedish school children. I. Prevalence. Acta Paediatr Scand 70: 441-444

Hagberg B, Hagberg G, Lewerth A et al. (1981b) Mild mental retardation in Swedish school children. II. Etiologic and pathogenetic aspects. Acta Paediatr Scand 70: 445-452

Henderson M, Goldstein H, Rogot E et al. (1964) Perinatal factors associated with epilepsy in negro children. Public Health Rep 17: 501-509

Holden J, Mellitz ED, Freeman JF (1982) Neonatal seizures. I. Correlation of prenatal and perinatal events with outcomes. Pediatrics 70: 168-176

Lilienfeld AM, Pasamanick B (1954) Association of maternal and fetal factors with the development of epilepsy. I. Abnormalities in the prenatal and perinatal periods. JAMA 155: 719-724

Little WJ (1862) On the influence of abnormal parturition, difficult labors, premature birth, and asphyxia neonatorum, on the mental and physical condition of the child, especially in relation to deformities. Trans Obstet Soc London 3: 283-344

McManus F, Rang M, Chanre G et al. (1977) Is cerebral palsy a preventable disease? Obstet Gynecol 50: 71-77
Nelson KB, Ellenberg JH (1984) Obstetrical complications as risk factors for cerebral palsy or seizure disorder. JAMA 25: 1843-1848
Nelson KB, Ellenberg JH (1985a) Antecedents of cerebral palsy. I. Univariate analysis of risks. Am J Dis Child 139: 1031-38
Nelson KB, Ellenberg JH (1985b) Predictors of very low birth weight and the relation of these to cerebral palsy. JAMA 254: 1473-9
Niswander K, Henson G, Elbourne D et al. (1984) Adverse outcomes of pregnancy and the quality of obstetric care. Lancet 2: 827-31
Peters TJ, Golding J, Lawrence CJ et al. (1984) Delayed onset of regular respiration and subsequent development. Early Hum Dev 9: 225-239
Ross EM, Peckham CS, West PB et al. (1980) Epilepsy in childhood. Findings from the national child development study. Br Med J 1: 207-210
Susser M (1973) Causal thinking in the health sciences: concepts and strategies in epidemiology. Oxford University Press, Oxford
Susser M, Stein Z (1982) Third variable analysis: application to causal sequences among nutrient intake, maternal weight, birth weight, placental weight and gestation. Stat Med 1: 105-20
Susser M, Hauser WA, Kiely J, Paneth N, Stein Z (1985) Quantitative estimates of prenatal and perinatal risk factors for perinatal mortality, cerebral palsy, mental retardation, and epilepsy. In: Freeman J (ed) Prenatal and perinatal factors associated with brain disorders. USDHHS, April
Van den Berg BJ, Yerushalmy J (1969) Studies on convulsive disorders in young children. I. Incidence of febrile and nonfebrile convulsions by age and other factors. Pediatr Res 3: 298-304

Epidemiologic Panorama of Brain Impairments and Causative Factors – Swedish Experiences

O. HJALMARSON, B. HAGBERG and G. HAGBERG

The rates of impairment of the CNS in children have been used as a measure of the quality of perinatal care. The relationship, however, between perinatal events and cerebral damage is frequently obscure. Data from selected high-risk groups have often been used to assess such associations. The possibility of selection bias makes results from studies of this kind difficult to interpret.

In this presentation, data from epidemiologic studies, based on total populations, on the prevalence of cerebral palsy (CP), mental retardation, and hearing deficiency will be given together with associated perinatal and other background factors.

Cerebral Palsy

There was astonishment and disappointment when Hagberg et al. (1984) recently showed that after a successive decrease in the prevalence rates of CP, in a total population in western Sweden, from 1.9 in 1959 to 1.4 per 1000 live births in 1970, the rates then rose significantly to 2.0 per 1000 in the cohort 1975–1978 (Fig. 1).

The puzzling feature is that this rise took place over a time period when there was a remarkable improvement in maternal health care, when deliveries were centralized in well-equipped hospitals, when fetal monitoring was improved and the

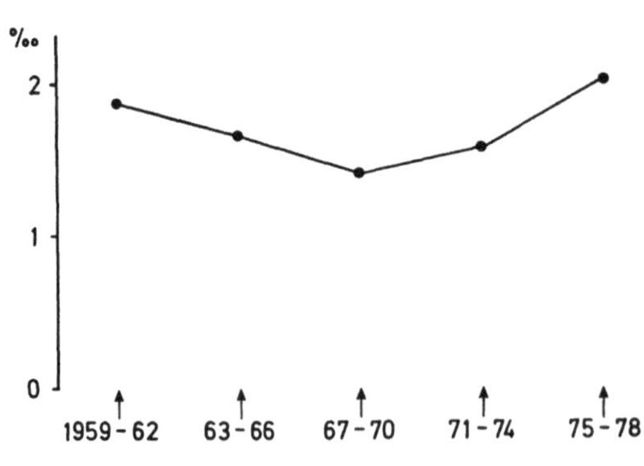

Fig. 1. Prevalence rate of CP per 1000 live births in western Sweden 1959–1978. (According to Hagberg et al. 1984)

practice of obstetrics became more active, when active cooperation between obstetricians and neonatologists in risk deliveries was developed, when a national program of resuscitation of newborns was generally accepted, and when neonatal intensive care was established.

At the same time, perinatal mortality rates decreased continuously as did the incidence rates of low Apgar scores. It was evident that the factors responsible for the rise in CP rates were either unrelated to those which caused mortality statistics to improve or represented an adverse effect of the same factors.

The population-based data cited here were collected for 30 years by Hagberg's group. In the project all cases with CP in Gothenburg and four counties in the western part of Sweden were identified. The area covers about 20% of all births in Sweden. Through close contact between the group of investigators and the local organizations caring for handicapped children, the identification of children with CP was made very effective. All the cases found were classified into CP syndromes according to the Swedish standard (Hagberg et al. 1975). All patients were at least 4 years of age when included. When the material was grouped into full-term and preterm cases it was evident that most of the dynamics over the time period, both the decline in 1959-1970 and the increase in 1971-1978 could be referred to preterm infants, although there was also a significant rise in 1971-1978 in term infants (Fig. 2).

When the change in prevalence rates for different CP syndromes was considered, a significant decrease in 1959-1970 and a significant rise in 1971-1978 was found for preterm infants with spastic or ataxic diplegia only, but dyskinetic syndromes in full-term infants also tended to follow the same pattern.

Mental retardation is not a rare concomitant to severe CP. It was therefore of considerable interest to study whether the change in the prevalence rates of CP had also affected the proportion of mentally retarded children. For children born preterm it was found that the prevalence rate of CP combined with an IQ below 70 had decreased and the increase in the CP rate had mainly generated affected

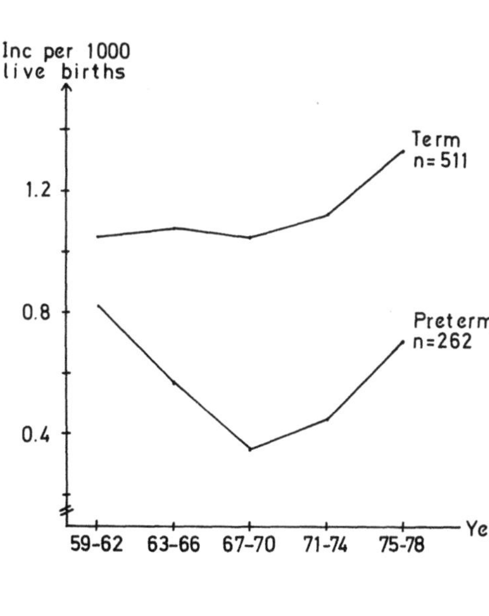

Fig. 2. Prevalence rate of CP per 1000 live births in western Sweden distributed by gestational age. (According to Hagberg et al. 1984)

children with an IQ above 70. For CP cases born at term, however, the trend was in the opposite direction.

The risk for CP increases sharply with low gestational age (Hagberg and Hagberg 1984). With a constant risk of CP among preterm survivors, the crude live-birth prevalence is bound to rise in parallel to increased survival rates. This is however not the only explanation. Figure 3 shows birthweight-specific prevalence rates per 1000 survivors of the perinatal period. Data from a recent, population-based, multi-center study of infants with birthweights below 1500 g in Sweden (Lagercrantz et al. 1985) is also included. There is a tendency for the rates for the group with the lowest birthweights to decrease. In all other weight groups an overall increase was visible but it was significant only among infants with birthweights between 2000 and 2500 g. Although difficult to discern in Fig. 3, the trend was the same for children with birthweights above 2500 g (from 1.06 per 1000 in 1967–1970 to 1.32 per 1000 in 1975–1978).

However, as indicated in Table 1, despite the high prevalence rate in the lowest weight group, less than 10% of all cases with CP had birthweights below 1500 g, while more than 60% of the cases were above 2500 g at birth, despite the low-risk figure in this weight group.

Different explanations for the increasing CP rates may be suggested.

Improved Capacity for Case Identification. This is not likely because of the way the study was organized. The same investigators examined all children and doubtful diagnoses were controlled. The same criteria for inclusion of cases were used throughout the periods. Special emphasis was laid on not changing the cut-off point in borderline cases.

Improved Survival After Severe Brain Damage Due to Intrauterine Asphyxia, Perinatal Brain Ischemia or Hemorrhage, or Other Causes. This potential explanation raises many more complicated problems. The early neonatal mortality rate (0–7 days) decreased remarkably over the period with an increasing CP rate. Official statistics from the whole country show a decrease from 6.5 per 1000 in 1973 to 3.4 per 1000 in 1981. The improvement was uniform at all gestational ages. This

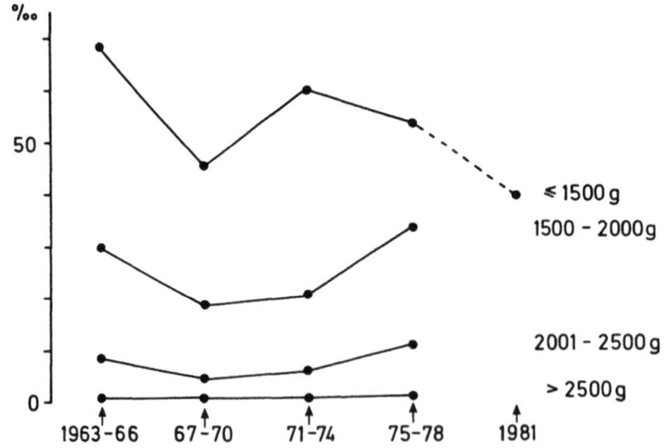

Fig. 3. Course of birthweight-specific prevalence rates of CP per 1000 infants surviving the 1 week of life in western Sweden 1963–1978. Numerical data on the rise in the group above 2500 g is given in the text. (Data from Hagberg et al. 1984 and from a Swedish multi-center study in 1981 – Lagercrantz et al. 1985)

Table 1. Prevalence of CP and distribution of CP cases by birthweight in Sweden during 1975-1978. (n=73842) According to Hagberg et al. 1984

Birthweight (g)	CP prevalence per 1000 survivors	CP (%)
<1500	54	9
1500-2500	17	29
>2500	13	62

means that despite the increase in CP rates from 1.4 per 1000 (1967-1970) to 2.0 per 1000 (1975-1978), there was still a considerable net gain of surviving newborns without CP. There is, however, no direct data to indicate that the increased proportion of infants with cerebral damage derive directly from the higher rate of surviving infants. In fact, the rate of very low Apgar scores decreased and in the most vulnerable group (below 1500 g) CP rates did not increase. Consequently, the strength of this possible explanation for the rising CP rate is still obscure.

Appearance of Detrimental Obstetric and/or Neonatal Procedures. This possibility is also difficult to evaluate. Neonatal intensive care and mechanical ventilation evidently contributed to the improved survival rates. However, they are also often considered to be risk factors for CP. Some complications in care, such as pneumothorax, are well known as carrying considerable risk for brain damage. But it is not known to what extent intensive care contributes to the CP rate by enabling infants already damaged to survive, or to what degree intensive care causes damage by complications in treatment.

Increasing Prevalence of Prenatal Etiologic Factors. This might give part of the explanation. A continuous but not statistically significant increase in obvious and defined prenatal causes has been observed (Hagberg et al. 1984). Improved diagnostic facilities and increased survival rates have contributed to this trend. It is a possibility of unknown relevance that prenatal causes, other than the defined ones and more difficult to reveal, exist and are increasing.

One way to elucidate possible etiologic mechanisms for brain damage in epidemiologic studies is to identify circumstances that might have direct associations with causative processes. Hagberg et al. analyzed the occurrence of sets of such "risk factors" (Table 2) (Hagberg et al. 1984; Hagberg and Hagberg 1984). Among the children with CP, perinatal risk factors dominated, but more prominently in preterm infants than in term ones. In preterm infants few distinct dissimilarities in risk factor distribution in different CP syndromes were found. In children born at term, dyskinetic syndromes were, however, associated with perinatal factors in about 85% of the cases in contrast to simple ataxia, which was associated with very few such risk factors. There was a time trend in the prevalence of risk factors in the cases studied. Obvious pre- or postnatal risk factors increased over the whole period of study (1959-1978) and this was almost exclusively confined to

Table 2. Pre- and perinatal risk factors for CP considered in the analysis of the study by Hagberg et al. (1984)

Prenatal	Perinatal
≥ Two abortions	Asphyxia
Significant maternal disorder	Cerebral hemorrhage
Bleeding during pregnancy (term births)	Ablatio placentae
Edema/proteinuria and blood pressure > 140/90	Respiratory disease
Small for gestational age	Hyperbilirubinemia
Placental infarction	CNS infection
Multiple birth	

Table 3. Relative risks for CP in infants with low Apgar scores at different gestational ages, calculated in a Swedish population (Hagberg et al. 1984)

Gestational age (weeks)	Relative risk for CP	
	Apgar score <7	Apgar score ≤3
≤31	0.9	0.9
32-36	4.6	10
≥37	19	27

term infants. Perinatal risk factors decreased during 1959-1970 and increased during 1971-1978 in term as well as preterm infants.

We have analyzed some risk factors from the last cohort (1975-1978) in Hagberg's study more closely. First we analyzed the Apgar score, which must not be regarded as a measure of perinatal asphyxia in any physiologic sense, but as a useful index of vitality at birth. Low Apgar scores and gestational age are closely related. We have used data from a total population of all 4629 surviving infants born in Gothenburg in 1978 as a reference and calculated relative risks for CP in surviving children born at different gestational ages. As shown in Table 3, low Apgar scores appear as an important risk factor only in more mature infants and the relative risks are highest in full-term infants. In absolute terms, however, the risk for CP was no higher than 2.1% when the Apgar score at 1 min was 3 or below.

The risk of neurologic sequelae - and mortality - increases if the criteria are made stricter. However, in a 2-year study of all infants in Sweden who had an Apgar score of only 0 or 1 at 5 min of age, 24% of the infants died but 76% of the survivors had no evident impairment at 2 years of age (Celander et al. 1985). Two recent Swedish publications have shown that only when asphyxia was so severe that mortality rates were around 50%, was the CP rate 75% among survivors (Ergander et al. 1983, Larsson et al. 1984) (Table 4).

Table 4. Mortality and prevalence rates of CP in full-term infants with severe perinatal asphyxia which required treatment by mechanical ventilation

Study	*n*	Mortality	CP rate in survivors
Ergander et al. (1983) 1973-1975 Stockholm	15	7/15	6/8
Larsson et al. (1985) 1979-1983 Gothenburg	18	10/18	6/8

Table 5. Calculated risk of CP after treatment by mechanical ventilation in the neonatal period

Gestational age (weeks)	CP risk in surviving infants treated by ventilator		Relative risk for CP after mechanical ventilation
	(*n*)	(%)	
≤31	10/71	14	4.4
32-36	8/81	10	15
≥37	4/50	8	81

In addition, a low Apgar score seldom appears as the only risk factor in affected children. In Hagberg's last cohort, 28 out of 30 term infants with Apgar scores below 7 at 1 min had at least one additional perinatal risk factor. This is in accordance with results from the Collaborative Perinatal Project as reported by Nelson and Ellenberg (1985).

Mechanical ventilation is also often considered as a risk factor for CP. In the last cohort in Hagberg's study (1975-1978) ten of the 29 children with CP who were born after 31 weeks of gestation or less were ventilated by a respirator in the neonatal period. Accepting the assumption that the reference population in Gothenburg in 1978 is valid for the whole cohort, the risk of CP after mechanical ventilation as well as the relative risk associated with this procedure (equals risk for CP in ventilated infants divided by risk for CP in nonventilated infants) can be calculated. As in the total population, the CP risk was higher in immature than in full-term infants but the relative risk was considerably higher in full-term infants (Table 5).

The same pattern was found for infants with birthweights below −2 SD (small for gestational age - SGA) (Table 6). Here SGA was significant as a risk factor only in term infants. This is in accordance with population-based results by Sabel and coworkers in Gothenburg, who found that the growth-retarded infants dominated among impaired children only if they were born after more than 36 weeks of gestation. So despite the fact that these risk factors were more common among preterm infants, their relative importance was much more pronounced in mature infants.

Table 6. Calculated risk of CP for children born as SGA

Gestational age (weeks)	CP risk in surviving SGA infants		Relative risk for CP when SGA
	(n)	(%)	
≤31	1/18	5.6	1.2
32-36	4/391	1.0	1.2
≥37	10/930	1.1	12

Mental Retardation

Large population-based series covering the years 1959-1970 and different regions in Sweden have showed fairly constant prevalence rates, 3.7-3.9 per 1000 for mild mental retardation (MMR) (IQ 50-70) and 2.8-3.5 per 1000 for severe mental retardation (SMR) (IQ <50) (Gustavson et al. 1977a, b; Hagberg et al. 1981a; Blomquist et al. 1981; Hagberg et al. 1986). No significant change has been noted for mental retardation over the time period, except for a significant decline in Down's syndrome in sparsely populated northern areas (Gustavson et al. 1977b).

In these series associated handicaps were found in 40%-50% of children with SMR and in about 25%-30% of those with MMR. Epilepsy and CP dominate. In term infants, perinatal complications, mainly severe birth asphyxia, are the likely cause of SMR in 10% of the cases. In this group virtually all the infants also have CP and 50% of them have epilepsy (Hagberg and Kyllerman 1983). The high frequency of associated handicaps illustrate the importance of biologic factors behind not only SMR but also MMR.

A careful search for obvious or potential etiology was made in a study in Gothenburg (Hagberg et al. 1981b) (Table 7). Early prenatal causative factors were found in more than half of the children with SMR and in one-quarter of those with MMR. Chromosomal aberrations dominated among the genetic causes. Eight percent of MMR had obvious alcohol fetopathy with stigmatization and a maternal history of heavy alcohol abuse. The total share of MMR due to alcohol might be greater.

A perinatal cause was considered likely in 15%-20% of both SMR and MMR when the perinatal period was broadly defined from 28 weeks' gestational age to the 28th postnatal day. This group comprised only children with additional neurologic signs together with signs of "fetal deprivation of supply," asphyxia, respiratory disease, or meningitis/encephalitis. If only negative events limited to delivery and the first 7 days of life were considered, the rate of perinatal causes decreased to about 10%.

More than half of the MMR cases and almost 20% of SMR cases lacked traces that would refer them to one of the etiologic groups shown. In a considerable number of cases, a familial disposition was suspected in MMR, as at least one other family member showed a subnormal school performance.

Table 7. Origin of mental retardation in Gothenburg, Sweden, according to Hagberg et al. (1981b)

Cause	SMR (%)	MMR (%)
Prenatal		
Genetic	34	5
Syndromes acquired	12	10
Alcohol	0	8
Infection	7	0
Perinatal[a]	15	18
Postnatal	11	2
Psychosis	1	2
Not traceable		
Familial	4	29
Nonfamilial	14	26

[a] Period from 28 weeks of gestation to 28th postnatal day

In summary, these series demonstrate that, regardless of the severity of mental retardation, about 15%-20% might have an origin due to identifiable factors operating from the 28th week of gestation until the end of the neonatal period.

Hearing Loss

Severe impairment of hearing is another handicap where perinatal factors are often assumed to play an important part. In Gothenburg, Thiringer et al. (1984) identified all children with substantial loss of hearing at 5-6 years of age in the population born during 1970-1979. The cases were found mainly by examination of risk groups according to sets of criteria in early infancy, by informing all mothers on the maternity wards about hereditary hearing deficits and examination of infants at risk, and finally by screening of 4-year-old children at postnatal clinics. The attendance rate at these 4-year examinations was more than 90%.

From the total population of 27425 6-year-old children over the study period, 146 cases were found to have loss of hearing. The investigators found a population-based rate of hearing impairment of 4.2 per 1000. If monoaural defects and those with a loss below 40 dB were excluded, the figure decreased to 1.5 per 1000, which is close to what has been found in other European countries.

As shown in Table 8, in 61% of the cases there were clear indications of a prenatal cause. The group was dominated by hereditary types of loss and malformations. A perinatal cause was considered likely in only 9%. Postnatal causes were exclusively infections, and in 12% no evident etiology could be traced.

We have calculated relative risks from Thiringer's data (Thiringer et al. 1984) to illustrate the impact of some perinatal factors (Table 9). Birthweight had a certain influence on the risk. However, the general risk for a baby with a very low

Table 8. Cause of hearing impairment in children born in Gothenburg 1970–1979 ($n=146$). (According to Thiringer et al. 1984)

	%	%
Prenatal causes		61
Hereditary forms	39	
Malformations	14	
Acquired forms		
Congenital infections	6	
Fetal alcohol syndrome	2	
Perinatal causes		9
Postnatal causes		18
Parotitis	7	
Meningitis	6	
Secretory otitis media	6	
Unknown etiology		12

Table 9. Risk factors for hearing impairment. Calculated from data from Thiringer et al. 1984

Risk factor	Relative risk
Birthweight <2500 g	2.0
<1500 g	5.0
Small for date (below −2 SD)	2.8
Apgar score (5 min) <7	0.9
Hyperbilirubinemia (>256 μmol/liter)	1.0
Neonatal intensive care	11
Mechanical ventilation	17

birthweight of having a hearing impairment was only about 1%. The most evident risk was associated with neonatal intensive care, especially mechanical ventilation. However, it must be remembered that very low birthweight, intensive care, and mechanical ventilation are highly correlated, so it is far from clear from these data whether artificial ventilation per se is an etiologic factor.

Concluding Remarks

Table 10 summarizes the major part of the panorama of CNS impairments in Sweden today. Epilepsy, MMR, and SMR dominate, followed by CP and severe hearing loss. There are marked differences among the groups according to rates of perinatal risk factors which are most prevalent in CP and simple hydrocephalus (hydrocephalus not associated with spina bifida cystica).

Table 10. Prevalence rates of various brain impairments in Swedish schoolchildren and proportion of perinatal origin according to population-based studies. Definitions used refer to Hagberg and Hagberg (1984)

	Prevalence per 1000	Perinatal origin (broad definition[a]) (%)	Perinatal origin (restricted definition[c]) (%)
Epilepsy	4	?	?
MMR (IQ 50-70)	4	18	10
SMR (IQ <50)	3	15	10
Cerebral palsy	2	65	45
Hearing loss (>40 dB)	1.5	9[b]	?
Simple hydrocephalus	0.4	?	40
Psychosis	0.2	?	?

[a] From 28 weeks of gestation to 28th postnatal day
[b] Refers to all degrees of hearing loss
[c] From delivery to 7th postnatal day

Provided that these figures also reflect the approximate distribution of etiologic factors, they give some understanding of the maximal potential effect of each group of measures taken to reduce perinatal risk factors.

From these population-based studies in Sweden it is evident that in some conditions perinatal risk factors are over-represented. The great majority of infants who are exposed to such factors have no discernible damage. Almost all factors discussed have low sensitivity, low specificity, and low power to predict CNS impairment. This reflects the complexity of the pathogenetic mechanisms involved.

There is an evident need to find more powerful predictors of cerebral function outcome. In the perinatal field, new clinical techniques to evaluate fetal condition and neonatal brain function may contribute. We might, on the other hand, already possess data or combinations of data with more power than those investigated so far. It is important to find them.

References

Celander O, Kjellmer I, Svenningsen N, Tunell R (1985) A Swedish national programme for resuscitation of newborn babies. In: Sterky G, Tafari N, Tunell R (eds) Breathing and warmth at birth. Judging the appropriateness of technology. Swedish agency for research cooperation with developing countries (Sarec report R2: 1985), Stockholm, pp 94-106

Ergander U, Eriksson M, Zetterström R (1983) Severe neonatal asphyxia. Incidence and prediction of outcome in the Stockholm area. Acta Paediatr Scand 72: 321-325

Gustavson KH, Hagberg B, Hagberg G, Sars K (1977a) Severe mental retardation in a Swedish county. I. Epidemiology, gestational age, birth weight and associated CNS handicaps in children born 1959-1970. Acta Paediatr Scand 66: 373-379

Gustavson KH, Hagberg B, Hagberg G, Sars K (1977b) Severe mental retardation in a Swedish county. II. Etiologic and pathogenetic aspects of children born 1959-1970. Neuropädiatric 8: 293-304

Hagberg B, Hagberg G (1984) Prenatal and perinatal risk factors in a survey of 681 Swedish cases. In: Stanley F, Alberman E (eds) Clinics in developmental medicine, vol 87. Blackwell, Oxford, pp 116-134

Hagberg B, Kyllerman M (1983) Epidemiology of mental retardation - a Swedish survey. Brain Dev 5: 441-449

Hagberg B, Hagberg G, Lewerth A, Lindberg U (1981a) Mild mental retardation in Swedish school children. I. Prevalence. Acta Paediatr Scand 70: 441-444

Hagberg B, Hagberg G, Lewerth A, Lindberg U (1981b) Mild mental retardation in Swedish school children. II. Etiologic and pathogenetic aspects. Acta Paediatr Scand 70: 445-452

Hagberg B, Hagberg G, Olow I (1975) The changing panorama of cerebral palsy in Sweden 1954-1970. II. Analysis of the general changes. Acta Paediatr Scand 64: 187-92

Hagberg B, Hagberg G, Olow I (1984) The changing panorama of cerebral palsy in Sweden. IV. Epidemiological trends 1959-1978. Acta Paediatr Scand 73: 433-440

Hagberg G, Lewerth A, Olsson E, Westerberg B (1986) Mild mental retardation in Gothenburg children born between 1966-70. Changes between two points of time. Paper at the 2nd European symposium on scientific studies in mental retardation. 24-26 June 1986, Uppsala

Lagercrantz H, Dahlström K, Lundberg A, Svenningsen N, Tunell R (1985) Follow-up of infants with birth-weight below 1500 g after two years. Report from a multi-centre study. Läkartidningen 82: 199-202

Larsson L, Ekström-Jodal B, Hjalmarson O (1984) Severe perinatal asphyxia requiring mechanical ventilation. Manuscript.

Nelson KB, Ellenberg JH (1984) Obstetric complications as risk factors for cerebral palsy or seizure disorders. JAMA 251: 1843-1848

Thiringer K, Kankkunen A, Liden G, Niklasson A (1984) Perinatal risk factors in the aetiology of hearing loss in preschool children. Dev Med Child Neurol 26: 799-807

Low Birthweight and Neurological Sequelae – A Summary of Some Swedish Studies

G. ROOTH

There is considerable concern amongst both laymen and doctors that the increased care of the small infants leads to increases in mental retardation and cerebral palsy. Results such as those described by Stewart (this volume) are clearly against this hypothesis, but there are three reasons for them:

1. The lower the birthweight, the higher the risk of cerebral lesions which increases with the degree of prematurity
2. Many more infants with low birthweight survive today than, say, 10 years ago
3. The results of the renowned studies by Hagberg et al. (this volume) show an increase in the frequency of cerebral palsy

The Hagberg studies are meticulous, covering a large population in south-western Sweden. It is interesting that he actually noticed a decrease in cerebral palsy in low birthweight infants, in spite of the increased number of survivals. There are so many more term infants and it is among these that Hagberg observed the increase. Unfortunately, few of those who quote Hagberg also take his birthweight distributions into account.

The total increase in cerebral palsy observed by the Hagberg group is not seen everywhere in Sweden. Studies from Lund in southern Sweden show a sharp decline in neurological sequelae in surviving infants. Ingemarsson et al. (1981), as shown in Table 1, found that, with improved obstetrical and neonatal care, the number of infants with neurological sequelae after at least 14 months was reduced from 1973-1974 to 1977-1979 from 25 to three, respectively. A more recent study, also from Lund (Westgren et al. 1985), reports on infants born before the 33rd week of gestation. Of the total of 108 infants, 83 survived at least 2 years after birth. Only 12, i.e., 14%, showed development of neurological abnormalities at 2 years of age. A recent study from the same group (Holmquist et al. 1986) refers

Table 1. Neurological sequelae in surviving infants

	1973-1974 (I) (n=71)	1975-1976 (II) (n=73)	1977-1979 (III) (n=66)
Cerebral palsy	9	6	2
Epilepsy	4	0	0
Psychomotor retardation	12	8	1
Total (n)	25	14	3
(%)	35.2	19.2	4.6

to all small-for-gestational-age infants born in Lund during 1977-1981. Of those born before the 34th week of gestation, 40% died and 16% showed major neurological handicap. If born in the 34th-36th week of gestation the corresponding figures were 8% and 8%, respectively. Among the term SCG infants only 0.5% died and 2% showed major handicaps.

In a multicenter study covering about 25% of the total births in Sweden, all infants with a birthweight below 1500 g born in 1981 participated in a follow-up study (Lagercrantz et al. 1985). The total mortality at 2 years was 36%, only 5% dying later than 1 month after birth. Out of 102 infants participating in the follow-up study, four had major disabilities and eight infants were classified as having immature development of their neurology and/or language.

This confirms the opinion expressed by Hagberg et al. (1984) that the net gain of survivals without cerebral palsy is in the group of infants with a birthweight below 1500 g.

In summary, the number of low birthweight infants with subsequent neurological sequelae has decreased in Sweden as well as in other countries, in spite of the increase in their survival rate. The increase in the rate of cerebral palsy in term or close-to-term infants seen by Hagberg stresses the importance of careful monitoring of labor in term infants.

Acknowledgements. Prof. N. Svenningsen and I. Ingermarsson generously supplied the material from Lund on which this review is based.

References

Holmqvist P, Ingemarsson E, Ingemarsson I (1986) Intrauterine growth retardation and gestational age. Acta Obstet Gynecol Scand (in press)

Ingemarsson E, Ingemarsson I, Swenningen NW (1981) Impact of routine fetal monitoring during labor on fetal outcome with long-term follow-up. Am J Obstet Gynecol 141: 29-38

Lagercrantz H, Dahlström K, Lundberg A et al. (1985) Multicenterstudie av lågviktiga barn visar god utveckling with tvååarsuppföljning. (Follow-up of infants with birth-weight below 1500 gram after two years. Report from a multi-center study) Läkartidningen 82: 199-202

Westgren LM, Malcus P, Svenningsen NW (1985) Intrauterine asphyxia and long-term outcome in preterm fetuses. Obstet Gynecol 67: 512-516

Biology and Pathogenetic Mechanisms

Genetic Factors Leading to Birth Defects and Diseases of the Newborn

F. VOGEL

Groups of Genetic Anomalies

It is my task to report on the genetic causes of defective health in newborns. And indeed, the *proportion* of genetically caused anomalies among newborns suffering from health problems has increased appreciably in recent years - not due to an increase in absolute numbers but because progress in monitoring pregnancy and, especially, delivery has led to a reduction of *exogenous* complications.

Genetic anomalies recognizable at birth can be subdivided into three groups:

1. Chromosomal aberrations
2. Hereditary diseases with simple modes of inheritance
3. So-called multifactorial birth defects

The first two groups are exclusively genetically determined; within the third, and very heterogeneous group, genetic susceptibilities and harmful environmental influences may act in an often obscure way. In many instances, there is no clearcut evidence either for a genetic susceptibility, or for an environmental factor.

Chromosomal Aberrations

In a number of chromosomal studies on consecutive series of newborns, incidence of major chromosomal aberrations has been established as 0.6%-0.7% (Nielsen and Sillessen 1975). Among prematurely born children and children with malformations of any type, this fraction is substantially higher (Bochkov et al. 1974). However, these chromosomal anomalies in living newborns are only a small fraction of all conceptuses carrying chromosomal aberrations. The great majority do not survive up to the time of delivery; most of them die during the first and, sometimes, second trimester of pregnancy (Hassold and Jacobs 1984; Lauritsen 1977). According to the obstetric literature, between 10% and 20% of all *recognized* pregnancies end with a spontaneous abortion; more than 50% of all spontaneously aborted embryos and fetuses show chromosomal aberrations. Moreover, there is very good evidence that many more chromosomally abnormal zygotes die within the first few days after fertilization (see Vogel and Motulsky 1986). They usually go unnoticed. On the other hand, chromosomally abnormal fetuses have a higher than normal risk of death even in the last trimester, as epitomized, for example, by

Table 1. Incidence of Down's syndrome in relation to maternal age, at birth and at amniocentesis. (Data from Harper 1984)

Maternal age (years)	Incidence per 1000	
	At birth	Amniocentesis
30	1.4	Not available
35	2.2	3.9
37	4.0	6.4
39	6.5	10.4
41	12.5	16.9
43	20	27.4
All ages	1.5	Not available

the well-known discrepancy between incidence of chromosomal aberrations such as Down's syndrome or amniocentesis (16th to 17th week) and at delivery (Table 1).

Due to the high prenatal mortality of chromosomally abnormal conceptuses, a small fraction of all possible types of numerical and structural chromosomal aberrations are seen at birth, trisomy 21 (Down's syndrome) and the gonosomal aneuploidies such as XXY (Klinefelter's syndrome), the XXX and XYY traits, and X0 (Turner's syndrome) being the most common ones.

In earlier times, a substantial fraction of Down's syndrome patients did not survive the first days or weeks of life; they died mostly from congenital heart disease or intestinal atresias. Many others, because of reduced resistance, fell victim to various infections during their first years of life. With the improvement in therapy, this has changed radically, and at present, the chances for a child with Down's syndrome to live into adult age are not much worse than those of chromosomally normal children.

Most numerical anomalies of the sex chromosomes cannot be recognized at birth. As a rule, they are diagnosed at puberty when the anomaly of sex development becomes apparent. According to recent, longitudinal studies, however, general and psychological development especially of children with XXY, XXX, and XYY karyotypes is often slightly retarded in several aspects but could be influenced favorably by appropriate education - sometimes in combination with hormonal therapy (Nielsen et al. 1979, 1981). Therefore, screening of *all* newborns for chromosomal abnormalities has often been suggested. At present, however, shortage of laboratory capacity prevents such screening. Moreover, acceptance in our population may meet with psychologic difficulties.

Only a small fraction of conceptuses with other, autosomal aberrations survive up to birth. Trisomies 13 and 18 are rare but well known. The number and variety of structural aberrations - all of them rare - are so great that probably nobody knows all of them, and could make a diagnosis on clinical evidence only (for an excellent survey of clinical and cytogenetic data, see Schinzel 1984). But a combination of several features is common to many of them. They helped medical geneticists to establish some rules on clinical signs that should induce the doctor to order a chromosome examination (Table 2). With refinement of our cytogenetic

Table 2. Main clinical signs that, if present in combination, may (but need not) point to presence of an autosomal chromosome aberration (Vogel and Motulsky 1986)

General signs	Low birthweight (small for date); failure to thrive; mental retardation (usually severe); short stature
Head and face	Microcephaly; incomplete ossification; micrognathia; anomalous positioning of eyes; "dysmorphic facies;" low-set, deformed ears
Hands and feet	Various anomalies; anomalous dermatoglyphic patterns
Internal organs	Congenital defects of heart and/or great vessels; cerebral malformations; malformations of the genitourinary system

methods - and especially with the perfection of high-resolution banding of chromosomes (see Vogel and Motulsky 1986) - small chromosomal aberrations, for example, deletions, are occasionally discovered in children showing less clear-cut symptoms; for example, newborns regarded as "small for date," with "failure to thrive," and with very minor clinical signs. By and large, however, these rules still apply.

In patients fulfilling the above-mentioned conditions, however, a chromosome study should not be omitted - even if the child has died before or during delivery. Lymphocytes from cord blood or fibroblasts very often permit a cytogenetic diagnosis. Such studies are necessary because the parents who have lost a child often want to have another one and require information as to the genetic risk involved (see Fuhrmann and Vogel 1983; Vogel 1982). A weak point in the Federal Republic of Germany - which I have tried to eliminate for many years but so far without success - is the lack of pediatric pathologists who are able to establish scientifically adequate diagnoses in deceased newborns.

Genetic Conditions with Simple Modes of Inheritance

The second group of genetic conditions recognizable in newborns are anomalies and diseases with simple monogenic modes of inheritance - the classical "hereditary diseases." According to a recent survey by McKusick (1986), about 4000 genetic variants with simple mendelian modes of inheritance are known to date - most of them herditary anomalies or diseases. Many of them can be recognized at birth. Not even the most excellent medical geneticist knows by personal experience even the majority of these diseases; much less can this be expected from the pediatrician. Not even the overall incidence of such cases among newborns can be estimated with confidence; suffice it to say that big obstetric centers will observe quite a few of these patients per year. Their number depends, among other factors, on the gentic structure of the population the center serves. In recent years, special knowledge in this field has increased tremendously, leading to improved opportunities for individual prevention or therapy by suitable therapeutic management (see, for example, Stanbury et al. 1983; Emery and Rimoin 1983; Vogel and Sperling 1987). The examples of phenylketonuria and galactosemia (see Bickel et al. 1980) are well known, but we must remember how important it is for a child with epileptic seizures and hypsarrhythmic EEG that we diagnose, for example, pyridoxine dependency in time for a suitable substitution before irreparable brain damage has occurred (see Scriver and Rosenberg 1973).

Here, close cooperation with pediatricians specially trained to recognize health problems in newborns is imperative. It is good to remember that, in highly developed industrial countries, pediatrics has undergone a shift in emphasis in recent decades. Whereas in earlier times, exogenous diseases such as infections and malnutrition occupied a major share of pediatric efforts, endogenous, and for the most part hereditary disease are now increasingly emphasized since, by and large, many exogenous problems are well under control. Big pediatric hospitals become more and more specialized for certain groups of hereditary metabolic diseases. As management centers for large areas, they cooperate with medical geneticists not only in diagnosis, but also in *prevention* of such diseases by genetic counseling and prenatal diagnosis. In recent years, methods from molecular biology, for example, the use of DNA polymorphisms (see Schmidtke and Cooper 1983, 1984) have enhanced our diagnostic potential (for details, see Vogel and Motulsky 1986). Gene therapy by introducing DNA into somatic cells is not yet possible but can be expected for one or a few genetic diseases in the near future (French-Anderson 1984).

Multifactorial Conditions

The third group of conditions to be considered are the birth defects for which neither a chromosomal aberration nor a monogenic mode of inheritance has been discovered. But in many of these instances, recurrence risk for sibs, when one child with such a birth defect has been born to unaffected parents, may be increased by a factor of about 10, often giving a risk of about 2%-5%. Many well-known conditions belong to this group, such as the majority of patients with neural tube defects, congenital heart disease, cleft lip and palate, hip dislocation, hydrocephalus, and malformations of the central nervous system (see, for example, Bergsma 1979; Nyhan and Sakati 1976; Salmon 1978; Smith 1982; Spranger et al. 1974; Warkany et al. 1981). But patients with multiple birth defects in which no chromosomal aberrations can be found are also fairly common. A preliminary explanation of this group is provided by the genetic model of "multifactorial inheritance in combination with a threshold" (Fig. 1). Disease "liability" (Falconer 1981) is conceived as a continuous variable that is normally distributed in the population. The birth defect occurs in individuals in whom this variable exceeds a certain threshold. This model provides a global description only, it poses questions instead of answering them (Vogel and Motulsky 1986). More specific answers can be found, for example, by isolating special types of birth defect or disease with more specific clinical features and single, genetic or environmental, major causes. This requires disentangling the causative networks with all available methods.

Some, more or less characteristic, malformation syndromes can be traced back to specific exogenous, teratogenic factors acting in early pregnancy. Fortunately, we do not see the thalidomide embryopathy any more. The most common exogenous malformation syndrome encountered at present is alcohol embryopathy, with

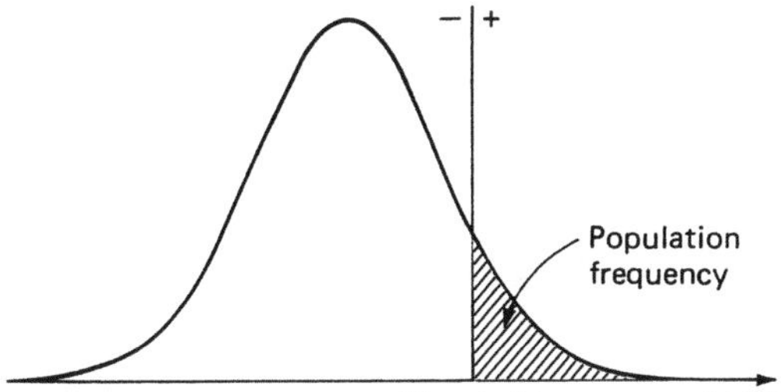

Fig. 1. The genetic model of multifactorial inheritance in combination with a threshold. Liability for a birth defect or disease is assumed to be normally distributed in the population. The birth defect becomes manifest when the liability exceeds a certain threshold. Position of this threshold determines incidence

its characteristic clinical features such as microcephaly, wide nasal bridge, long philtrum and small lips (see Majewski 1980).

In other malformation syndromes, genetic and environmental factors appear to cooperate. As to neural tube defects, for example, there is now fairly good evidence that the high incidence in parts of Great Britain has *not only* genetic reasons but may, in part, be nutritional. Administration of multivitamin preparations in combination with folic acid during pregnancy prevents many occurrences (see, for example, Laurence et al. 1982).

In a substantial fraction of birth defects, however, neither genetic nor environmental factors can be reasonably held responsible for the occurrence of a specific birth defect. It is not unreasonable to assume that, in a certain fraction, *random* combination of poorly defined factors during embryonic development may lead to a malformation of the child. The famous British mouse geneticist and developmental biologist Grüneberg (personal communication) has likened the situation with that of porcelain plates in a dishwasher: a small fraction of all plates will always break but there is no way of analyzing why a specific plate was broken.

Total Number of Birth Defects

So far in my paper you may have missed a *number* - an estimate of the fraction of all newborns who are severely damaged at birth for genetic or partially genetic reasons. Such figures are available from several sources (see, for example, the UNSCEAR report, Anonymous 1982). But only one of them is fairly reliable - the incidence of patients showing major chromosomal aberrations. All other figures are unreliable; they might indicate at best an order of magnitude. Depending on definition, literature data on incidence of birth defects in living newborns, irrespective of their cause, range from 1%-2% to more than 10%.

In has almost become a commonplace statement that genetic causation of an anomaly or birth defect does not necessarily exclude the chances for efficient therapy. Our therapeutic chances do *not* depend on the causation of a condition but on our insights into pathogenetic mechanisms and our ability of influencing them. Therefore, the medical geneticist is not only the counterpart of the therapist, offering *counseling* and *prevention* whenever therapy is limited or even impossible. He is increasingly becoming the *partner* of the therapist who uses his diagnostic skills to help in making therapy more efficient.

Summary

Three groups of genetic anomalies can be distinguished in newborns:

1. Chromosomal aberration, numerical, and structural - they are observed in about 0.6%-0.7% of all newborns.
2. Hereditary diseases with simple mendelian modes of inheritance - more than 3000 such conditions have been described. Most of them are rare or very rare.
3. So-called multifactorial birth defects - their cause is sometimes genetic, sometimes environmental; in other instances, genetic and environmental factors cooperate. For many malformations, no causative factor can be identified.

References

Anonymous (1982) Ionizing radiation: sources and biological effects. United Nations scientific committee on the effects of atomic radiation. United Nations, New York

Bergsma D (1979) Birth defects compendium, 2nd edn. An encyclopedic guide to birth defects. Liss, New York

Bickel H, Guthrie R, Hammersen G (eds) (1980) Neonatal screening for inborn errors of metabolism. Springer, Berlin Heidelberg New York

Bochkov NP, Kuleshov NP, Chebotarev AN, Alekhin VI, Midian SA (1974) Population cytogenetic investigation of newborns in Moscow. Hum Genet 22: 139-152

Emery AEH, Rimoin DL (1983) Principles and practice of medical genetics, 2 vols. Churchill Livingstone, Edinburgh

Falconer DS (1981) Introduction to quantitative genetics, 2nd edn. Oliver and Boyd, Edinburgh

French-Anderson W (1984) Prospects for human gene therapy. Science 229: 401-409

Fuhrmann W, Vogel F (1983) Genetic counseling, 3rd edn. Heidelberg Science Library vol 10. Springer, Berlin Heidelberg New York

Harper PS (1984) Practical genetic counseling, 2nd edn. Wright, Bristol

Hassold TJ, Jacobs PA (1984) Trisomy in man. Ann Rev Genet 18: 69-77

Laurence KM, James N, Miller M, Campbell H, Tennant GB (1982) A double randomised control trial for preconceptional folic acid supplementation for the prevention of recurrence of neural tube defects in high risk pregnancies. J Med Genet 19: 66

Lauritsen JG (1977) Genetic aspects of spontaneous abortion. University of Aarhus, Laegeforeninges.

Majewski F (1980) Untersuchungen zur Alkoholembryopathie. Thieme, Stuttgart

McKusick VA (1986) Mendelian inheritance in man, 7th edn. Johns Hopkins University Press, Baltimore

Nielsen J, Sillesen I (1975) Incidence of chromosome aberrations among 11, 148 newborn children. Hum Genet 30: 1-12

Nielsen J, Sillesen I, Sørensen AM, Sørensen K (1979) Follow-up until age 4 to 8 of 25 unselected children with sex chromosome abnormalities, compared with sibs and controls. Birth Defects XV: 15-73
Nielsen J, Sørensen AM, Sørensen K (1981) Mental development of unselected children with sex chromosome abnormalities. Hum Genet 59: 324-332
Nyhan EL, Sakati NO (1976) Genetic and malformation syndromes in clinical medicine. Year Book Medical, Chicago
Salmon MA (1978) Developmental defects and syndromes. HM + M Publishers, Aylesbury
Scriver CA, Rosenberg LE (1973) Amino acid metabolism and its disorders. Saunders, Philadelphia
Schinzel A (1984) Catalogue of unbalanced chromosome aberrations in man. De Gruyter, Berlin
Schmidtke J, Cooper DN (1983) A list of cloned DNA sequences. Hum Genet 65: 19-26
Schmidtke J, Cooper DN (1984) A list of cloned human DNA sequences - Supplement. Hum Genet 67: 111-114
Smith DW (1982) Recognizable patterns of human malformations, 3rd edn. Saunders, Philadelphia
Spranger JW, Langer LO, Wiedemann HR (1974) Bone dysplasias. Fischer, Stuttgart
Stanbury JB, Wyngaarden JB, Frederickson DS, Goldstein JL, Brown MS (1983) The metabolic basis of inherited disease, 5th edn. Mc Graw-Hill, New York
Vogel F (1982) Die Bedeutung der Humangenetik für eine Theorie der Krankheit. Verh Dtsch Ges Pathol 66: 1-15
Vogel F, Motulsky AG (1986) Human genetics - problems and approaches, 2nd edn. Springer, Berlin Heidelberg New York Tokyo
Vogel F, Sperling K (1987) Proceedings of the 7th international congress of human genetics, September 1986, Berlin. Springer, Berlin Heidelberg New York Tokyo
Warkany J, Lemire RJ, Cohen MM (1981) Mental retardation and congenital malformations of the central nervous system. Year Book Medical, Chicago

Developmental Neurology of the Fetus and Newborn

H. F. R. PRECHTL

Introduction

There is no doubt that obstetrical dilemmas can lead to damage to the fetal and neonatal brain. Why damage occurs in some cases but not in others in apparently comparable situations of hazard is something we do not yet understand. All we know is that statistical relationships can be demonstrated between certain obstetrical complications and neurological outcome. At its earliest, neurological assessment is carried out in the neonatal period. However, it is often delayed until weeks, months, or years later. Many factors can intervene with the passage of time to distort the relationship between the original insult and neurological function at a later age. The relationships found will of necessity be rather loose and will generally only emerge if large groups are studied. Another problem ensuing from taking the results of late evaluations to monitor outcome is the unacceptably long delay this implies for the obstetrician interested in evaluating his management regimes. Since obstetrical and neonatal care practices change rapidly, long-term neurological results are often only of historical interest.

This dilemma would be partly resolved if the neurological condition of the fetus could be evaluated at the time of exposure to a potentially compromising prenatal hazard. Such an evaluation would avoid the necessity of having to wait until much later to tell if the fetus had sustained any functional impairment. Three phenomena which are now available for study reflect the functional integrity of the fetal nervous system. These are: (a) fetal movements; (b) fetal behavioral states; and (c) fetal responses to sensory stimuli.

An attempt will be made in the following to critically scrutinize such possibilities and to compare them with findings in the newborn infant.

Fetal Movements

The old desire to observe the undisturbed fetus in utero has been fulfilled with modern ultrasound equipment. Dynamics and resolution have improved so much that real-time scanning now reveals sufficient detail to detect even small and delicate fetal movements. With this advancement, the classical studies of reflex responses in exteriorized fetuses in terminal condition (Hooker 1952; Humphrey 1978) became of historical interest only.

Maternal counting of fetal movements or repeated mechanical recordings of fetal movements through the maternal abdominal wall provide only crude estimates of motility. Only if there are major changes in the developmental course of motility, can a clinical significance be attributed. However, more refined differentiation of movements is not possible.

What can be seen with modern real-time ultrasound equipment with linear array transducers are specific motor patterns which emerge at an early age. From 7½–8 weeks postmenstrual age onwards, the fetus moves spontaneously. Within a few weeks the repertoire of movements becomes rich, comprising a variety of distinct patterns (see Fig. 1).

Several attempts have been made in the past with varying success to categorize fetal movements (e.g., Birnholz et al. 1978; Van Dongen et al. 1980; Ianniruberto and Tajani 1981). Our own attempts in Groningen are based on long experience of infant observations. My personal hope at the beginning of our ultrasound studies of fetal movements was that familiarity with motor patterns in the preterm and term infant might help us to recognize similar patterns in the fetus. It came some-

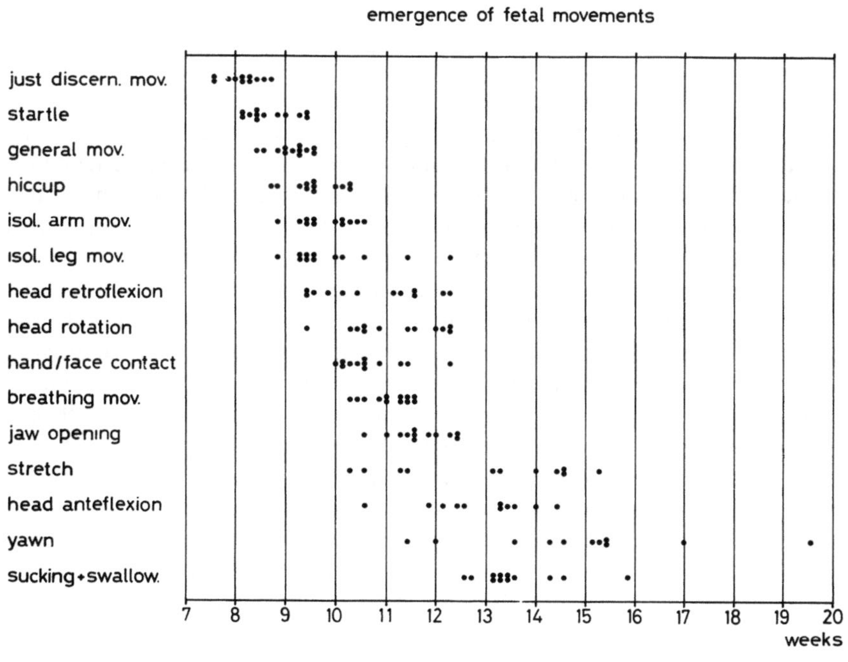

Fig. 1. Timetable of emergence of specific movement patterns in a longitudinal study of 12 fetuses. Each *dot* indicates the first observation of a particular pattern in an individual from the weekly observation. Postmenstrual age is given in weeks and days. *HRP*, heart rate pattern. (From De Vries et al. 1982)

what as a surprise that the repertoire of fetal movements consists exclusively of motor patterns which can also be observed postnatally. The striking similarity of fetal movements with postnatal motor patterns, which can be seen directly after birth or after some delay, greatly facilitates a consistent and comprehensive descriptive classification and terminology.

The emergence of these various movement patterns closely follows a timetable in normal fetuses (De Vries et al. 1982). Once developed, movements hardly change their pattern until birth and are consequently easily recognizable at various gestational ages. However, the rate at which they occur during the observation period is, for most of the patterns, dependent on age (De Vries et al. 1985). For example, the incidence of those short movements, involving all limbs and trunk, which have been called "startles" reach a peak at 9 weeks, followed by a gradual decline until term. Isolated arm movements, on the other hand, show a gradual increase from 10 weeks to mid-pregnancy while the rate of occurrence of general movements stabilizes around 10-11 weeks without major changes afterwards.

Which aspects of fetal movements could be used for the assessment of the neurological condition of the fetus exposed to complications which might have affected the nervous system? The most obvious approach might seem to be to count the various movements and eventually also to assess their strength and forcefulness. The latter has actually been included in Manning's (1980, 1986) scale termed "biophysical profile." The strength of leg movements is scored as "fetal tone" which carries a different connotation than in neurology.

In most severe, especially in terminal, conditions fetal movements decrease. They are also low in certain cases of muscle diseases. Coordination patterns and temporal sequence of occurrence is grossly distorted in anencephalic fetuses (Visser et al. 1985), and leg movements are affected in cases with spina bifida. In many other conditions the diagnostic power of quantification of fetal movements is rather disappointing. This observation is in line with our experience in preterm infants (Prechtl and Nolte 1984). Differences between the amount of the various movement patterns, observed in a carefully selected low-risk group (Prechtl et al. 1979) and in a high-risk group, developing later neurological handicaps, are minimal. It seems likely that we can expect similar findings in the fetus. More striking are changes in the execution of the fetal movements. Preterm infants and fetuses with brain impairment may move monotonously, lacking subtle fluctuations in speed, force, and amplitude of their spontaneous movements. There may also be a restriction in the repertoire of movements, with a drop-out of small movements. Such complex phenomena can be easily recognized, especially when observed from videotape replays, but are very difficult to describe in terms other than fluency, variability, and smoothness. Our visual gestalt perception is a powerful and sensitive instrument enabling us to grasp the simultaneous multifaceted complexity of such phenomena. Such features easily escape the transformation into a linear sequence of verbal descriptions. Attempts to measure quantitatively certain components of movements such as amplitude, acceleration, etc. miss the important complexity and have insufficient discriminative power. A reductionistic approach to solving this problem is not helpful. On the other hand, the validity of such subjective judgements based on gestalt perception made with the unaided eye must be tested. Only a high degree of intersubjectivity between different observers guarantees satisfactory objectivity. Our experience so far is most encouraging. Bekedam et al. (1985) have employed this method in a study of growth-retarded fetuses and demonstrated high interobserver agreement in the recognition of qualitatively abnormal movements. Although further elaboration of this technique will be necessary, this method is one of the most promising approaches for the assessment of the neurological condition of the compromised fetus. It is important to note that recordings of actual movements of a few minutes' duration are sufficient for assessment. This makes this method suitable for clinical application.

Behavioral States

By behavioral states are meant temporary stable conditions of neural and autonomic functions, known as sleep and wakefulness. They are characterized by a distinct behavior of certain variables in concert. Such variables comprise breathing patterns, variability of heart rate, body motility, eye movements, EEG patterns, and tonic activity in certain muscles. These variables can be observed or recorded over long periods, leading to a state profile. There exist extensive studies in the full-term neonate (see Prechtl 1974) and several attempts have been made to define states in the preterm infant (e.g., Parmelee 1975; Stefansky et al. 1984). In the healthy full-term newborn, transitions from the one state to the other last no longer than 2-3 min, which means that all variables have changed their parameters to the characteristics of the new state. It is this phenomenon of alignment between variables at transitions which develops at around 36-38 weeks conceptional age in the preterm infant. Before this age, states are "poorly organized" (Parmelee 1975). An essential aspect is the development of simultaneity in the change of the state variables. Periods of congruency between state variables which fit the state definition do exist at earlier ages but as they do not start and end at the same time, they are called periods of coincidence and must not be considered as "true behavioral states." It is clear from this argument that state assessment can never be carried out properly by the analysis of only one or two variables.

Early attempts to describe behavioral states in the fetus have indeed been made on fetal heart rate patterns alone (Junge 1979) or on motility and heart rate (Timor-Tritsch et al. 1978). These investigators have missed the opportunity of discovering the phenomenon of synchronization of transitions as an ontogenetic event. Nijhuis et al. (1982) were able to show that fetuses of 36-38 weeks had developed behavioral states which, in their organization, are fully comparable to the full-term newborn. The criteria are given in Fig. 2. Of course, the selection of state criteria had to be adapted to the particular situation in utero and differ from those employed in the neonate. Three independent variables were chosen: eye movements present or absent, gross body movements present or absent, and fetal heart rate pattern. For the latter it is crucial to consider only those parts of the record which lie between fetal movements, as accelerations during movements must be excluded for judging the heart rate pattern, except in "pattern D."

STATE CRITERIA

State criteria	State 1F	State 2F	State 3F	State 4F
Body movements	Incidental	Periodic	Absent	Continuous
Eye movements	Absent	Present	Present	Present
Heart rate pattern	A	B	C	D

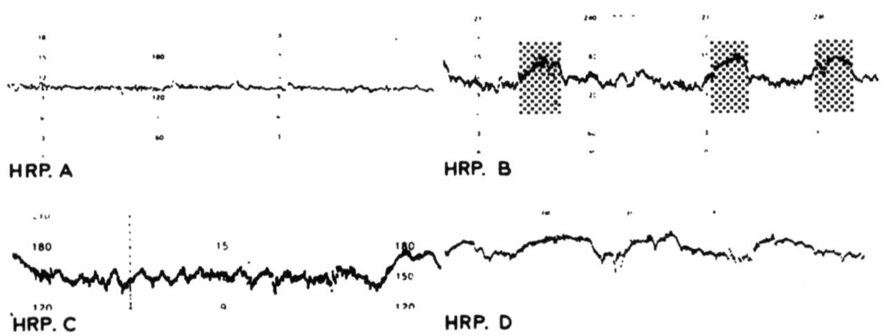

Fig. 2. State criteria in the near-term fetus. *Dotted areas* in heart rate pattern B are excluded, because of movement-induced accelerations. *mov.*, movement. (After Van Vliet et al. 1985)

An important step was achieved by the differentiation between "coincidence" and true "behavioral states" in the fetus. The synchronization of the transitions, lasting no longer than 3 min, is a sensitive indicator of proper maturation of this neural function. The assessment of behavioral states in the near-term fetus is important in two respects. First, states must be assessed when physiological parameters are investigated in the fetus. For example, regularity and amount of breathing movements differ in different behavioral states (Nijhuis et al. 1983; Van Vliet et al. 1985); pulsatility index in the aorta descendente undergoes state-dependent changes (Van Eyck et al. 1985). Hence, for standardization of physiological measures, the simultaneous monitoring of fetal behavioral states is mandatory, a fact long since recognized for the newborn infant (see Prechtl 1974). The second aspect concerns state assessment as a neurological index of fetal wellbeing. Recent studies have discovered that states are poorly developed in growth-retarded fetuses (Bekedam et al. 1985) and a similar finding was obtained in fetuses of diabetic mothers (Mulder et al. 1987). Although coincidence may remain unimpaired, the mechanisms of synchronization of the transitions between states are in many cases lacking. However, in more severe cases, the cyclical organization of single variables (e.g., heart rate pattern) may be abnormal, consequently also affecting the expression of coincidences.

State assessment and the measure of coincidence have turned out to be important aspects for the evaluation of the neurological condition in the near-term fetus.

Fetal Responses to Sensory Stimuli

Although it may be tempting to assess the neurological condition of the fetus in a simple and quick stimulus-response experiment, this hope is in vain. All that we know from the neurological examination of preterm and full-term infants contraindicates such a reductionistic approach. The nervous system is much too complicated to permit reliable answers to be obtained using simplistic methods (see Prechtl 1977, 1982). Another difficulty in the study of fetal reactions to external stimuli is the high base rate of spontaneous fetal movements. It needs great methodological precautions to prove that fetal movements following stimuli are true answers and not spontaneous movements which would have occurred even without the stimulus. For these reasons this method is unsuitable for routine clinical assessment. A third point is the state dependency of many responses which is different for different stimulus modalities. Again, extrapolating from findings in the neonate, auditory reactions may be the most interesting to study. They are present in the fetus in state 2F but are absent during state 1F (Schmidt et al. 1985; Lecanuet et al. 1986). For any clinically useful test with pure auditory stimuli, simultaneous monitoring of behavioral states is necessary (as it is in the newborn).

Stimuli of other modalities have not yet been studied in sufficient detail. For example, it is not clear which receptors are stimulated when the fetus is exposed to "shaking" (Paul and Keegan 1979). But even this response is state dependent, as has been shown by Visser et al. (1983).

In the neonate, responses to mild "pain" stimuli are nearly independent of state (Prechtl and O'Brien 1982). The results by Birnholz and Benacerraf (1983) and Ohel et al. (1986) on stimulation of fetuses with an electro-larynx (vibroacoustic) may consist of "pain" responses as they are apparently very consistent and state independent. The forceful reactions seem a major disturbance to the fetus and it is not at all certain that they are not potentially harmful (e.g., sudden rise in fetal blood pressure).

In summary, it can be said that "shot gun" approaches in testing fetal responses is mistaken because they are much too simplistic. Systematic testing with auditory stimuli is methodologically difficult and very time consuming and is therefore not easy to employ as a routine clinical method.

Conclusions

Modern ultrasound equipment has opened the way toward fetal neurology. The aim is to provide the obstetrician with standardized and comprehensive methods to evaluate the neurological condition in compromised fetuses. Such possibilities will greatly improve assessments which have so far been based on fetal heart rate monitoring and quantitative counts of fetal motility. The most important candidates for neurological assessment are the quality of fetal movements and the organization of behavioral states, the latter only in the near-term fetus. Tests for fetal responses to sensory stimuli (e.g., sound, vibration) are less suitable because of their state dependency and the problem of the high rate of spontaneous movements. Moreover, these tests do not correspond with a comprehensive assessment of the complex nervous system.

References

Bekedam DJ, Visser GHA, de Vries JJ, Prechtl HFR (1985) Motor behaviour in the growth retarded fetus. Early Hum Dev 12: 155-166
Birnholz JC, Benacerraf BR (1983) The development of human fetal hearing. Science 222: 516-518
Birnholz JC, Stephens JC, Faria M (1978) Fetal movement patterns: a possible means of defining neurologic developmental milestones in utero. Am J Roentgenol 130: 537-540
de Vries JIP, Visser GHA, Prechtl HFR (1982) The emergence of fetal behaviour. I. Qualitative aspects. Early Hum Dev 7: 301-322
de Vries JIP, Visser GHA, Prechtl HFR (1985) The emergence of fetal behaviour. II. Quantitative aspects. Early Hum Dev 12: 99-120
Hooker D (1952) The prenatal origin of behaviour. University of Kansas Press, Lawrence
Humphrey T (1978) Function of the nervous system during prenatal life. In: Stave U (ed) Perinatal physiology. Plenum, New York, pp 651-683
Ianniruberto A, Tajani E (1981) Ultrasonographic study of fetal movements. Semin Perinatol 5: 175-181
Junge HD (1979) Behavioral states and state related heart rate and motor activity patterns in the newborn infant and the fetus antepartum - comparative study. 1. Technique, illustration of recordings and general results. J Perinat Med 7: 85-107
Lecanuet JP, Granier-Deferre C, Cohen H, le Houezec R, Busnel MC (1986) Fetal responses to acoustic stimulation depend on heart rate variability pattern, stimulus intensity and repetition. Early Hum Dev 13: 269-283
Manning FA, Platt LD, Sipos L (1980) Antepartum fetal evaluation: development of a fetal biophysical profile. Am J Obstet Gynecol 136: 787-795
Manning FA, Harman CR, Lange IR, Morrison I (1986) Fetal assessment by biophysical profile scoring: 1985 update. Eur J Obstet Gynecol Reprod Biol 21: 331-339
Mulder EJH, Visser GHA, Bekedam DJ, Prechtl HFR (1987) Emergence of behavioural states in fetuses of type-1-diabetic women. Early Hum Dev 15: 231-251
Nijhuis JG, Prechtl HFR, Martin CB Jr, Bots RSGM (1982) Are there behavioural states in the human fetus? Early Hum Dev 6: 177-195
Nijhuis JG, Martin CB Jr, Gommers S, Bouws P, Bots RSGM, Jongsma HW (1983) The rhythmicity of fetal breathing varies with behavioural state in the human fetus. Early Hum Dev 9: 1-7
Ohel G, Birkenfeld A, Rabinowitz R, Sadovsky E (1986) Fetal response to vibratory acoustic stimulation in periods of low heart rate reactivity and low activity. Am J Obstet Gynecol 154: 619-621
Parmelee AH (1975) Neurophysiological and behavioral organization of premature infants in the first months of life. Biol Psychiatry 10: 501-512
Paul RH, Keegan KA (1979) Nonstress antepartum fetal monitoring. Clin Obstet Gynecol 6: 351-358
Prechtl HFR (1974) The behavioural states of the newborn infant (a review). Brain Research 76: 185-212
Prechtl HFR (1977) The neurological examination of the full-term newborn infant. Second edition. Clin Dev Med 63: 65. Heinemann, London
Prechtl HFR (1982) Assessment methods for the newborn infant, a critical evaluation. In: Stratton P (ed) Psychobiology of the human newborn. Wiley, Chichester, pp 21-52

Prechtl HFR, Nolte R (1984) Motor behaviour of preterm infants. In: Prechtl HFR (ed) Continuity of neural functions from prenatal to postnatal life. Clin Dev Med 94: 79-92. Blackwell, Oxford

Prechtl HFR, O'Brien MJ (1982) Behavioural states of the full-term newborn. The emergence of a concept. In: Stratton P (ed) Psychobiology of the newborn infant. Wiley, Chichester, pp 53-73

Prechtl HFR, Fargel JW, Weinmann HM, Bakker HH (1979) Posture, motility and respiration in low-risk preterm infants. Dev Med Child Neurol 21: 3-27

Schmidt W, Boos R, Gnirs J, Auer L, Schulze S (1985) Fetal behavioural states and controlled sound stimulation. Early Hum Dev 12: 245-254

Stefanski M, Schulze K, Bateman D, Kairam R, Pedley TA, Masterson J, James LS (1984) A scoring system for states of sleep and wakefulness in term and preterm infants. Pediatr Res 18: 58-63

Timor-Tritsch IE, Dierker LJ, Hertz RH, Deagan NC, Rosen MG (1978) Studies of antepartum behavioral state in human fetus at term. Am J Obstet Gynecol 132: 524-528

van Dongen LGR, Goudie EG (1980) Fetal movement patterns in the first trimester of pregnancy. Br J Obstet Gynaecol 87: 191-193

van Eyck J, Wladimiroff JW, Noordam MJ, Tonge HM, Prechtl HFR (1985) The blood flow velocity waveform in the fetal descending aorta: its relationship to fetal behavioural states in normal pregnancy at 37/38 weeks. Early Hum Dev 12: 137-143

van Vliet MAT, Martin CB Jr, Nijhuis JG, Prechtl HFR (1985) Behavioural states in growth retarded human fetuses. Early Hum Dev 12: 183-198

Visser GHA, Zeelenburg HJ, de Vries JIP, Dawes GS (1983) External physical stimulation of the human fetus during episodes of low heart rate variation. Am J Obstet Gynecol 145: 579-584

Visser GHA, Laurini RN, de Vries JIP, Bekedam DJ, Prechtl HFR (1985) Abnormal motor behaviour in anencephalic fetuses. Early Hum Dev 12: 173-182

Pathophysiological Mechanisms Leading to Permanent Brain Damage in Surviving Children

F. J. SCHULTE

According to our present state of knowledge, there are four principally different pathophysiological mechanisms which can lead to permanent brain dysfunction (Table 1). In some specific disorders of the nervous system, brain dysfunction is mainly due to one or other of these mechanisms but it is hardly ever exclusively caused by only one. Perinatal brain damage is most frequently caused by either hypoxia, ischemia, bleeding, or trauma. Thus, direct cell injury leading to nerve cell death is a most important pathogenetic mechanism (Friede 1975; Myers 1977).

However, impairment of protein synthesis with structural abnormalities of the dendritic tree and an abnormal time course of synaptogenesis have also definitely been encountered in infants after pathological events in the neonatal period. Since legal aspects of perinatal medicine are becoming more and more important, it is necessary to keep in mind that almost every adverse factor during pregnancy can cause developmental delay or even gross structural abnormality of the brain which, in turn, can be responsible for hypoxia and/or ischemia in the peri- and postnatal period.

It has been one of the most striking results of fetal brain pathology during the recent past that placental insufficiency with intrauterine malnutrition and/or chronic hypoxia, maternal alcoholism, smoking and drug addiction, intrauterine and perinatal infections, as well as perhaps many other still unknown adverse factors which are operative during the most vulnerable period of brain development result in a measurable paucity of nerve cells, dendrites, and synapses (Dobbing 1981; Fabregues and Ferrer 1983; Huttenlocher 1974; Jones 1975; Machado-Salas 1984; Purpura 1974; Schapiro et al. 1984; Wisniewski et al. 1983).

Table 1. Pathophysiological mechanisms of permanent neonatal brain damage

1. Direct cell injury Nerve cell death	Hypoxia/ischemia/trauma/bleeding
2. Impairment of protein synthesis (a) Structural abnormality of the dendritic tree (b) Interference with endoplasmatic reticulum and Golgi apparatus	Malnutrition/toxic agents Hypothyroidism Storage disorders
3. Abnormality of synaptogenesis (a) Abnormal time course (b) Impaired neuronal geometry	Developmental retardation and defects Storage disorders
4. Imbalance of transmitters	Metabolic disturbances, e.g., phenylketonuria

We have to consider that much below the level of gross brain pathology the reduction of dendrites and synapses together with anomalies of the endoplasmatic reticulum and/or Golgi apparatus might be the morphological correlate of numerous forms of both minimal and major brain dysfunction. This has been beautifully shown in the brain of infants with prolonged sleep apnea with recurrent hypoxia finally leading to the sudden infant death syndrome where a developmental delay and/or anomaly of the synpatification of brain stem neurons have been found (Takashima et al. 1985). A similar correlate might be responsible for difficulties in the acquisition of language, for clumsiness of motor function as well as for impaired sensitivity in the different sensory qualities. The distortion of the axo-dendritic and synaptic geometry leads to an imbalance of excitatory vs. inhibitory influences in a given neuronal pool with a possible result of hyperirritability and epilepsy on one side or apathy and coma on the other (Purpura et al. 1980).

The development of the endoplasmatic reticulum is another essential part of nerve cell maturation and differentiation, i.e., the acquisition of certain functional properties (Hammerschlag 1983). Moreover, the endoplasmatic reticulum and the Golgi apparatus are necessary for dendritic growth and for the formation of synapses, the two main prerequisites of normal brain function. Finally, total loss of the endoplasmatic reticulum leads to loss of dendrites and synapses as well as to cell death (Table 2). Hypoxia, toxic agents, as well as storage material (gangliosidoses) apparently interfere with the development of the endoplasmatic reticulum and finally destroy it (Adachi and Volk 1975).

Thus, in summary, the chief "baby killers" (Table 2) are usually operative as a team rather than as single factors although hypoxia/ischemia is the most prominent cause of perinatal brain damage and, therefore, selective nerve cell necrosis (Table 3) is the fundamental morphological correlate of perinatally caused brain

Table 2. Pathophysiological mechanisms of permanent neonatal brain damage - causative factors of brain dysfunction (chief "baby killers")

Hypoxic/ischemic brain injury
Malnutrition of the nervous system, placental insufficiency
Toxic encephalopathies drugs, smoking, alcohol, etc.
Intracranial hemorrhage
Infectious encephalopathies
Metabolic encephalopathies
Hemolytic disorder and kernicterus

Table 3. Anoxic nerve cell damage in infancy - cell death

Cytoplasmatic swelling
Chromatolysis
Nuclear pyknosis
Karyorrhexis

Table 4. Impairment of brain function in hypoxemia/ischemia

Stupor - coma - depressed bioelectric activity as a protective mechanism with maintained ATP levels
Accumulation of extracellular potassium
Intracellular acidosis: lactate accumulation
Diminuition of high-energy compounds
Increased glycogenolysis and glycolysis
Decrease of brain glucose
↓
"No reflow phenomenon"
(Impairment of microvascular perfusion)

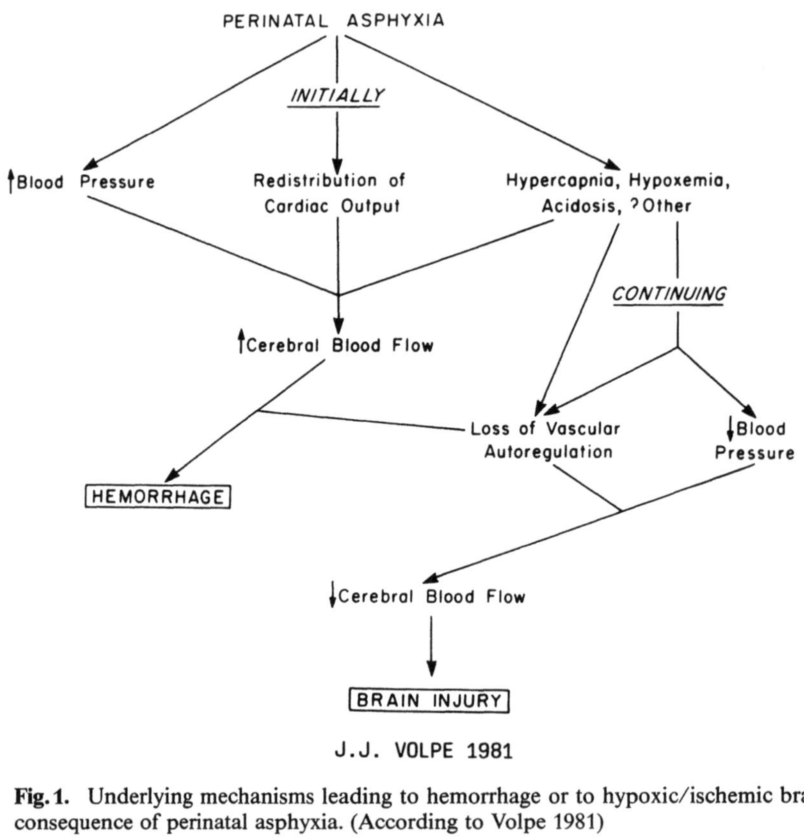

Fig. 1. Underlying mechanisms leading to hemorrhage or to hypoxic/ischemic brain damage in consequence of perinatal asphyxia. (According to Volpe 1981)

dysfunction. The biochemical changes which occur in the hypoxic/ischemic brain are compatible with accelerated anaerobic glycolysis and glycogenolysis. Brain concentration of glucose and glycogen decreases. Initially, ATP levels are preserved at the expense of phosphocreatine, the principal storage form of high-energy phosphate in the brain (Holowach-Thurston and McDougal 1969). The accumulation of lactate is initially a beneficial adaptive response to oxygen deprivation. Tissue acidosis leads to the generation of ATP from phosphocreatine and also to an increase in cerebral blood flow. With progression of lactate accumulation, however, the vascular autoregulation is impaired and enzyme activity (phosphofructokinase) is inhibited (Table 4). In the process of hypoxic/ischemic brain damage this impairment of the microcirculation plays an important role (Lou et al. 1979; Milligan and Bryan 1979).

The underlying mechanisms leading to either hemorrhage or to hypoxic/ischemic brain damage in consequence of perinatal asphyxia are summarized in Fig. 1.

Table 5. Pathophysiological mechanisms of permanent neonatal brain damage - selective neuronal necroses

Cerebral cortex (including hippocampus)
Ulegyria/sclerotic microgyria
Porencephaly
Multicystic encephalomalacia
Parasagittal cerebral injury
Cerebellar cortex
Loss of Purkinje cells and granular layer
Crossed cerebrocerebellar atrophy
Transneuronal necroses
Diencephalon - thalamus - hypothalamus
Basal ganglia
Status marmoratus
White matter infarcts and myelin breakdown
Periventricular leukomalacia
(Cavitated lesions)
Lower brain stem
Pontosubicular neuronal necroses
Medulla
Nucleus ambiguus (IX and X)
Cardiorespiratory neurones

Table 6. Pathophysiological mechanisms of permanent neonatal brain damage - neurological residuals of neonatal encephalopathies

Motor syndromes	Spasticity
	Rigidity - dystonia
	Hyperkinesia (chorea/athetosis)
	Ataxia
Psychological syndromes	Psycho-intellectual and behavioral defects
	Hearing loss
	Visual defects
Abnormal excitability	Convulsions
	Prolonged apnea

As explained in Table 4, depressed central nervous system activity, both mental/motor and bioelectric (electroencephalogram; evoked responses) is a protective mechanism which can still lead to either complete recovery or to incomplete recovery with selective neuronal necroses. Depending on the localization as well as on the extension of the lesion, typical sequelae and residual syndromes can be encountered (Tables 5 and 6).

Summary

I, that am curtail'd of this fair proportion,
Cheated of feature by dissembling Nature,
Deform'd, unfinish'd, sent before my time
Into this breathing world, scarce half made up,
And that so lamely and unfashionable,
That dogs bark at me as I halt by them.

Shakespeare: *King Richard III*

References

Adachi M, Volk BW (1975) Pathology of GM2-Gangliosidoses. In: Volk BW, Scheck L (eds) The gangliosidoses. Plenum, New York

Dobbing J (1981) The later development of the brain and its vulnerability. In: Davis JA (eds) Scientific foundation in pediatrics, 2nd edn. Heinemann, p 744

Fábregues I, Ferrer I (1983) Abnormal perisomatic structures in non-pyramidal neurons in the cerebral cortex in Down's syndrome. Neuropathol Appl Neurobiol 9: 165-170

Friede RL (1975) Developmental neuropathology. Springer, Vienna New York

Hammerschlag R (1983) How do neuronal proteins know where they are going? Speculations on the role of molecular address markers. Dev Neurosci 6: 2-17

Holowach-Thurston J, McDougal DB Jr (1969) Effect of ischemia on metabolism of the brain of the newborn mouse. Am J Physiol 216: 348

Huttenlocher PR (1974) Dendritic development in neocortex of children with mental defect and infantile spasms. Neurology 24: 203-210

Jones KL (1975) Aberrant neuronal migration in the fetal alcohol syndrome. Birth Defects 11 (7): 131-132

Lou HC, Lassen NA, Tweed WA, Johnson G, Jones M, Palahniuk RJ (1979) Pressure passive cerebral blood flow and breakdown of the blood-brain barrier in experimental fetal asphyxia. Acta Paediatr Scand 68: 35

Machado-Salas JP (1984) Abnormal, dendritic patterns and aberrant spine development in Bourneville's disease - a Golgi survey. Clin Neuropathol 3: 52-58

Milligan DW, Bryan MH (1979) Failure of autoregulation of the cerebral circulation in the sick newborn infant. Pediatr Res 13: 527

Myers RE (1977) Experimental models of perinatal brain damage: relevance to human pathology. In: Gluck L (ed) Intrauterine asphyxia and the developing fetal brain. Reprinted by the US Department of Health, Education, and Welfare, NIH 4: 37-97

Purpura DP (1974) Dendritic spine dysgenesis and mental retardation. Science 186: 1126-1128

Purpura DP, Highstein SM, Karabelas AB, Walkley SU (1980) Intracellular recording and HRP-staining of cortical neurons in feline ganglioside storage disease. Brain Res 181: 446-449

Schapiro MB, Rosman NP, Kemper TL (1984) Effects of chronic exposure to alcohol on the developing brain. Neurobehav Toxicol Teratol 6: 351-356

Takashima S, Mitro T, Becker LW (1985) Neuronal development in the medullary reticular formation in sudden infant death syndrome and premature infants. Neuropediatrics 16: 76

Volpe JJ (1981) Neurology of the newborn. Saunders, Philadelphia

Wisniewski K, Dambska M, Sher JH, Quazi Q (1983) A clinical neuropathological study of the fetal alcohol syndrome. Neuropediatrics 14: 197-201

Trauma and the Developing Brain

J. S. Wigglesworth

Introduction

Cranial birth trauma is generally considered to be an uncommon condition and is certainly one that is diagnosed in few infants in life and by few pathologists at perinatal autopsy. However, it is apparent that trauma is inseparable from the birth process and few adults would willingly allow their heads to be submitted to the forms of mechanical stress involved in spontaneous or forceps-aided vaginal delivery.

Since some degree of trauma, with cranial moulding, tissue oedema or capillary haemorrhages, is an inevitable result of the birth process, the questions to be addressed in this presentation are related to the frequency and nature of significant forms of trauma. The viewpoint which I shall adopt is that of a perinatal pathologist whose suspicions about the frequency of trauma became aroused some 12 years ago.

Historical Aspects

A number of classical anatomical studies on cranial trauma published in the first half of this century stressed the importance of the tentorium cerebelli in the genesis of obstetrically induced subdural haemorrhage (Holland 1922; Rydberg 1932; Craig 1938). During this period the associated processes of asphyxia and trauma far outweighed all other forms of pathology as contributors to the enormous perinatal mortality of the times. The most important aspect of examination of the cranial contents was dissection in a manner which would demonstrate traumatic lesions. Hemsath (1934) alone in this period recognised the frequency of injury to the occipital bone as a significant form of cranial trauma. In the British Perinatal Mortality Survey of 1958 (Fedrick and Butler 1971), the incidence of death associated with intracranial trauma had fallen to 3.1 per 1000 births, including 9.5% of stillbirths and 10.9% of first-week neonatal deaths. A 12% incidence was noted in infants who were small for date. Since that time, the overall incidence has fallen steadily (Chamberlain et al. 1975), with an increasing proportion of cases involving preterm infants. Larroche (1977), reviewing 700 necropsies during the period

1967-1973, found subdural bleeds in 18% of infants of more than 36 weeks' gestation who died and in 11% of preterm infants who died. Wigglesworth and Husemeyer (1977) confirmed the previous observations of Hemsath (1934) as to the importance of suboccipital osteodiastasis as a traumatic lesion and the ease with which it could be overlooked in life and at autopsy.

Sites and Mechanisms of Trauma

Extracranial Haemorrhage. This includes caput succedaneum, subaponeurotic haemorrhage, and subperiosteal cephalhaematoma. Caput succedaneum and subperiosteal cephalhaematoma are relatively common minor traumatic lesions, not usually by themselves of serious significance. Occasionally cephalhaematoma is associated with underlying fracture of a cranial bone. More important, although rare, is subaponeurotic or subgaleal haemorrhage, in which the bleeding may extend insidiously beneath the epicranial aponeurosis and into the muscles of the neck resulting in eventual collapse from haemorrhagic shock (Robinson and Rossiter 1968).

Damage to Cranial Bones. The lesions seen include linear or depressed fractures of individual bones and separation of the squamous and lateral parts of the occipital bone. The presence of linear or depressed fractures may, like the presence of a severe caput succedaneum or cephalhaematoma, indicate the possibility of significant cerebral trauma but are not often of great importance per se. Separation of the squamous and lateral parts of the occipital bone is a lesion of major importance (Wigglesworth and Husemeyer 1977). The squamous and lateral parts of the occipital bone develop from a number of separate ossification centres and remain widely separated by cartilage until about 36 weeks' gestation. Bony fusion does not occur until the 2nd year of life. The lower margin of the squamous occipital bone forms the posterior boundary of the foramen magnum centrally and is closely related to the occipital sinuses on each side. Traumatic separation of the cartilaginous joints between the squamous and lateral parts on one or both sides may readily be caused by pressure exerted on the suboccipital region during birth. The lower edge of the squamous occipital bone may then be rotated forwards and tear the occipital sinuses or impinge on the cerebellum and brain stem.

Disruption of Dural Folds. The most well-recognised lesions are tears of the tentorium and falx, with or without associated tears of veins and sinuses. Tears of the tentorium have long been recognised as being due to excessive fronto-occipital or oblique compression during delivery. Tentorial tears usually involve the free margin near the junction with the falx. Tears of the falx are usually oval in form and occur in the posterior part. Bleeding into the subdural or subarachnoid spaces in association with tentorial tears is usually attributed to rupture of the groups of veins which drain the superficial cerebral veins into the sagittal and lateral sinuses (Pape and Wigglesworth 1979). Occasionally there is disruption of the vein of

Galen or extension of a tentorial tear into the lateral or straight sinuses. However, it has recently been pointed out that the tentorium has an artery supplying it which runs near the free border and is thus at risk of disruption (Welch and Strand 1986).

Subdural and Subarachnoid Haemorrhage. These forms of bleeding often occur, as mentioned above, in association with tentorial tears. Frequently such bleeds occur without damage to the dural folds. In many cases it can be assumed that the bleeding is due to traumatic rupture of bridging veins within either the subdural or subarachnoid part of their course. Subarachnoid haemorrhage is however usually of non-traumatic cause and subdural haemorrhage is common in cases of massive intracranial haemorrhage associated with haemostatic failure.

Direct Trauma to the CNS. This is most commonly described in the form of spinal cord transection in the lower cervical region associated with breech delivery. Rarely, transection of the upper cervical cord has been described in cephalic deliveries (Shulman et al. 1971). Damage to the cerebellum has been described in cases of occipital osteodiastasis (Wigglesworth and Husemeyer 1977).

Current Frequency and Variety of Cranial Birth Trauma

Most recent surveys of perinatal mortality or morbidity dismiss cranial trauma as of exceptionally low frequency and hardly worthy of report, if indeed they even mention the occurrence. Welch and Strand (1986) have recently published a series of 25 cases of traumatic intracranial haemorrhage recognised on computerised tomography (CT). These were nearly all well-grown mature infants who presented with signs referable to the CNS. They were estimated to have been derived from a population of about 130000 births.

In order to assess the range of cranial trauma currently occurring and its likely significance for mortality and morbidity, the pathology records of infants examined postmortem at Hammersmith Hospital over the 10 years 1976–1985 have been analysed.

Of 515 infants who died intrapartum or in the 1st week of life, 47 were reported as having significant cranial or intracranial trauma at postmortem, a frequency of 9.1%. Trauma was considered to be a major factor leading to death in 13 cases. Fifteen of the infants had been born at Hammersmith Hospital; the rest were transferred from other hospitals to the Hammersmith Hospital neonatal intensive care unit after birth or were referred after death for specialist perinatal autopsy. All postmortems were performed or closely supervised by one pathologist. The integrity of the occipital bone was assessed in all cases, with dissection of the suboccipital region in those infants in whom trauma could not be excluded on initial external palpation.

Thirty-three of the infants were below 2.5 kg in weight and 28 were of less than 36 weeks' gestation, a similar distribution to that of perinatal deaths in general.

Eighteen of the infants (38%) were delivered vaginally by the breech, only nine (19%) had spontaneous vertex delivery and only six (13%) were delivered by Caesarean section.

Nine of the infants were stillborn, and a further 17 died at under 12 h of age. All had died by 8 days of age.

Ten of the infants had significant malformations, most of them being related to the head or neck (e.g. short neck syndromes or cerebral anomalies associated with thin cranium). Particularly striking was the severe trauma seen in four infants with congenital muscle disorders associated with flexion deformities.

The lesion most frequently seen was occipital osteodiastasis in 32 cases (68%). Other common findings were subdural haemorrhage in 27 cases (57%) with involvement of the posterior fossa in six, tears of the tentorium in 20 (43%) and of the falx in seven (15%).

Mechanisms of trauma were indicated by the patterns of lesion that were found to occur together. Important findings in association with occipital osteodiastasis were tentorial tears in nine cases, haemorrhagic necrosis or laceration of the cerebellum in five instances and transection of the lower medulla in two. The infants with medullary transection had both been maintained alive on the ventilator, for 10 h in one instance and 2 days in the other. Each had a tentorial tear in addition to the other lesions. One of these cases has been previously described and illustrated (Pape and Wigglesworth 1979).

Significance of Postmortem Findings for Cerebral Development in Survivors

The frequency with which cranial trauma has been observed at postmortem in our own series could be interpreted in a number of different ways. There will inevitably be a tendency to dismiss the findings as unrepresentative of infants dying after modern obstetric management since other pathologists do not report such lesions. Of the lesions described here it is probable that less than half would have been recognised by pathologists carrying out a standard form of autopsy. In many cases the lesions are unlikely to cause death and may not present the infant with any problem. However, the most minor lesions may be an indication of cranial deformation which would be expected to result in changes recognisable only as asphyxia. Occipital osteodiastasis without displacement of the squamous occipital bone in the immature infant is an example of this. Disturbance of the integrity of the occiput indicates that significant deformation of the cranium has occurred irrespective of whether or not there is any haemorrhage or cerebral laceration. Such deformation is likely to cause temporary impairment of cerebral circulation and might be expected to affect the posterior fossa in particular. Support for this view of cerebral ischaemia as a consequence of cranial trauma was provided by one case in which a dramatic clinical deterioration followed reintubation in an infant of 37 weeks' gestation who developed respiratory distress syndrome following an uncomplicated spontaneous vertex delivery. At postmortem following death at 72 h of age, bilateral occipital osteodiastasis was found to be associated with kinking of the lateral sinuses by the margin of the occipital bone and petechiae over the occipital lobes. At the sight of the unexpected trauma, the resident who intubated the infant made the spontaneous suggestion that the lesion had occurred during the intubation procedure which had been made difficult by the infant's abnormally short neck. Dissection of the fixed brain revealed early periventricular leucomalacia, indicating episodes of severe hypotension.

Follow-up of infants recognised on CT to have traumatic cranial haemorrhage showed various sequelae including microcephaly, frontal porencephaly with seizures, clumsiness (following cerebellar haemorrhage), hemiparesis, visual disturbances, spastic diplegia and shunt dependency (Welch and Strand 1986). These will represent the severe end of the spectrum as the infants were sufficiently ill in the neonatal period to justify CT. Most infants who suffer cranial trauma are assumed to have birth asphyxia unless they present unequivocal evidence of haemorrhage. In fact the distinction is extremely difficult in life. The infant with asphyxia may develop haemorrhagic cerebral infarcts mimicking trauma while the traumatised infant may appear shocked and asphyxiated. It seems unlikely that it will ever be possible to differentiate fully the effects of trauma from those of the associated asphyxia or preterm birth.

Postmortem diagnosis is also relatively difficult. The occiput has to be dissected externally before opening the cranium if occipital osteodiastasis is to be recognised routinely, and it is necessary to look specifically for evidence of trauma in every case if it is not to be missed in the small preterm infant.

Although gross trauma in mature infants is now relatively uncommon it appears from these postmortem studies that trauma may occur far more frequently in small preterm infants than is suspected clinically. Vaginal breech delivery appears particularly hazardous. Infants with congenital neuromuscular problems and those with cerebral anomalies may also be at undue risk of trauma. These risks should be taken into account when planning the perinatal management of such infants.

References

Chamberlain et al (1975) British births 1970, vol 1. The first week of life. Heinemann, London

Craig WS (1938) Intracranial hemorrhage in the newborn. Arch Dis Child 13: 89-124

Fedrick J, Butler NR (1971) Certain causes of neonatal death. V. Cerebral birth trauma. Biol Neonate 18: 321-329

Hemsath FA (1934) Birth injury of the occipital bone with a report of thirty-two cases. Am J Obstet Gynecol 27: 194-203

Holland EL (1922) Cranial stress in the foetus during labour. J Obstet Gynaecol Br Empire 29: 551-571

Larroche JC (1977) Developmental pathology of the neonate. Excerpta Medica, Amsterdam

Pape KE, Wigglesworth JS (1979) Haemorrhage, ischaemia and the perinatal brain. Heinemann, London; Lippincott, Philadelphia

Robinson RJ, Rossiter MA (1968) Massive subaponeurotic haemorrhage in babies of African origin. Arch Dis Child 43: 684-687

Rydberg E (1932) Cerebral injuries in newborn children consequent on birth trauma. Acta Pathol Microbiol Scand [Suppl] 10

Shulman et al (1971) Transection of the spinal cord: a rare obstetrical complication of cephalic delivery. Arch Dis Child 46: 291-294

Welch K, Strand R (1986) Traumatic parturitional intracranial hemorrhage. Dev Med Child Neurol 28: 156-164

Wigglesworth JS, Husemeyer RP (1977) Intracranial birth trauma in vaginal breech delivery: the continued importance of injury to the occipital bone. Br J Obstet Gynaecol 84: 684-691

How and When Does Antenatal Hypoxia Damage Fetal Brains?

R. L. Naeye

Introduction

Many seem to believe that asphyxia during labor and delivery is a frequent cause of non-progressive neurologic impairments. This assumption needs close examination because very few impaired individuals have placental abruptions, umbilical cord compression, or any other cause of intrapartum asphyxia diagnosed at birth, and only a small minority are in coma or have kidney failure in the neonatal period (Naeye 1986; Niswander 1983; Tack et al. 1986). Stupor or coma would be frequent if intrapartum asphyxia caused their impairments because the cerebral edema and uneven blood flow that damage the brain in these circumstances markedly depress brain function (Van Bel et al. 1984). Renal failure would also be frequent because severe intrapartum hypoxia almost always produces renal failure (Tack et al. 1986).

A history of intrapartum fetal distress is another factor that is often cited as evidence that many individuals with neurologic impairments are asphyxiated during labor and delivery. It now appears that fetal distress in these individuals is probably the result of already damaged brains malfunctioning when subjected to the stress of normal labor. This can be inferred from the many studies that have found no quantitative correlations between markers of fetal distress, biochemical evidences of intrapartum hypoxia, and subsequent neurologic impairments (Dijxhoorn et al. 1986; Low et al. 1978; Niswander 1983). Niswander and others have cited this as evidence that acute intrapartum hypoxia is less likely to be a cause of neurologic impairments than is subacute and chronic hypoxia that occurred earlier in gestation (Chiswick et al. 1977; Gross et al. 1968; Niswander 1983).

Many are convinced that intrapartum asphyxia is a frequent cause of neurologic abnormalities because Myers produced severe brain damage in monkeys by asphyxiating them in the fetal and newborn periods (Myers 1972; Myers and Adamsons 1981; Myers et al. 1981). What is less well known is that many of these monkeys died and most of the survivors had no neurologic impairments, even when the degree and duration of asphyxia were carefully controlled (Myers 1972; Adamsons 1981). This suggests that the oxygenation level at which monkeys were brain damaged and survived was just below the level at which the damage was fatal.

The present study looked for new mechanisms to explain how brain damage takes place before birth. Pregnancy, intrapartum, and neonatal findings in neurologically impaired individuals were analyzed to try to determine whether their impairments originated before, during, or after the intrapartum period. Disorders that can make fetuses hypoxic during pregnancy, the intrapartum, and neonatal periods were analyzed to see if they explain any of the impairments.

Patients and Methods

The data for our analyses came from the Collaborative Perinatal Study (NCPS) of the National Institute of Neurological and Communicative Disorders and Stroke. The NCPS was set up to identify fetal, intrapartum, and neonatal events that affect children's development. It prospectively followed the course of over 56000 pregnancies in 12 medical school-affiliated hospitals in different regions of the United States between 1959 and 1966. Events of gestation, labor, delivery, and the neonatal period were recorded, as well as children's subsequent psychomotor, sensory, and physical development (Naeye and Tafari 1983; Anonymous 1966). The analyses of the present study included 35419 of these children who had complete developmental evaluations at 7 years of age. The present study focuses on the results of the 7-year neurologic examination that recorded abnormalities in motor and sensory performance. Details of the methods used to evaluate psychomotor and sensory performance in the NCPS have been previously published (Anonymous 1966).

If a large proportion of the NCPS children who have unexplained neurologic abnormalities were growth retarded at birth, the growth retardation might be evidence that they experienced adverse influences during pregnancy that affected their brains as well as their overall growth. Our first analyses were designed to identify children who were growth retarded at birth. We calculated the growth percentiles for birthweight, length, head circumference, umbilical cord length and placental weight for each NCPS newborn based on growth charts that take into consideration maternal pregravid body weight as well as gestational age at delivery and the sex of the infant (Naeye 1986). Gestational age was computed at birth from the 1st day of the mother's last menstrual period. The socioeconomic scores used in many of the analyses combined values for family income, education, and occupation of the head of household (Myrianthopolous and French 1968). Scores from a nonverbal intelligence test (SRA test), given to each gravida, were included in many analyses (Anonymous 1966).

Efforts were made to determine if fetal, intrapartum, or neonatal hypoxia could explain some of the neurologic abnormalities that were present at 7 years of age. The various causes of acute, subacute, and chronic hypoxia are listed in Table 1. Each cause of hypoxia was placed in the category that we judged most often represents its action, recognizing that some could be placed in more than one category. The causes of acute antenatal, intrapartum, and neonatal hypoxia are well known (Naeye and Tafari 1983). The mechanisms of subacute and chronic hypoxia may not be as widely understood, so some brief explanations may be useful. Subacute and chronic fetal hypoxia are most often caused by low

Table 1. Classification of antenatal and neonatal hypoxia

A. Causes of acute hypoxia
Vaginal bleeding
Placenta previa
Abruptio placentae
Tight knot in umbilical cord
Cord tight around neck
Cord prolapse
Long labor
Persistent high uterine tone during labor
Tumultuous labor
Maternal shock
Gaseous anesthesia
B. Causes of subacute and chronic hypoxia
(a) Anemia
Fetal blood loss
Rh erythroblastosis
Severe maternal anemia
(b) Low uteroplacental blood flow
Third trimester hypotension
Severe hypertension
Multiple births
Cigarette smoking
(c) Other causes
Neonatal respiratory distress syndrome

uteroplacental blood flow and by maternal or fetal anemia (Naeye and Tafari 1983). The most frequent causes of low uteroplacental blood flow are low maternal blood volume expansion during pregnancy, relative maternal hypotension, hypertension, damage to the uterine arteries, and cigarette smoking (Gallery et al. 1979; Goodlin et al. 1983; Grunberger et al. 1979; Lehtovirta and Forss 1978; Naeye and Tafari 1983). Twins and triplets have long been known to have a lower uteroplacental blood flow per fetus than the single born (Morris et al. 1955). Smoking a cigarette frequently reduces uteroplacental blood flow for 5-20 min (Lehtovirta and Forss 1978).

Low 1-min Apgar scores, the need for prolonged resuscitation at birth, and neonatal seizures were added to the analyses because they are characteristic consequences of intrapartum hypoxia. They are also manifestations of brain dysfunction, so in some circumstances they could be the consequence of brain damage or maldevelopment that had originated earlier in gestation. Neonatal seizures, in particular, are often considered an indicator that intrapartum asphyxia adversely affected a child's brain (Low et al. 1985). If true, adding another marker of intrapartum asphyxia, such as 1-min Apgar scores, should reduce the correlation of the seizures with subsequent neurologic abnormalities in regression analyses. We undertook such analyses to see if the correlation between neonatal seizures and subsequent neurologic abnormalities is strongly correlated with intrapartum asphyxia or hypoxia.

To compare the possible effects of hypoxia with the established effects of nonhypoxia factors that damage fetal brains, the following nonhypoxia factors were

Table 2. Relationship of fetal growth and demographic factors to the frequency of neurologic abnormalities at 7 years of age

Growth and Demographic factors	Beta values	Neurologic abnormalities associated with:
Down's syndrome	+.076[a]	Down's syndrome
Sex of child, female	−.073[a]	Males
Congenital malformations	+.054[a]	Congenital malformations
Socioeconomic index scores	−.046[a]	Low socioeconomic status
Maternal intelligence test scores	+.044[a]	Low maternal IQ
Gestational age at birth	−0.38[a]	Low preterm gestational age
Race, non-white	−.031[a]	Being white
Head circumference, percentiles	−.027[a]	Small head size
Birth length, percentiles	−.024[a]	Low birth length
Single born, twins, triplets	+.018[a]	Being a twin or triplet
Birthweight, percentiles	−.009[b]	-
Umbilical cord length, percentiles	−.007[b]	-
Placental weights, percentiles	−.001[b]	-

This is a single multiple regression analysis that includes all of the factors in the list.
[a] $p<.001$
[b] $p>.1$

Table 3. Relationship of various maternal pregnancy factors to the frequency of neurologic abnormalities in children at 7 years of age

Maternal Pregnancy factors	Beta values	Neurologic abnormalities associated with:
Alcoholism	+.032[a]	Alcoholism
Albuminuria, absent to 4+	+.025[a]	Albuminuria
Peak third trimester diastolic blood pressure		
40-79 mmHg	−.015[b]	Relative hypotension
71-200 mmHg	+.020[c]	Hypertension
Cigarettes smoked/day	+.019[a]	Smoked cigarettes
Pregnancy weight gain	−.012[d]	-
Edema on hands and face	−.013[d]	-
Urinary tract infection, + culture	+.012[d]	-
Diabetes mellitus, insulin reaction	+.006[d]	-
ketoacidosis	+.011[e]	-
Chronic hypertension	+.010[d]	-
Vaginal bleeding, first trimester	+.007[d]	-
Second trimester	+.007[d]	-
Third trimester	+.001[d]	-
Lowest third trimester hemoglobin value		
3.0-12.0 gm/dl	−.004[d]	-
Pregravid weight	+.004[d]	-
Hyperemesis with acetonuria	+.003[d]	-
Irregular menses	+.001[d]	-
Seizure disorder	+.001[d]	-

[a] $p<.001$
[b] $p<.05$
[c] $p<.01$
[d] $p>.1$
[e] $p<.1$

included in the analyses: congenital malformations, Down's syndrome, maternal alcoholism, neonatal hyperbilirubinemia, symptomatic hypoglycemia. Neonatal hypoglycemia can be the consequence of intrapartum hypoxia but it has many additional causes.

Stepwise multiple regression analysis was used to control for interactions between factors that might affect or correlate with neurologic abnormalities. The dependent variable was the result of the neurologic examination undertaken at 7 years of age. It was treated as a three-step variable: neurologically normal, suspicious for neurologic abnormalities, definite neurologic abnormalities. Each analysis included a selected list of sociohereditary, demographic, and fetal growth parameters (Table 2) to which was added one cause of acute hypoxia (Tables 3-5). This approach was adopted to try to determine if individual acute hypoxia factors correlated with neurologic impairments independently of the effects of the sociohereditary, demographic, and fetal growth influences. The same approach was used to determine if subacute and chronic hypoxia predisposed to neurologic

Table 4. Relationship of fetal, prelabor, labor, and delivery factors to neurologic abnormalities at 7 years of age

Fetal Factors	Beta values	Neurologic abnormalities associated with:
Fetal blood loss	$+.028^{a}$	Fetal blood loss
Rh erythroblastosis fetalis	$+.013^{b}$	Rh disease
Fetal aspiration	$+.010^{c}$	-
Cord tight around neck	$+.006^{c}$	-
Tight knot, umbilical cord	$+.003^{c}$	-
Prelabor and Labor factors		
Duration second stage labor	$-.015^{d}$	Very short labor
Reaction to uterine stimulation	$+.008^{c}$	-
Persistent high uterine tone		
Tumultous labor	$+.006^{c}$	-
Placenta previa	$+.004^{c}$	-
Umbilical cord prolapse	$-.004^{c}$	-
Abruptio placentae	$+.004^{c}$	-
Used oxytocin	$+.002^{c}$	-
Arrested progress of active labor	$+.001^{c}$	-
Delivery Factors		
Forceps, outlet, low, mid, high	$-.008^{c}$	-
Fractured skull	$+.006^{c}$	-
Used gas anesthesia	$-.006^{c}$	-
Breech delivery	$+.002^{c}$	-
Podalic version	$-.006^{c}$	-
Maternal shock		
Due to anesthesia	$+.004^{c}$	-
Due to hemorrhage	$+.001^{c}$	-
Due to other causes	$-.007^{c}$	-

[a] $p<.001$
[b] $p<.05$
[c] $p>.1$
[d] $p<.02$

abnormalities, except that fetal growth parameters were not included in these analyses because most of the disorders that produce subacute or chronic hypoxia also retard fetal growth (Naeye and Tafari 1983) (Tables 3-5).

The factors that proved to be most significant in the initial analyses were put into a single regression analysis to see how independent they were of each other (Table 6). Several of the disorders that presumably cause chronic hypoxia, as well

Table 5. Relationship of neonatal factors to neurologic abnormalities at 7 years of age

Neonatal factors	Beta values	Neurologic abnormalities associated with:
Seizures	+.074[a]	Seizures
1-min Apgar scores	−.048[a]	Low Apgar scores
Required > 5 min resuscitation	+.030[a]	Prolonged resuscitation
Symptomatic hypoglycemia	+.029[a]	Hypoglycemia
Peak serum bilirubin 0-40 mg/dl	+.028[a]	Hyperbilirubinemia
Respiratory distress syndrome	+.023[a]	Neonatal respiratory distress syndrome

[a] $p < .001$

Table 6. Relationship of maternal and fetal factors to 7-year neurologic abnormalities when those found most significant in Tables 3-5 are included in a single analysis

	Beta values	Neurologic abnormalities associated with:	Cumulative R^2values
Down's syndrome	+.075[a]	Down's syndrome	.0048
Sex of child, female	−.069[a]	Males	.0090
Congenital malformations	+.056[a]	Congenital malformations	.0102
Socioeconomic index scores	−.047[a]	Low socioeconomic status	.0214
Maternal intelligence test score	−.039[a]	Low maternal IQ	.0229
Fetal blood loss	+.034[a]	Fetal blood loss	.0233
Neonatal respiratory distress syndrome	+.032[a]	Neonatal respiratory distress	.0238
Neonatal symptomatic hypoglycemia	+.026[a]	Symptomatic hypoglycemia	.0245
Alcoholism	+.025[a]	Mother alcoholic	.0251
Race, non-white	−.023[a]	Whites	.0258
Single born, twins, triplets	+.019[a]		.0262
Gestational albuminuria, 0 to 4+	+.018[b]	Albuminuria	.0266
Neonatal hypobilirubinemia	+.015[c]	Hyperbilirubinemia	.0274
Peak third trimester diastolic blood pressure			
40-79 mmHg	+.012[d]	Relative hypotension	.0276
71-200 mmHg	−.011[e]	-	.0278
Gestational age	−.005[f]	-	.0279

[a] $p < .001$
[b] $p < .005$
[c] $p < .02$
[d] $p < .05$
[e] $p < .1$
[f] $p > .1$

Table 7. Interaction of fetal growth with perinatal factors on the frequency of neurologic abnormalities at 7 years of age

	Beta values
Pregnancy	
Lowest maternal third trimester hemoglobin value 3.0 to 12.0 gm/dl	
Birthweight percentile 1-10	−.039[a]
Birthweight percentile 11-30	−.024[b]
Birthweight percentile > 30	+.014[c]
Peak third trimester diastolic blood pressure 40-79 mmHg	
Birthweight percentile 1-10	−.039[a]
Birthweight percentile 11-30	−.029[a]
Birthweight percentile > 30	+.004[c]
Single born, twins, triplets	
Birthweight percentile 1-10	+.035[a]
Birthweight percentile 11-30	+.030[d]
Birthweight percentile > 30	+.001[c]
Neonatal period	
1-min Apgar score	
Birthweight percentile 1-10	−.080[e]
Birthweight percentile 11-30	−.059[e]
Birthweight percentile > 30	−.025[e]
Resuscitation > 5 min	
Birthweight percentile 1-10	+.078[e]
Birthweight percentile 11-30	+.025[a]
Birthweight percentile > 30	+.010[c]
Neonatal seizures	
Birthweight percentile 1-10	+.091[e]
Birthweight percentile 11-30	+.033[f]
Birthweight percentile > 30	+.018[a]

[a] $p < .05$
[b] $p < .1$
[c] $p > .1$
[d] $p < .02$
[e] $p < .001$
[f] $p < .01$

as low 1-min Apgar scores, the need for prolonged resuscitation at birth, and neonatal seizures were further analyzed by birthweight percentiles to see if their correlation with neurologic impairments was greater when children had been growth retarded at birth (Table 7).

Results

At 7 years of age, 1437 (4.1%) of the children had one or more definite neurologic abnormalities. The sociohereditary and demographic factors selected for analysis

Table 8. Correlation of neonatal seizures with subsequent neurologic abnormalities, with and without preceding 1-min Apgar scores in stepwise multiple regression analysis

	Beta values
Neonatal seizures	+.047[a]
After adding 1-min Apgar scores	
Neonatal seizures	+.046[a]
Analysis limited to children whose birthweights were in the 1-20th percentile	
Neonatal seizures	+.074[a]
After adding 1-min Apgar scores	
Neonatal seizures	+.073[a]

[a] $p<.001$

had a significant correlation with the neurologic abnormalities (Table 2). Short body length and small head circumference at birth also had a positive correlation with neurologic abnormalities. All of the presumed causes of subacute and chronic fetal hypoxia except maternal anemia had a positive correlation with the neurologic impairments, whereas none of the causes of acute hypoxia had such a correlation (Tables 3-7). Low 1-min Apgar scores, the need for prolonged resuscitation at birth, and neonatal seizures also correlated with neurologic abnormalities, particularly when the neonate was growth retarded (Tables 5, 7). Most of the chronic hypoxia factors as well as low Apgar scores, the need to resuscitate, and neonatal seizures had a much stronger correlation with neurologic abnormalities when children had been growth retarded than when they were normally grown at birth (Table 7). In a separate analysis, the addition of 1-min Apgar scores to multiple regression analyses did not decrease the correlation of neonatal seizures with neurologic abnormalities (Table 8). All of the nonhypoxic factors that were anticipated to correlate with neurologic abnormalities had such correlations (Tables 2, 3, 5, 6).

Discussion

Results of the present study confirm previous reports that neurologic abnormalities in older children are more frequent when growth retardation was present at birth (Naeye 1986; Niswander 1983). When such growth retardation was absent, none of the disorders or clinical managements of labor and delivery that can produce intrapartum asphyxia were associated with subsequent long-term neurologic abnormalities. This greatly strengthens the possibility that intrapartum hypoxia that is severe enough to damage fetal brains is an uncommon cause of neurologic abnormalities in surviving children. This is compatible with evidence that the neonate's brain is better protected from the effects of acute hypoxia than are some other organs (Oh et al. 1986).

Most of the factors that correlated with long-term neurologic abnormalities appear to have exerted their influence long before labor and delivery. The antenatal factors fall into three categories: factors that limit oxygen delivery to the fetus, factors that restrict the delivery of oxygen to the fetal brain, and nonhypoxic factors such as congenital malformations, Down's syndrome, and maternal alcoholism (Table 1). Low uteroplacental blood flow appears to be the most frequent factor that limits oxygen delivery to the fetus while fetal blood loss and anemia are the factors that most often restrict oxygen delivery to fetal brains.

None of the disorders or factors that produce intrapartum hypoxia correlated with subsequent neurologic abnormalities and there is evidence that intrapartum hypoxia did not potentiate already existing brain damage. Children who had neonatal seizures, commonly recognized evidence of intrapartum asphyxia, had no weakening of the correlation between such seizures and subsequent neurologic abnormalities when 1-min Apgar scores were added to the analysis. This indicates that the relationship of seizures to subsequent neurologic abnormalities was unrelated to intrapartum hypoxia because intrapartum asphyxia characteristically depresses 1-min Apgar scores.

One of the noteworthy findings of the present study is that perinatal hypoxia, as reflected by low 1-min Apgar scores, the need for prolonged resuscitation at birth, and the presence of the neonatal respiratory distress syndrome, explains less than 1% of the long-term neurologic abnormalities in the NCPS population (Table 5). Many children who died as the result of perinatal hypoxia in the NCPS would probably have lived if they had been born during the last few years. This would not necessarily make perinatal hypoxia a more important cause of neurologic abnormalities in children now being born because the effect of more survivors would, to some extent, be counterbalanced by modern obstetrical and neonatal managements that appear to lower the frequency of central nervous system damage in high-risk fetuses and neonates. Whatever the net effect of these two trends, intrapartum and neonatal hypoxia had such a small role in the genesis of neurologic abnormalities in the NCPS that it is difficult to see how any changes in obstetric and medical management in the intervening years could much affect the frequency of neurologic impairments in children now being born.

There are still other reasons to think that the obstetric and medical managements of labor, delivery, and the neonate have a very small role in the genesis of neurologic impairments in society. More than 95% of the morbidity and mortality we currently see in newborns who do not have congenital malformations is due to the hypoxia produced by placental villous edema or low uteroplacental blood flow (Naeye 1985; Naeye and Tafari 1983; Naeye et al. 1983). Both of these disorders antedate labor and delivery, villous edema most often by several days and low uteroplacental blood flow by days or weeks. Obstetric and medical interventions in such circumstances take place after prolonged fetal hypoxia. Since the threshold at which intrapartum asphyxia begins to damage brains is apparently very close to the level at which asphyxia is fatal, it is doubtful that early interventions, such as early cesarean section, prevent many neurologic impairments. Very gentle handling of the preterm infant during delivery and the neonatal period is another matter. It may prevent some neurologic abnormalities because it seems to reduce the frequency of the respiratory distress syndrome and its central nervous system complications in preterm neonates.

Findings of the present study provide strong support for the possibility that many neurologic abnormalities currently attributed to severe intrapartum and neonatal hypoxia are due instead to other causes. Several mechanisms are identified by which some of this brain damage most likely takes place. These mechanisms explain only a small percentage of the total neurologic abnormalities in the current analyses but this could be an underestimate of their full role because they most likely operated for days or weeks before they were recognized at regular antenatal medical visits, and even when they were recognized there was no way to quantitate their duration, severity, or effects on the fetus. Medical and obstetric advances since the NCPS have not solved this problem because almost all of the neurologic impairments are still originating in a setting where the danger cannot be recognized before the damage has most likely taken place.

Summary

Analyses were undertaken to evalute the role of antenatal and neonatal hypoxia in causing neurologic abnormalities. In a prospective study, 4.1% (1437) of 35419 children had neurologic (motor or sensory) abnormalities at 7 years of age. All but one of the disorders that can produce subacute or chronic fetal hypoxia had a positive correlation with these neurologic abnormalities while none of the disorders that can produce acute antenatal hypoxia had such a correlation. The correlation of subacute and chronic hypoxic disorders with neurologic abnormalities was much stronger when children were growth retarded at birth than when they were normally grown. These findings suggest that subacute and chronic fetal hypoxia are causes of long-term neurologic abnormalities while acute hypoxia rarely plays such a role.

References

Anonymous (1966) The collaborative study on cerebral palsy, mental retardation and other neurological and sensory disorders of infancy and childhood manual. US Department of Health, Education and Welfare, Bethesda

Chiswick M, D'Sousa S, Occleshaw J (1977) Computerized transverse axial tomography in the newborn. Early Hum Dev 1: 171-9

Dijxhoorn MJ, Visser GHA, Fidler VJ, Touwen CL, Huisjes HJ (1986) Apgar score, meconium and acidaemia at birth in relation to neonatal neurological morbidity in term infants. Br J Obstet Gynaecol 93: 217-22

Gallery EDM, Hunyor SN, Gyory AZ (1979) Plasma volume contraction, a significant factor in both pregnancy-associated hypertension and chronic hypertension in pregnancy. Q J Med 48: 593-602

Goodlin RC, Dobry CA, Anderson JC, Woods RE, Quaife M (1983) Clinical signs of normal plasma volume expansion during pregnancy. Am J Obstet Gynecol 145: 1001-9

Gross H, Jellinger J, Kaltenback E et al. (1968) Infantile cerebral disorders. J Neuro Sci 7: 551-64

Grunberger W, Leodolter S, Parschalk O (1979) Maternal hypotension: fetal outcome in treated and untreated cases. Gynecol Obstet Invest 10: 32-8
Lehtovirta P, Forss M (1978) The acute effect of smoking on intervillous blood flow of the placenta. Br J Obstet Gynaecol 85: 729-31
Low JA, Galbraith RS, Muir DW et al. (1978) Intrapartum fetal asphyxia, a preliminary report in regard to long-term morbidity. Am J Obstet Gynecol 130: 525-33
Low JA, Galbraith RS, Muir DW et al. (1985) The relationship between perinatal hypoxia and newborn encephalopathy. Am J Obstet Gynecol 152: 256-60
Morris N, Osborn SB, Wright HP (1955) Effective circulation of the uterine wall in late pregnancy. Lancet 1: 323-4
Myers RE (1972) Two patterns of perinatal brain damage and their conditions of occurrence. Am J Obstet Gynecol 112: 246-76
Myers RE, Adamsons K (1981) Obstetric considerations of perinatal brain injury. Rev Perinatal Med 4: 221-45
Myers RE, Wagner KR, DeCourten GM (1981) Lactic acid accumulation in tissue as cause of brain injury and death in cardiogenic shock from asphyxia. In: Lauerser NH, Hockberg HM (eds) Perinatal biochemical monitoring. Williams and Wilkins, Baltimore, p 11
Myrianthopolous NC, French KS (1968) An application of the US Bureau of the Census socioeconomic index to a large, diversified patient population. Soc Sci Med 2: 283-99
Naeye RL (1986) When and how does antenatal brain damage occur? In: Iffy L (ed) Second perinatal practice and malpractice Symposium, Healthmark Comm, New York, p 125
Naeye RL (1985) Standardizing the mortality risk for newborns with very low birth weights. Am J Dis Child 139: 445-6
Naeye RL, Tafari N (1983) Risk factors in pregnancy and diseases of the fetus and newborn. Williams and Wilkins, Baltimore
Naeye RL, Maisels MJ, Lorenz RP et al. (1983) The clinical significance of placental villous edema. Pediatrics 71: 588-94
Niswander KR (1983) Asphyxia in the fetus and cerebral palsy. Yearbook Medical, Chicago, pp 107-25
Oh W, Piva DL, Gulati R, Stonestreet BS (1986) The effects of hypoxia and hyperviscosity on the cerebral cortex and gastrointestinal tract oxygenation and glucose metabolism. Pediatr Res 20: 348 A
Tack E, Perlman JM, Hause C, Griften M, Margin T (1986) Systemic manifestations of perinatal asphyxia in the newborn. Pediatr Res 20: 362 A
Van Bel, Hirasing RA, Grimberg MT (1984) Can perinatal asphyxia cause cerebral edema and affect cerebral blod flow velocity? Eur J Pediatr 142: 29-32

Intrauterine Deprivation – Growth Retardation and Chronic Hypoxia

Antepartum Events and Cerebral Handicap

R. L. NAEYE and E. C. PETERS

Introduction

Twenty years ago Penrose, Drillien and others developed the two-population theory to explain the causes of mental retardation (Drillien et al. 1966; Penrose 1983; Zigler 1967). In this model, heredity and sociocultural deprivation are the major causes of mild retardation while brain damage and maldevelopment cause most severe retardation. This two-population model has been challenged in recent years by reports that disorders that might damage fetal brains are as frequent in the histories of mildly as of severely retarded individuals (Costeff et al. 1983; Drillien 1968; Hagberg et al. 1981; Lilienfeld and Pasamanick 1956). The identity of these damaging disorders has not usually been determined, but a few of the retarded children reportedly had mothers who were hypertensive or bled during pregnancy (Broman et al. 1975; Drillien 1968; Hagberg et al. 1981). Other children had placental infarcts, clinical evidences of asphyxia at birth, a history of kernicterus or cyanotic disorders in the neonatal period (Broman et al. 1975; Costeff et al. 1983; Drillien 1968; Drillien et al. 1966; Hagberg et al. 1981).

The present study analyzed 19117 children from a prospective study to determine if hypoxia during labor, delivery, or the neonatal period affected their IQ scores at 7 years of age. The analyses took into consideration sociohereditary and demographic factors that strongly affect IQ values.

Patients and Methods

The data for the analyses came from the Collaborative Perinatal Study (NCPS) of the National Institute of Neurological and Communicative Disorders and Stroke. The NCPS was set up to identify fetal, intrapartum, and neonatal events that affect children's development. It prospectively followed the course of over 56000 pregnancies in 12 medical school-affiliated hospitals in different regions of the United States between 1959 and 1966. Events of gestation, labor, delivery, and the neonatal period were recorded as well as children's mental, motor, sensory and physical development to 7 years of age (Broman et al. 1975; Naeye and Tafari 1983; The Collaborative Study 1966). The last child was examined in 1973 and the complete data set for the study became available for analysis in 1976.

We selected results of the Wechsler intelligence scale (1949) test for analysis because it was administered at 7 years of age when mental impairments are more often permanent than at earlier ages. Two percent of the children had IQ scores between 50 and 70 and 8% had scores under 80.

Maternal IQ values were obtained from a nonverbal intelligence test (SRA test) that was given to most gravidas (The Collaborative Study 1966). Socioeconomic scores combined values for family income, education, and occupation of the head of household (Myrianthopolous and French 1968). Definitions and detailed descriptions of the other hereditary and sociocultural factors included in the analyses have been published (Broman et al. 1975; The Collaborative Study 1966).

Efforts were made to determine if fetal, intrapartum, or neonatal hypoxia lowered IQ values. The various analyzed causes of acute, subacute, and chronic hypoxia are listed in Table 1. Each cause of hypoxia was placed in the category that we judged most often represents its action, recognizing that some could be placed in more than one category. The causes of acute antenatal, intrapartum, and neonatal hypoxia are well known (Naeye and Tafari 1983). The mechanisms of subacute and chronic hypoxia may not be as widely understood, so some brief explanations are in order. Subacute and chronic fetal hypoxia are most often caused by low uteroplacental blood flow and by maternal anemia (Naeye and Tafari 1983). The most frequent causes of low uteroplacental blood flow are low maternal blood volume expansion during pregnancy, relative maternal hypotension and hypertension (Gallery et al. 1979; Gant et al. 1976; Garn et al. 1978; Goodlin et al. 1983; Grunberger et al. 1979; Naeye and Tafari 1983). Twins and triplets have long been known to have a lower uteroplacental blood flow per fetus than the single born (Morris et al. 1955). Smoking a cigarette frequently reduces

Table 1. Classification of antenatal and neonatal hypoxia

A. Causes of acute hypoxia:
Vaginal bleeding
Placenta previa
Abruptio placentae
Maternal shock
Tight knot in umbilical cord
Cord tight around neck
Cord prolapse
Long labor
Persistent high uterine tone during labor
Tumultuous labor
Neonatal apneic episodes
B. Causes of subacute and chronic hypoxia:
(a) Anemia
Severe maternal anemia
(b) Low uteroplacental blood flow
Third trimester hypotension
Hypertension
Multiple births
(c) Other causes
Neonatal respiratory distress syndrome

uteroplacental blood flow for 5-20 min but it is not known how often this produces fetal hypoxia (Lehtovirta and Forss 1978). Abnormally high hemoglobin levels in neonates are sometimes the result of protracted or intermittent fetal hypoxia (Garn et al. 1978).

The neonatal respiratory distress syndrome and apneic episodes are the most frequent causes of neonatal hypoxia. With both disorders, cerebral blood flow can be reduced or uneven, which sometimes leads to cerebral ischemia (Perlman and Volpe 1985; Perlman et al. 1984).

Low 1-min Apgar scores, the need for prolonged resuscitation at birth, and neonatal seizures were added to the analyses because they are characteristic consequences of intrapartum hypoxia. They are also manifestations of brain dysfunction, so in some circumstances they could be the consequence of brain damage or maldevelopment that had originated long before labor and delivery.

To compare the possible effects of hypoxia with the effects of nonhypoxic factors that are known to damage fetal brains, the following nonhypoxic factors were included in the analyses: congenital malformations, Down's syndrome, maternal alcoholism, and neonatal hyperbilirubinemia.

Fetal growth retardation can be the consequence of antenatal adversity that affects the fetus' brain as well as overall growth so fetal growth parameters were included in the analyses. We calculated the growth percentiles for birthweight, length, head circumference, umbilical cord length and placental weight for each newborn based on growth charts that take into consideration maternal pregravid body weight as well as gestational age at delivery and the sex of the infant. Gestational age was computed at birth from the first day of the mother's last menstrual period.

Stepwise multiple regression analysis was the analytic tool used in the study. Each analysis included one of the factors that are possible causes of hypoxia as well as all of the sociohereditary and demographic factors that influence IQ values. This approach was adopted to try to determine if individual hypoxia factors affected IQ values independently of the effects of the sociohereditary and demographic factors. In a final analysis the disorders that were most significant in the various individual analyses were put into a single regression analysis to see how independent they were from each other.

Results

Maternal IQ scores, sociocultural, and demographic factors had a strong influence on the children's IQ values (Table 2). Antenatal, intrapartum, and neonatal factors that can produce acute hypoxia were followed by normal IQ values, whereas factors that can produce subacute or chronic fetal hypoxia were associated with low IQ values (Tables 3-7). These subacute and chronic hypoxia factors were: maternal gestational anemia, relative hypotension, hypertension, multiple births, and fetal growth retardation. As a group, the subacute and chronic hypoxia factors had a weaker correlation with low IQ values than did most of the sociohereditary and demographic factors. As expected, congenital malformations, Down's syndrome, and maternal alcoholism correlated with low IQ values (Tables 3, 4).

Table 2. Relationship of sociodemographic, lifestyle, and hereditary factors to IQ values of 7-year-old children

Demographic, hereditary, and lifestyle factors	Beta values	Low IQ values associated with:
Socioeconomic score[a]	+.201[b]	Low socioeconomic status
Race, black[a]	−.200[b]	Being black
Maternal or surrogate IQ value[a]	+.160[b]	Low maternal IQ
Maternal education (years)[a]	+.139[b]	Few years of education
Maternal age[a]	+.097[b]	Very young mothers
Birth order[a]	−.088[b]	High birth order
Breast feeding, duration[a]	+.074[b]	No breast feeding
Gestational age at birth[a]	+.035[b]	Preterm birth
Singletons, twins, triplets[a]	−.039[b]	Multiple births
Sex of infant, female	−.004[c]	-
Mental retardation, siblings	+.009[c]	-
Consanguinity, parents of child	−.005[c]	-

[a] Items included in every analysis in tables 3-6.
[b] $p < .001$
[c] $p > .1$

Table 3. Relationship of maternal pregravid and pregnancy factors to IQ values

Neurologic abnormalities present	Beta values	Low IQ values associated with:
Maternal pregravid factors		
Prior stillbirths, neonatal deaths	−.020[a]	Prior losses
Pregravid weight	+.003[a]	-
Irregular menses	+.001[a]	-
Pregnancy factors		
Lowest third trimester hemoglobin level		
4.0-11.5 gm/dl	+.053[b]	Maternal anemia
11.6-16.0 gm/dl	+.007[a]	-
Peak diastolic blood pressure third trimester		
40-79 mmHg	+.017[a]	Relative hypotension
71-200 mmHg	−.016[a]	-
Alcoholism	−.015[c]	Alcoholism
Vaginal bleeding	+.008	-
Abruptio placentae	+.008	-
Edema on hands and face	+.007[a]	-
Hypothyroidism	+.007[a]	-
Hyperemesis with acetonuria	+.006[a]	-
Seizure disorder	−.006[a]	-
Pregnancy weight gain	+.004[a]	-
Cigarettes/day	−.004[a]	-
Placenta previa	+.004[a]	-
Syphilis	−.004[a]	-
Hyperthyroidism	+.003[a]	-
Albuminuria, 0-4+	−.011[b]	-
Diabetes mellitus, ketoacidosis	−.001[a]	-

Items marked[a] in Table 2 are included in the analysis of every factor in this table.
[a] $p > .1$
[b] $p < .01$
[c] $p < .001$

Table 4. Relationship of fetal factors to IQ values of 7-year-old children

	Beta value	Low IQ values associated with:
Fetal growth		
Growth (percentiles)		
Head circumference	+.068[a]	Small head circumference
Birthweight	+.067[a]	Low birthweight
Birth length	+.055[a]	Short at birth
Placental weight	+.040[a]	Low placental weight
Umbilical cord length	+.034[a]	Short umbilical cord
Other fetal factors		
Down's syndrome	−.054[a]	Down's syndrome
Congenital malformations	−.021[a]	Congenital malformations
Fetus aspirated amniotic fluid	+.007[b]	-
Large placental infarct	+.004[b]	-
Tight knot in umbilical cord	+.003[b]	-
Fetal blood loss	+.002[b]	-
Cord tight around neck	+.001[b]	-

Items marked[a] in Table 2 are included in the analysis of every factor in this table.
[a] $p < .001$
[b] $p > .1$

Table 5. Relationship of intrapartum factors to IQ values of 7-year-old children

	Beta values	Low IQ values associated with:
Labor factors		
Umbilical cord prolapse	−.006[a]	-
Arrested progress of active labor	+.006[a]	-
Meconium in the amniotic fluid	−.006[a]	-
Reaction to uterine stimulation		
Persistent high uterine tone	−.002[a]	-
Tumultuous labor	−.001[a]	-
Delivery factors		
Severe ecchymoses	−.010[b]	-
Breech delivery	−.008[a]	-
Fetal skull fractured	+.004[a]	-
Maternal shock	+.002[a]	-

Items marked[a] in Table 2 are included in the analysis of every factor in this table.
[a] $p > .1$
[b] $p < .1$

Table 6. Relationship of newborn and childhood findings to IQ values of 7-year-old children

	Beta values	Low IQ values associated with:
Neonatal factors		
Hemoglobin value at 48 h of age, 17.0–24.0 gm/dl	$-.026^{a}$	High hemoglobin values
1-min Apgar score	$+.016^{a}$	Low Apgar scores
Respiratory distress syndrome	$-.012^{b}$	Respiratory distress syndrome
Required resuscitation > 5 min	$+.007^{c}$	-
Symptomatic hypoglycemia	$+.007^{c}$	-
Multiple apneic episodes	$-.007^{c}$	-
Seizures	$+.005^{c}$	-
Peak serum bilirubin level	$+.002^{c}$	-
Any time before 7 years of age		
Head trauma	$-.008^{d}$	Head trauma
Central nervous system infection	$-.002^{c}$	Infection
Lead poisoning	$+.001^{c}$	-

Items marked[a] in Table 2 are included in the analysis of every factor in this table.
[a] $p<.001$
[b] $p<.005$
[c] $p>.1$
[d] $p<.05$

Table 7. Relationship of maternal, fetal, and perinatal findings to IQ values of 7-year-old children when the most significant factors from previous tables are included in the same analysis

Maternal, fetal and perinatal factors in same analysis	Beta values	Low IQ values associated with:	Cumulative R^2 values
Socioeconomic score	$+.219^{a}$	Low socioeconomic status	.203
Race, black	$-.218^{a}$	Being black	.320
Maternal education (years)	$+.153^{a}$	Few years of education	.342
Maternal age	$+.153^{a}$	Very young mothers	.357
Maternal IQ value	$+.142^{a}$	Low maternal IQ	.370
Breast feeding, duration	$+.078^{a}$	No breast feeding	.378
Singletons, twins, triplets	$-.039^{a}$	Multiple births	.380
Gestational age at birth	$+.035^{a}$	Preterm birth	.381
Birth order	$-.024^{a}$	High birth order	.382
Birthweight percentile	$+.060^{a}$	Low birth weight	.389
Head circumference percentiles	$+.047^{a}$	Small head	.392
Down's syndrome	$-.047^{a}$	Down's syndrome	.395
Lowest maternal third trimester hemoglobin level 4.0–11.5 gm/dl	$+.040^{a}$	Maternal anemia	.397
Peak maternal diastolic blood pressure during pregnancy 40–79 mmHg	$+.020^{a}$	Hypertension	.398
Neonatal respiratory distress syndrome	$-.012^{b}$	Respiratory distress syndrome	.399
Newborn's hemoglobin value at 48 h of age, 17.0–24.0 gm/dl	$-.009^{b}$	High hemoglobin value	.399

[a] $p<.001$
[b] $p<.05$

Discussion

The present study tried to determine if fetal and neonatal hypoxia sometimes lower children's IQ values. Taking sociohereditary and demographic influences into consideration, antenatal disorders and factors that can produce subacute or chronic hypoxia correlated with low IQ scores, whereas disorders that can produce acute hypoxia did not have this correlation. This raises the possibility that subacute and chronic fetal hypoxia can impair children's cognitive development. A deficiency of nutrients that the fetal brain uses for energy and growth could also contribute to the low IQ values because most of the factors that restrict the delivery of oxygen to the fetal brain also limit the delivery of glucose and other nutrients.

It is unlikely that chronic hypoxia is a proxy for nonhypoxic factors in the current analyses because all of the subacute and chronic hypoxic factors were followed by low IQ scores whereas none of the acute hypoxic factors, including those that exert their influence during labor and delivery, correlated with low IQ scores.

IQ values in the present study increased with increasing maternal gestational blood pressures until the hypertensive range was reached. The simplest explanation is that the lower pressures limited uteroplacental blood flows which in turn retarded brain development by restricting the delivery of oxygen and nutrients to the fetus. This explanation is consistent with the progressive increase in newborn head circumference that occurred with increasing maternal blood pressures in the NCPS (Naeye 1981). The studies by Grunberger et al. (1979) also demonstrate that low blood pressures that persist into late gestation have unfavorable effects. Grunberger et al. found that uteroplacental blood flow was low and full-term neonates markedly undergrown (<2.9 kg birthweight) when maternal blood pressures did not exceed 110/65 mmHg during pregnancy. Birthweights increased to a mean of 3.3 kg after blood pressures and uteroplacental blood flows had been increased in a second group of hypotensive gravidas by the administration of desoxycorticosterone.

If chronically low uteroplacental blood flow can lower IQ values, the children of women who were hypertensive during pregnancy should have lower than expected IQ values because uteroplacental blood flow is often persistently low after gravidas became hypertensive (Gallery et al. 1979). Gestational hypertension correlated with low IQ values in the present study.

Are the findings of the present study obsolete because there have been many improvements in the management of pregnancy, labor, delivery, and the neonate since the NCPS data were collected? A striking finding of the present study is that intrapartum and neonatal factors that can produce acute hypoxia accounted for less than 1% of the IQ variance in the NCPS population (Table 7). Since their effect was so small it is most unlikely that advances in the management of labor, delivery, and the neonate since the NCPS data were collected have produced a measurable improvement in IQ values. Among the causes of low uteroplacental blood flow, only gestational hypertension is much better managed now than at the time of the NCPS. There are no data available to know whether this better management is improving the cognitive development of some children whose mothers were hypertensive during pregnancy.

Another factor that needs to be considered is the fragile-X syndrome. It is an important cause of mental retardation that was not recognized at the time the NCPS data were collected. Its omission from the current analyses would not change their conclusions because with a frequency of only one per 2000 births, fragile-X could account for only about one in 200 of the < 80 IQ values in the NCPS (Turner and Jacobs 1983).

Findings of the present study indicate that maintaining a large maternal blood volume during pregnancy and preventing maternal anemia might sometimes prevent the fetal brain from being adversely affected by low uteroplacental blood flow. A large maternal blood volume usually ensures a large uteroplacental blood flow, which in turn protects the fetus from the adverse effects of abnormally low maternal blood pressures and other factors that might otherwise restrict uteroplacental blood flow (Grunberger et al. 1979; Naeye 1981; Naeye and Tafari 1983). Goodlin et al. (1983) have reviewed the clinical and laboratory methods that are available for recognizing low maternal blood volume during pregnancy.

Summary

Analyses were undertaken to determine if fetal, intrapartum, and neonatal hypoxia are important causes of low IQ values. Prospectively collected pregnancy, perinatal, and subsequent developmental data were analyzed for 19117 children. As expected, sociohereditary and demographic factors had a large influence on IQ scores. Taking these latter influences into consideration, nothing that happened during labor, delivery, or the neonatal period affected subsequent IQ values. The same was true for antenatal disorders that can produce acute fetal hypoxia. By contrast, antenatal disorders and conditions that can produce subacute or chronic fetal hypoxia correlated with low IQ values. These antenatal disorders and conditions were: maternal gestational anemia, relative gestational hypotension, hypertension, multiple births, and fetal growth retardation.

References

Broman SH, Nichols PL, Kennedy WA (1975) Preschool IQ, prenatal and early developmental correlates. Erlbaum, New York

Costeff H, Cohen BE, Weller LE (1983) Biological factors in mild mental retardation. Dev Med Child Neurol 25: 580-587

Drillien CM (1968) Studies in mental handicap. II. Some obstetric factors of possible aetiological significance. Arch Dis Child 43: 283-294

Drillien CM, Jameson S, Wilkinson EM (1966) Studies in mental handicap. I. Prevalence and distribution by clinical type and severity of defect. Arch Dis Child 41: 528-538

Gallery EDM, Hunyor SN, Gyorgy AZ (1979) Plasma volume contraction, a significant factor in both pregnancy-associated hypertension (preeclampsia) and chronic hypertension in pregnancy. QJ Med 48: 593-602
Gant NF, Madden JS, Chand S, Worley RJ, Strong JD, MacDonald PC (1976) Metabolic clearance rate of dehydroisoandrosterone sulfate. V. Studies of essential hypertension complicating pregnancy. Obstet Gynecol 47: 319-326
Garn SM, Shaw HA, McCabe KD (1978) Effect of maternal smoking on hemoglobins and hematocrits of the newborn. Am J Clin Nutr 31: 557-558
Goodlin RC, Dobry CA, Anderson JC, Woods RE, Quaife M (1983) Clinical signs of normal plasma volume expansion during pregnancy. Am J Obstet Gynecol 145: 1001-1007
Grunberger W, Leodolter S, Parschalk O (1979) Maternal hypotension, fetal outcome in treated and untreated cases. Gynecol Obstet Invest 10: 32-38
Hagberg B, Hagberg G, Lewerth A, Lindberg (1981) Mild mental retardation in Swedish school children. II. Etiologic and pathogenetic aspects. Acta Paediatr Scand 70: 445-452
Lehtovirta P, Forss M (1978) The acute effect of smoking on intervillous blood flow of the placenta. Br J Obstet Gynaecol 85: 729-731
Lilienfeld AM, Pasamanick B (1956) The association of maternal and fetal factors with the development of mental deficiency. II. Relationship to maternal age, birth order, previous reproductive loss and degree of maternal deficiency. Am J Ment Defic 60: 557-569
Morris N, Osborn SB, Wright HP (1955) Effective circulation of the uterine wall in late pregnancy. Lancet 1: 323-324
Myrianthopolous NC, French KS (1968) An application of the US Bureau of the Census socioeconomic index to a large, diversified patient population. Soc Sci Med 2: 283-299
Naeye RL (1981) Maternal blood pressure and fetal growth. Am J Obstet Gynecol 141: 780-787
Naeye RL (1985) Umbilical cord length. J Pediatr 107: 278-282
Naeye RL, Tafari N (1983) Risk factors in pregnancy and diseases of the fetus and newborn. Williams and Wilkins, Baltimore
Penrose LS (1983) The biology of mental defect, 3rd edn. Sidgwick and Jackson, London
Perlman JM, Volpe JJ (1985) Episodes of apnea and bradycardia in the preterm newborn: impact on cerebral circulation. Pediatrics 76: 333-338
Perlman JM, McMenamin JB, Volpe JJ (1984) Fluctuating cerebral blood flow velocity in the respiratory distress syndrome. N Engl J Med 310: 204-209
The Collaborative Study (1966) on cerebral palsy, mental retardation and other neurological and sensory disorders of infancy and childhood manual. US Department of Health, Education and Welfare, Bethesda
Turner G, Jacobs P (1983) Marker X-linked mental retardation. Adv Hum Genet 13: 83-112
Wechsler Intelligence Scales for Children (1949) Psychological, New York
Zigler E (1967) Familial mental retardation, a continuing dilemma. Science 155: 292-298

Available Evidence Relating Intrauterine Growth Retardation to Neuromotor Dysfunction and Mental Handicap

G. BREART

This paper is based on a review of the recent (since 1980) English and French literature. Its aim is, first, to look at the level of risk of unfavorable long-term outcome for full-term (>36 weeks of gestation) intrauterine growth-retarded (IUGR) babies (defined, most of the time, as small for gestational age, SGA) and then to look at the antenatal determinants in order to discuss the possible means of prevention and the current state of their evaluation.

Level of Risk

In their paper published in 1972, Fitzhardinge and Steven gave one of the most dramatic figures for SGA babies. Among 96 full-term babies whose weights were below the mean −2 SD, they observed: 6% convulsions, 25% minimal brain damage, a two-fold increase in EEG anomalies, and a five-fold increase in speech defects. Since this publication, several surveys on long-term outcome of SGA babies have been reported with, sometimes, conflicting results. Rantakallio (1985) reported the 14-year outcome of an entire cohort of 12000 children from northern Finland. She showed (Table 1) that the number of children with major neurological handicaps but normal school performance did not vary significantly by birthweight percentiles, whereas educational subnormality, including mental retardation, was highly significantly more frequent in all the percentile classes lower than the median.

In another survey (Table 2), Ounsted et al. (1984) compared the 7-year outcome of 138 neonates whose birthweight was below the mean −2 SD (SGA) with the outcome of 138 neonates whose birthweight was average for gestational age

Table 1. Fourteen-year outcome by birthweight centiles (Rantakallio 1985)

	Birthweight centiles		
	Mean − 2 SD	−2 SD − 10th	25th − 75th
n	214	869	5661
Low school performance (per 1000)	135.5	105.9	52.1
Handicapped (per 1000)	18.7	18.4	14.0

Table 2. Seven-year outcome by fetal growth (Ounsted et al. 1984)

	SGA	AGA
n	138	138
Handicap (moderate or severe)	7	2
Gross or fine motor incoordination	10	9
Developmental score (mean + SD) Boys	36.8 + 7.0	38.2 + 6.7
Girls	39.2 + 8.3	41.6 + 7.1

(AGA). Seven infants in the SGA group had a handicap (moderate or severe) compared to two in the AGA group, this difference is due to congenital or genetically determined conditions. There were no differences between the groups for chronic or specific ill health, hearing, sight, and speech defects or motor incoordination, however SGA children had a lower total developmental score than the AGA group.

In 1982, Low et al. published the long-term outcome (1 and 5 years) of two groups of neonates. Sixty-one were growth retarded (< 10th percentile) and 70 had an AGA birthweight. They found no significant difference in the frequency of handicap (minor or major) or delay in motor or cognitive development.

These three surveys published since 1980 show some discrepancies concerning the actual level of risks of unfavorable long-term outcome for SGA babies. The discrepancies are even more apparent if we look at other published results: Hill et al. (1984), MacGee et al. (1984), Villar et al. (1984), and Westwood et al. (1983) found an increased risk among SGA whereas Nilsen et al. (1984), Drew et al. (1983), and Vohr and Oh (1983) did not. Since there is no agreement among the authors of the various papers, it is important to try to understand the reasons for the differences in reported results.

Reasons for Discrepancies Between Surveys

The discrepancies between the reported results of the different surveys might be due to methodological problems which can be classified into two categories: statistical power and confounding variables, or differences in populations studied.

Statistical Power

The sample size of most of the studies is not very large and therefore can only detect important differences. For instance (Schwartz et al. 1970), in a survey comparing a group of SGA babies to a group of AGA babies, in order to detect a twofold increase in the frequency of any bad outcome, the required sample size is 600 per group if the frequency of bad outcome among AGA babies is 5%, 270 if the frequency is 10%, 160 if the frequency is 15%.

If the comparison is carried out on a quantitative variable (IQ for instance) instead of a qualitative variable, the required sample size depends on the expected difference expressed as a fraction of standard deviation. If the expected difference is equivalent to one-third of the SD, the required sample size is 240, if it is one-half, the sample size is 100, and if the expected difference is equivalent to 1 SD the required sample size is 26. These figures show that very few published surveys could have shown a significant difference in frequency of handicap, but rather in mean IQ. And because of the low number of subjects enrolled in certain surveys the significant differences observed are more likely to be an overestimation of the true difference. This is the reason why the results of a comparison should not only be expressed with the *p* value but also with the confidence interval of either the difference or the relative risk in order to have a better estimate of the actual difference between the groups compared.

Confounding Variables

When comparing AGA and SGA babies, three types of confounding variables may be misleading. The first one is linked to the risk factors of IUGR which can also be risk factors of long-term handicap. In this category the most common is social class. Since the percentage of parents belonging to low social class is, in most countries, higher among the SGA babies, and since development is linked to social class, social class might explain part of the differences observed.

The second is linked to perinatal consequences of IUGR. IUGR babies are more likely than others to have perinatal problems (fetal distress, hypoglycemia, respiratory distress syndrome, Chiswick 1985). Unfavorable outcomes might be due to perinatal problems rather than IUGR per se. Therefore it is particularly important that any comparison looking at the long-term outcome of SGA babies is made controlling these factors.

In this respect, the study made by Westwood et al. in 1983 (Table 3) is very demonstrative. They compared 33 SGA infants to 33 controls matched by gestational age, gender, race, and ethnic origin; none of these infants had perinatal asphyxia. In neurological and cognitive testing, the SGA infants tended toward

Table 3. Fourteen-year outcome by fetal growth (Westwood et al. 1983)

	SGA	Control	p^a
n	33	33	
WISC			
Verbal IQ (mean)	101.6	108.6	.09
Performance IQ (mean)	104.5	106.8	NS
Full scale (mean)	103.6	108.7	.07
WRAT			
Reading (mean)	99.7	105.9	.08
Spelling (mean)	94.5	99.0	NS
Arithmetic (mean)	87.8	94.5	.01

[a] After controlling for socioeconomical status.
WISC, Wechsler intelligence scale for children; WRAT, wide range achievement test.

Table 4. IQ of twins of different birthweights (Taylor 1984)

Author	n	Weight difference	IQ difference	p value
Babson et al. (1964)	12	25%	6.5 + 2.4	0.02
Churchill (1965)	17	> 300 g	5.8 + 2.2	0.02
Kaelber and Pugh (1969)				
Dyzygous	16	> 300 g	− 1.9 + 3.3	NS
Monozygous	17	> 300 g	5.8 + 2.5	0.05
Hohenauer (1971)	16	> 300 g	7.7	0.001

Table 5. Type of handicap by fetal growth (Ounsted et al. 1984)

	SGA	AGA
Babies *(n)*	138	138
Handicaps *(n)*	7	2
Cri du chat	1	
Trisomy 21	1	
Severe infantile hypercalcemia	2	
Duchenne muscular dystrophy	1	
Bilateral hearing defect	1	
Global retardation		1
Severe talipes		1

lower scores but scores were well within the normal range (Table 3). It must be noted that the infants belonged to the cohort studied by Fitzhardinge and Steven (1972). Another way of matching environment is to study twins with different birthweights. Table 4 presents the results of different surveys conducted on twins. It shows that the difference in IQ is around 6 when the difference in birthweight is > 300 g.

The third type of confounding is linked *to the etiology of IUGR* (Doyen et al. 1985). In their study Ounsted et al. (1984) observed seven moderate or severe handicaps among the 138 SGA babies, compared to two among the 138 AGA babies, diagnoses are noted in Table 5. Winer et al. (1982) reported the results of testing for intellectual and neurological development of 55 SGA neonates at 4-7 years of age (Table 6). When infants of mothers who had hypertensive disease (group A) were compared with those who had no such disease (group B), it was found that group A babies had better scores than group B babies.

Differences in Population

Beside the confounding factors which have been discussed, the type of IUGR must be taken into account in determining the prognosis. Three parameters seem

Table 6. Outcome by type of IUGR (Winer et al. 1982)

	Group A[a]	Group B[b]	p value[c]
n	20	34	
Verbal IQ (mean)	105.8	93.7	0.05
Performance IQ (mean)	99.4	93.9	
Full scale IQ (mean)	102.7	93.2	

[a] SGA + high blood pressures (HBP).
[b] SGA without HBP.
[c] After controlling for socioeconomic status.

Table 7. Outcome by type of IUGR (Harvey et al. 1982)

	Intrauterine <26 weeks	Head growth >26 weeks	p value
Verbal[a]	53.4	56.7	NS
Performance[a]	51.5	58.0	.05
Quantitative[a]	49.2	55.7	.02
Motor[a]	45.1	51.1	.05
Memory[a]	46.8	52.2	NS
General cognitive index[a]	102.9	113.2	.05

[a] McCarthy scale.

to be of particular importance: the importance of the IUGR, the head circumference, and the duration of IUGR.

The *importance of IUGR* seems to play a role since, in the Rantakallio study (Table 1), the frequency of low school performance is correlated to the birthweight centiles class: the lower the centiles class, the higher the rate of low school performance. The *head circumference* appears to be negatively correlated with IQ in several studies. The *duration of IUGR* and the moment it started also have a prognostic value. Harvey et al., in a study published in 1982, reported the 5-year follow up of 51 SGA babies. Children whose head growth began to slow before 26 weeks of gestation had significantly lower scores for the general cognitive index than the children whose head growth began to slow later in gestation (Table 7). In their study, Winer et al. (1982), found that in group B (SGA babies whose mothers had no hypertensive disease) heavier neonates of more advanced gestational ages scored higher, whereas in group A (SGA babies whose mothers had a hypertensive disease) lighter neonates who had been delivered earlier scored better.

Prospect for Prevention

To study the implications of these different results for prevention, the first step is to try to make a summary. For full-term SGA babies, the level of handicap seems to be quite low, even if it is higher than the level of handicap for AGA babies. The mean reduction in IQ for SGA babies considered as a whole appears to be between 5 and 10 points. If we assume firstly that this reduction is equivalent to half the SD of the distribution of IQ, and secondly that the distribution of IQ is gaussian, the frequency of SGA babies with low IQ (below the mean −2 SD) is twice as high as the frequency among AGA babies. However, this rather optimistic view regarding the risk for SGA babies as a whole does not apply in every case and the individual prognosis should take into account the etiology of IUGR, its type, its importance, the head circumference, the gestational age when the head growth began to slow, and the perinatal events.

Because of the prognostic value of the above-mentioned factors, early intervention, especially for babies with assymetric IUGR, has been proposed to prevent long-term handicap (Pearce and Campbell 1985). However, it should be stressed that this attitude is based on observational surveys which give statistical association and do not prove a causal relationship. Therefore policies of early intervention remain to be evaluated in order to be sure that the additional risk linked to an induced preterm birth does not exceed the gain due to early intervention.

For this reason, evaluative studies in this field should define precisely the population studied especially regarding the factors known to influence the outcome. It should also be defined prospectively in order to reproduce the situation when the decision has to be made during the pregnancy and must not be limited to full-term or preterm babies. As a matter of fact, if a given "new" attitude toward SGA babies leads to increased preterm births, it is likely that the SGA babies born preterm because of this new attitude have a better prognosis than the SGA babies born preterm previously. Therefore, if one compares separately the evolution of the prognosis for preterm and full-term babies, an improvement will be observed in each group even if there is no improvement when considering all SGA babies. The study should be very carefully designed and as close as possible to the experimental design. And if for certain groups of SGA babies there is current disagreement among the perinatal community regarding what is the best attitude, there is certainly room for randomized controlled trials. Whereas for groups where there is consensus it might be necessary to perform evaluative studies based upon observational data.

References

Chiswick ML (1985) Intrauterine growth retardation. Br Med J 291: 845–847

Doyen J, Thoumsin H, Lambotte R (1985) Rôle des facteurs gestationels dans la constitution de handicaps neurologiques irréversibles. J Gynecol Obstet Biol Reprod (Paris) 14: 431–438

Drew JH, Bayly J, Beischer NA (1983) Prospective follow-up of growth retarded infants and of those from pregnancies complicated by low oestriol excretion. Aust NZ J Obstet Gynaecol 23: 150–154

Fitzhardinge PM, Steven EM (1972) The small for date infant. II. Neurological and intellectual sequellae. Pediatrics 50: 50–57

Harvey D, Prince J, Bunton J, Parkinson C, Campbell S (1982) Abilities of children who were small for gestational age babies. Pediatrics 69: 296–300

Hill RM, Verniaud M, Deter RL, Tennyson LM, Rettig GM, Zion TE, Vorderman AL, Helms PG, McCulley LB, Hill LL (1984) The effect of intrauterine malnutrition on the term infant, a 14 year progressive study. Acta Paediatr Scand 73: 482-487
Low JA, Galbraith RS, Muir D, Killen H, Pater B, Karchmar J (1982) Intrauterine growth retardation: a study of long-term morbidity. Am J Obstet Gynecol 142: 670-677
MacGee R, Silva PA, Williams S (1984) Perinatal, neurological, environmental and developmental characteristics of seven-year children with stable behaviour problems. J Child Psychol Psychiatry 25: 573-586
Nilsen ST, Finne PN, Bergjso P, Stamnes O (1984) Males with low birthweight examined at 18 years of age. Acta Paediatr Scand 73: 168-175
Ounsted MK, Moar VA, Scott A (1984) Children of deviant birthweight at the age of seven years: health, handicap, size and developmental status. Early Hum Dev 9: 323-340
Pearce JM, Campbell S (1985) Intrauterine growth retardation. Birth Defects 21: 109-130
Rantakallio P (1985) A 14 year follow-up of children with normal and abnormal birthweight for their gestational age. Acta Paediatr Scand 74: 62-69
Schwartz D, Lellouch J, Flamant R (1970) L'essai thérapeutique chez l'homme. Flammarion, Paris
Taylor DJ (1984) Low birthweight and neurodevelopmental handicap. Clin Obstet Gynaecol 11: 525-542
Villar J, Smeriglio V, Martorell R, Brown CH, Klein RE (1984) Heterogeneous growth and mental development of intrauterine growth-retarded infants during the first 3 years of life. Pediatrics 74: 783-791
Vohr BR, Oh W (1983) Growth and development in preterm infants small for gestational age. J Pediatr 103: 941-945
Westwood M, Kramer MS, Munz D, Lovett JM, Watters GV (1983) Growth and development of full-term nonasphyxiated small for gestational age newborns: follow-up through adolescence. Pediatrics 71: 376-382
Winer EK, Tejani NA, Atluru V, Digiuseppe R, Borofsky LG (1982) Four to seven year evaluation in two groups of small for gestational age infants. Am J Obstet Gynecol 143: 425-429

Growth Retardation: Individual Risk Assessment During Pregnancy

G. PONTONNIER, H. GRANDJEAN, A. FOURNIE and M.-F. SARRAMON

Is it possible to assess the individual risk of brain damage in case of intrauterine growth retardation? It is difficult to give a clear, straightforward, and conclusive answer to this question. Yet, it is well worth answering. Indeed, obstetricians now tend to extract small for date infants more and more frequently and earlier for fear of perinatal death or psychomotor sequelae. If this attitude is generally accepted in cases of early and severe growth retardation, it can be considered in less severe cases. As an example, Table 1 reports the results of our department over a 5-year period. When considering the whole population, the rate of cesarean sections in small for date infants decreased. But if we look more precisely, we can see that the rate of cesarean sections increased slighty from 33% to 46% in early growth retardation but decreased significantly in late growth retardation.

The attitude of obstetricians is influenced by papers in which a positive correlation is found between growth retardation and psychomotor sequelae (Collins and Turner 1971; Ellenberg and Nelson 1979; Francis-Williams and Davies 1974; Heidelise et al. 1976; Henrichsen et al. 1986; Nickel et al. 1982; Sabel et al. 1976). However, a review of the main papers on this subject yields conflicting results. The risk of sequelae in small for date infants is highly variable on the qualitative and quantitative level (Allen 1984). Several factors account for this discrepancy (Voyer and Dehan 1985; Prechtl 1981).

Table 1. Evolution of cesarean section rate in IUGR in our department

	1980 ($n=3139$)	1985 ($n=3083$)	Statistical comparison
Whole population			
Cesarean section in IUGR (%)	23.5	19.5	NS
Relative risk/non-IUGR	2.2	1.6	
Premature infants			
Cesarean section in IUGR (%)	33	46	NS
Relative risk/non-IUGR	3.1	3.8	
Term infants			
Cesarean section in IUGR (%)	22	14	$p<0.05$
Relative risk/non-IUGR	2.1	1.2	
Premature infants in IUGR (%)	17	15	NS

One main factor is the diversity of the populations involved in follow-up studies. First, considerable differences arise from the period in which the studies were published. A distinction should be made between results concerning infants born before 1970 (Collins and Turner 1971; Fitzhardinge and Steven 1972; Lubchenco et al. 1972; Michaelis et al. 1970; Papaevangelou et al. 1972) or after (Ounsted et al. 1984; Starfield et al. 1982). Substantial advances were indeed observed in obstetrical and neonatal management during the latter period (Stanley 1981). Secondly, the severity of growth retardation differs from one center to another because of their specific recruitment. Thirdly, wide variations exist in definitions with a frequent lack of distinction between premature, small for date premature, and term small for date infants. Results are often devoid of statistical significance because of the small number of cases involved. Besides, the duration of these follow-up studies is highly variable, ranging from 1 (Starfield et al. 1982) to over 20 years (Westwood et al. 1983).

Another factor in conflicting results concerns the difficulty of evaluating the fetal condition and interpreting the child's condition at school age. Such fuzziness in the assessment of two situations one is striving to correlate is probably one essential reason for discrepant opinions. The severity of growth retardation in pregnancy cannot be evaluated except indirectly by tests that are quite often of poor sensitivity and specificity. Furthermore, the use of these tests is recent and very few of the available follow-up studies are initiated during pregnancy. Most studies begin after birth. This is of interest to the pediatrician but has less value for the obstetrician who is concerned with evaluating brain damage risks during gestation, but not after birth when it is generally too late.

This fuzziness also affects the interpretation of the condition of school-age or even 2-year-old children. This condition is not solely determined by pregnancy events. Correlations are often warped by other interference factors such as complications of labor and delivery, and of the neonatal period.

Many sequelae attributed to growth retardation are really due to per- or postpartum asphyxia (Calame et al. 1976). In a review of Fitzhardinge's follow-up study, Westwood et al. (1983) showed that most of the sequelae reported about small for date infants were linked to perinatal asphyxia and neonatal complications. The quality of obstetrical and neonatal care is fundamental and advances made in this area during the last decade should improve the long-term prognosis of fetal growth retardation.

Environment also plays a part as sequelae are more severe with a lower socioeconomic status (Drillien 1970; Low et al. 1982; Neligan et al. 1976; Parkinson et al. 1981). Authors sometimes disregard this notion. The importance of genetic determination is probably considerable as was shown by studies of twins; it is now known that individual cognitive faculties are more dependent on genetic factors than on environmental events.

In spite of inadequacies, some conclusions cans be drawn from these follow-up studies:

- Most term small for date infants will not be severely motor or mentally handicapped (Harvey et al. 1982; Lubchenco et al. 1972; Wiener 1970; Winer et al. 1982). But increased brain damage risks do exist that will result in neurological

sequelae, difficulties at school, speech or language abnormalities (Heidelise et al. 1976; Henrichsen et al. 1986; Michaelis et al. 1970; Rantakallio 1985). The frequency of these abnormalities varies from study to study, but is in any case higher than in normal birthweight infants.
- The more severe the growth retardation, the higher the risk of sequelae (Fitzardinghe and Steven 1972; Hagberg 1979; Low et al. 1978).
- Small for date infants are more liable than other infants to asphyxia during and after delivery (Commey and Fitzardinghe 1979).

The obstetrician must define his policy from these conclusions. No proof exists that all small for date infants should be extracted before term. The difficulty lies in ascertaining cases at risk of brain damage if pregnancy goes to term. From this viewpoint, an evaluation of the degree of malnutrition and fetal vitality should be attempted. Premature extraction or abstention should depend on these evaluations and on the degree of fetal maturity.

Evaluation of the Degree of Malnutrition

The evaluation of the degree of malnutrition is important because the risk damage is inversely proportional to birthweight for gestational age. There are three ways of evaluating the degree of growth retardation:

- Clinical examination
- Ultrasonography
- Hormonal measurements

The clinical assessment of the degree of growth retardation is commonly considered as inaccurate (Persson et al. 1986). But as was shown in several studies on fundus height (Belizan et al. 1978; Calvert et al. 1982; Cnattingius et al. 1985; Daikoku et al. 1979), the value of clinical examinations should not be neglected and a growth retardation diagnosis should never be dropped because of normal ultrasound measurements as the clinical impression is sometimes right.

The monitoring of head growth is essential. The prognosis value of head size and its postnatal evolution in small for date infants has been surveyed in several follow-up studies (Babson et Henderson 1974; Gross et al. 1978, 1983; Lipper et al. 1981; Nelson and Broman 1977; Nelson and Ellenberg 1979; Westwood et al. 1983). Gross et al. (1978) studied the outcome of newborns with a head size below the 10th centile and found a higher rate of neurodevelopmental sequelae than in normal infants. Lipper et al. (1981) went further into this notion with an analysis of the respective importance of birthweight, gestational age, and head size. Their conclusion was that head size was probably the most adequate prognosis parameter and perhaps the only one, weight and gestational age being only indirectly correlated with sequelae via their correlation with head size. Finally, several authors have shown that risks of subsequent sequelae are influenced even more by initial growth speed than by initial head size, slowly growing infants being at a higher risk than infants whose head growth catches up (Brandt 1981; Gross et al. 1983).

These concepts enhance the importance of the findings of the authors (Fancourt et al. 1976; Harvey et al. 1982; Parkinson et al. 1981) who observed a decrease in development quotient, perceptual performance, and coordination activity in infants whose biparietal diameter was below the 10th centile from the 34th week. The statistical significance of this decrease in performances was, however, limited to those in whom the biparietal decrease had started as early as the 26th week (Fancourt et al. 1976). Furthermore, they have shown that head growth would remain abnormal after birth in cases of early impairment. The high prognosis value of impairment of in utero head growth can be inferred from these data. The earlier the impairment, the higher the risk of brain damage. This is not surprising given the chronology of fetal brain development and the relationship between biparietal diameter and brain volume (Brandt 1981; Dobbing and Sand 1978). It should follow that inasmuch as immaturity is not excessive, biparietal diameter impairment must lead to premature extraction. But this should be discussed given that even if early impairment of biparietal diameter is a cause for subsequent sequelae, no proof exists that an early intervention would improve postnatal evolution of biparietal diameter and reduce risks of sequelae. A randomized prospective study should be attempted on this subject. However, Westwood et al. (1983) found that decreased cephalic diameter in the small for date infant was not correlated to sequelae insofar as no asphyxia had occurred. But his series is short and lacks data as to antenatal head growth.

An interesting study could be made about the outcome of infants with respect to abdominal diameter growth in utero, since this parameter is altered earlier than biparietal diameter, however it it less directly linked to brain volume.

Results of investigations on the prognosis value of hormonal dosages with regard to the further development and neurological condition of the infants are conflicting (Drillien 1970; Greene et al. 1969; Jörgensen 1978; Leijon et al. 1980; Wade et al. 1978; Wallace and Michiel 1966; Yogman et al. 1972). Leijon et al. (1980) concluded from a prospective study with control series that low urinary estriol is an indicator of infants who will have a head growth retardation and thus increased risks of psychomotor sequelae. In our own experience (Pontonnier et al. 1985), these tests have only an auxiliary value for the prediction of neonatal infant condition, thus we doubt their predictive value for long-term sequelae. Moreover, to be interpretable they require a curve comprising at least three values.

Evaluation of Fetal Vitality

Except for malformations, genetic abnormalities, or infectious fetopathies which are beyond therapy, intrauterine growth retardation may be considered as being caused by insufficient placental exchange. The first result is impairment of growth. But if the nutritional deficit persists or worsens, two consequences follow: first, decreasing fetal vitality probably linked to brain depression, and then terminal anoxia in the perinatal period. The impaired fetus will be unable to pass the critical period of birth without brain damage. Clinical examinations, ultrasonography, and hormonal assays, which are fetal denutrition tests, are inadequate indicators of fetal vitality. Other tests should be used.

Until recently, the only paraclinical examination used to evaluate fetal vitality was fetal heart rate monitoring. By correlating antenatal fetal heart rate and the infant's condition during the neonatal period, the prognosis value of several types of tracings was determined (Breart et al. 1981; Holmqvist et al. 1984; Kubli 1984; Pontonnier et al. 1982). These tracings allow the evaluation of the risk of imminent death with good accuracy. An attempt is now being made to extend this predictive value to the risk of brain damage although correlations are much more difficult to establish in this case. It may be considered that:

- A T2 tracing is indicative of a good vitality at the time of the recording but does not give information about fetal oxygen reserves. Thus, it cannot predict how long the fetus will be out of danger, especially at the beginning of labor.
- The risk of fetal distress and consequently of brain damage is real with a predominantly T0 tracing over several recordings. This risk is probably greater with a higher T0 percentage.
- Reactivity impairment in fetal heart rate tracings has a negative significance. The disappearance of reactivity is an earlier indicator of fetal distress than the disappearance of oscillations. At this stage, preventive intervention might be envisaged but, unfortunately, many hyporeactive tracings are false alarms.
- If repeated, late deceleration occurrences with spontaneous contractions have a bad prognosis (Visser et al. 1980).

The nonstress test is far from solving all the difficulties. A doubt often remains either because other fetal monitoring parameters are contradict the fetal heart rate, or because tracings are difficult to interpret. In such cases, the nonstress test will have to be used on its own, at more or less close intervals, and/or an oxytocin challenge test performed.

Few needless interventions will occur if cardiotocographic signs of imminent death are awaited before extracting the infant; but a number of brain-damaged infants will be born. The tendency will then be to intervene upon signs of moderate fetal heart rate disorders, thus risking needless intervention. The fetal heart rate recording test does not constitute a way out of this dilemma. Other recently developed paraclinical examinations should be used.

With their score, Manning et al. (1985) reduced perinatal mortality by half in their department. We now use this score. Unquestionably, this is an additional method of assessing in utero fetal vitality. But its use is too recent for the value in the prevention of psychomotor sequelae to have been assessed by follow-up studies.

Fetal blood velocity measurements using Doppler ultrasound are the most recent exploratory means. To assess its value in monitoring of intrauterine growth, we have measured the index of placental resistance on the umbilical artery in 62 pregnancies at risk of growth retardation (Table 2). Doppler, biparietal and abdominal diameter measurements, and a fetal heart rate recording were performed on the same day. The sensitivity and specificity of each test was assessed.

Table 2. Sensitivity and specificity of Doppler, ultrasound, and FHR in 62 pregnancies

	IUGR			Perinatal death		
	Sensitivity	Specificity	Exact diagnosis (%)	Sensitivity	Specificity	Exact diagnosis (%)
Doppler	61	100	77	90	73	76
Ultrasound	81	65	74	100	65	71
FHR	31	100	61	100	92	92
Statistical comparison	$p<0.01$	$p<0.01$	NS	NS	$p<0.01$	$p<0.05$

IUGR (<10th percentiles) = 36 cases (58%). Perinatal deaths = 10 cases (16%).

In the case of growth retardation, the Doppler measurement is more frequently pathological than fetal heart rate measurements but less so than ultrasonography. The reverse is seen with perinatal deaths: a change in Doppler measurement is seen more often than in ultrasound measurement but less so than in fetal heart rate tracings. A pathological Doppler measurement is always accompanied by growth retardation and the only instance where a death in utero occurred with a normal Doppler measurement happened with an 8-day-old measurement. Therefore, we check cases at risk twice a week. The Doppler measurement plays a distinct part in the fetal vitality assessment: the fetal heart rate recording shows the risk of acute fetal distress, ultrasonography shows the risk of growth retardation, Doppler measurements are in between. They are certainly valuable as a predictor of long-term brain damage, but follow-up studies should determine this.

Conclusion

In conclusion, we wish to summarize a few essential ideas. Brain damage risks in the small for date infant are low and usually minor. However, fetuses rendered very small for date and microcephalic by malnutrition are at high risk of perinatal complications. These considerations lead to very eclectic policies:

- If the intrauterine growth retardation seems moderate and if there is no sign of decreasing fetal vitality and, naturally, of imminent death, the pregnancy should be allowed to go to term. Labor and delivery should receive particular attention with monitoring of fetal heart rate and periodical measurements of the pH on the scalp.
- If growth retardation is estimated to be severe by clinical and ultrasound examinations (especially with reduced biparietal diameter) and/or if signs of fetal distress are present, preterm extraction is advisable except in cases of excessive immaturity.

In order to prevent the severe consequences of growth retardation we must intervene before signs of imminent death appear. From this viewpoint, paraclinical examinations should be developed for use before fetal heart rate monitoring or Manning's score. Their aim would be the successful detection of fetuses which, owing to a pathological in utero environment, were in distress. The measurement of the umbilical blood flow, and possibly of the cerebral blood flow, would be advances toward this goal. For even earlier action, means of evaluating mother-to-fetus transplacental exchanges would be required. This is our challenge for the future.

References

Allen MC (1984) Developmental outcome and follow-up of small for gestational age infant. Semin Perinatol 2: 123-156

Babson SG, Henderson NB (1974) Fetal undergrowth: relation of head growth to later intellectual performance. Pediatrics 53: 890-894

Belizan JM, Villar JC, Nordin J, Malamud J, de Vicuna LS (1978) Diagnosis of intrauterine growth retardation by a simple clinical method: measurement of uterine height. Am J Obstet Gynecol 13: 643-647

Brandt I (1981) Brain growth, fetal malnutrition and clinical consequence. J Perinat Med 9: 3-26

Breart G, Goupil F, Legrand H, Vaquier J, Rochart F, Milliez J, Sureau C (1981) Antepartum fetal heart rate monitoring. I. A semi quantitative evaluation of the "non stressed" fetal heart rate. Eur J Obstet Gynecol Reprod Biol 11: 227-237

Calame A, Reymond-Goni I, Maherzi M, Roulet M, Marchand C, Prod'hom LS (1976) Psychological and neurodevelopmental outcome of high risk newborn infants. Helv Paediatr Acta 31: 287-297

Calvert JP, Crean EE, Newcombe RG, Pearson JF (1982) Antenatal screening by measurements of symphysis-fundus height. Br Med J 285: 846-849

Cnattingius S, Axelsson O, Lindmark G (1985) The clinical value of measurements of the symphysis-fundus distance and ultrasonic measurements of the biparietal diameter in the diagnosis of intrauterine growth retardation. J Perinat Med 13: 227-232

Collins E, Turner G (1971) The importance of the "small-for-dates" baby to the problem of mental retardation. Med J Aust 2: 313-315

Commey JOO, Fitzhardinge PM (1979) Handicap in the preterm small-for-gestational age infant. J Pediatr 94: 779-786

Daikoku NH, Johnson JWC, Graf C, Kearney K, Tyson JE, King TM (1979) Patterns of intrauterine growth retardation. Obstet Gynecol 54: 211-219

Dobbing J, Sand J (1978) Head circumference biparietal diameter and brain growth in fetal and postnatal life. Early Hum Dev 2: 81-89

Drillien CM (1970) The small-for-date infant: etiology and prognosis. Pediatr Clin North Am 17: 9-24

Drillien CM, Thomson AJM, Burgoyne K (1980) Low-birthweight children at early school-age: a longitudinal study. Dev Med Child Neurol 22: 26-47

Ellenberg JH, Nelson KB (1979) Birthweight and gestational age in children with cerebral palsy or seizure disorders. Am J Dis Child 133: 1044-1048

Fancourt R, Campbell S, Harvey D, Norman AP (1976) Follow-up study of small-for-dates babies. Br Med J 1: 1435-1437

Fitzhardinge PM, Steven EM (1972) The small-for-date infant. II. Neurological and intellectual sequelae. Pediatrics 50: 50-57

Francis-Williams J, Davies PA (1974) Very low birthweight and later intelligence. Dev Med Child Neurol 16: 709-728

Greene JW, Beargie RA, Clark BK, Smith K (1969) Correlation of estriol excretion patterns of pregnant women with subsequent development of their children. Am J Obstet Gynecol 105: 730-745

Gross SJ, Kosmetatos N, Grimes CT, Williams ML (1978) Newborn head size and neurological status. Am J Dis Child 132: 753-756
Gross SJ, Oehler JM, Eckerman CO (1983) Head growth and developmental outcome in very-low-birthweight infants. Pediatrics 71: 70-75
Hagberg B (1979) Epidemiological and preventive aspects of cerebral palsy and severe mental retardation in Sweden. Eur J Pediatr 130: 71-78
Harvey D, Prince J, Bunton J (1982) Abilities of children who were small-for-gestational-age babies. Pediatrics 69: 296-300
Heidelise ALS, Tronick E, Adamson L, Brazelton TB (1976) The behavior of the full-term but underweight newborn infant. Dev Med Child Neurol 18: 590-602
Henrichsen L, Skinhy K, Andersen GE (1986) Delayed growth and reduced intelligence in 9-17 year old intrauterine growth retarded children compared with their monozygous cotwins. Acta Paediatr Scand 75: 31-35
Holmqvist P, Svenningsen NW, Ingemarsson I (1984) Neurodevelopmental outcome and electronic fetal heart rate monitoring in a neonatal intensive care population. Acta Obstet Gynecol Scand 63: 527-532
Jorgensen PI (1978) Prognostic value of urinary oestriol studies during the last trimester of pregnancy. Medical Dissertation, University of Copenhagen
Kubli F (1984) Antepartum monitoring of fetal heart rate. In: Beard RW, Nathaniels PW (eds) Fetal physiology and medicine, 2nd edn. Dekker, New-York, pp 655-677
Leijon I, Billström G, Lind I (1980) An 18-month follow-up study of growth-retarded neonates. Relation to biochemical tests of placental function in late pregnancy and neurobehavioural condition in the newborn period. Early Hum Dev 4 (3): 271-285
Lipper E, Lee KS, Gariner LM, Grellong B (1981) Determinants of neurobehavioral outcome in low-birth-weight infants. Pediatrics 67: 502-505
Low JA, Galbraith RS, Muir D, Killen H, Pater B, Karchmar J (1978) Intrauterine growth retardation: a preliminary report of long-term morbidity. Am J Obstet Gynecol 130: 534-545
Low JA, Galbraith RS, Muir D, Killen H, Pater B, Karchmar J (1982) Intrauterine growth retardation: a study of long term morbidity. Am J Obstet Gynecol 142: 670-677
Lubchenco LO, Delivoria-Papadopoulos M, Searls D (1972) Long-term follow-up studies of prematurely born infants. II. Influence of birthweight and gestational age on sequelae. J Pediatr 80: 509-512
Manning FA, Morrisson I, Lange IR, Chamberlain PF (1985) Fetal assessment based on fetal biophysical profile score: experience in 12620 referred high-risk pregnancies. Am J Obstet Gynecol 151: 343-350
Michaelis R, Schulte FJ, Nolte R (1970) Motor behavior of small for gestational age newborn infants. J Pediatr 76: 208-213
Neligan GA, Kolvin I, Scott DM, Garside RF (1976) Born too soon or born too small. A follow-up study to seven years of age. Clin Dev Med 61
Nelson KB, Broman SH (1977) Perinatal risk factors in children with serious motor and mental handicaps. Ann Neurol 2: 371-377
Nelson KB, Ellenberg JH (1979) Neonatal signs as predictors of cerebral palsy. Pediatrics 64: 225-232
Nickel RE, Bennett FC, Lamson FN (1982) School performance of children with birthweights of 1000 g or less. Am J Dis Child 136: 105-110
Ounsted MK, Moar VA, Scott A (1984) Children of deviant birthweight at the age of seven years: health, size and developmental status. Early Hum Dev 9: 323-340
Papaevangelou G, Papadatos C, Alexiou D (1972) Perinatal mortality and morbidity in "small-for-dates" newborns. Helv Paediatr Acta 27: 415-424
Parkinson CE, Wallis S, Harvey D (1981) School achievement and behaviour of children who were small-for-dates at birth. Dev Med Child Neurol 23: 41-50
Persson B, Stangenberg M, Lunell NO, Brodin U, Holmberg NG, Vaclavinkova V (1986) Prediction of size of infants at birth by measurement of symphysis fundus height. Br J Obstet Gynecol 93: 206-211
Pontonnier G, Mandry J, Grandjean H, Reme JM (1982) La signification pronostique du rythme cardiaque foetal au cours de la grossesse. Rev Fr Gynecol Obstet 77: 373-375
Pontonnier G, Grandjean H, Halasz A, Fournie A (1985) A critical assessment of antenatal tests of fetal well being. In: Stern L, Xanthou M, Friis-Hansen B (eds) Praeger, New-York, pp 1-11

Prechtl HFR (1981) Risk factors and neurological follow-up. In: Manciaux M, Tomkiewicz S (eds) Deficience mentale chez les jeunes. INSERM, Paris, pp 173-179

Rantakallio P (1985) A 14-year follow-up of children with normal and abnormal birthweight for their gestational age. A population study. Acta Paediatr Scand 74: 62-69

Sabel KG, Olegard R, Victorin L (1976) Remaining sequelae with modern perinatal care. Pediatrics 57: 652-658

Stanley FJ (1981) Spatic cerebral palsy: changes in birthweight and gestational age. Early Hum Dev 5: 167-178

Starfield B, Shapiro S, McCormick M, Bros D (1982) Mortality and morbidity in infants with intrauterine growth retardation. J Pediatr 101: 978-893

Visser GHA, Redman CWG, Huisjes HJ, Turnbull AC (1980) Nonstressed antepartum heart rate monitoring: implications of decelerations after spontaneous contractions. Am J Obstet Gynecol 138: 429-435

Voyer M, Dehan M (1985) Quel est le pronostic des enfants nés avant terme? II. Devenir jusqu'à l'âge scolaire. Arch Fr Pediatr 42: 795-802

Wade RW, Pepperell RJ, Kitchen WH, Whiteside U, Cameron SE, Townsend L (1978) Paediatric follow-up of pregnancies complicated by subnormal oestriol excretion. Med J Aust 1: 525-530

Wallace SJ, Michiel EA (1966) A follow-up study of infants born to mothers with low oestriol excretion during pregnancy. Lancet 2: 560-563

Westwood M, Kramer MS, Munz D, Lovett JM, Watters GV (1983) Growth and developmentent of full-term nonasphyxiated small-for-gestational-age newborns: follow-up through adolescence. Pediatrics 71: 376-382

Wiener G (1970) The relationship of birthweight and length of gestation to intellectual development at ages 8 to 10 years. J Pediatr 76: 694-699

Winer EK, Tejani NA, Atluru VL, DiGiuseppe R, Borofsky LG (1982) Four-to-seven-year evaluations in two groups of small for gestational age infants. Am J Obstet Gynecol 143: 425-429

Yogman MW, Speroff L, Huttenlocher PR, Kase NG (1972) Child development after pregnancies complicated by low urinary estriol excretion and preeclampsia. Am J Obstet Gynecol 114: 1069-1077

Management of Growth Retardation with a View to Preventing Neuromotor Dysfunction and Mental Handicaps

K. R. NISWANDER

My remarks will be based on several uncertain assumptions and these need to be briefly discussed before proceeding to my topic. The first assumption is that we usually know what causes cerebral palsy in an individual case. Clearly this is not so. We can make certain generalizations about the etiology if we analyze groups of cases rather than try to arrive at a cause in an individual patient. Hagberg and Hagberg (1984), for example, did not try to find a single cause for each case of cerebral palsy. Rather, they listed all of the prenatal, perinatal (intrapartum plus neonatal), and postnatal "factors" that they felt *might* have contributed to the cause. With this exercise, they were able to suggest that certain types of cerebral palsy (e.g., dyskinesia) are more likely than not to be related to perinatal events, while other types (e.g., spastic/ataxic diplegia in term children) are more than likely to be due to prenatal events. They emphasized, however, the likelihood of multiple causes in an individual patient, e.g., a prenatal disposition to the ill effects of a perinatal event.

This leads to another generalization I should mention. Obstetricians and neonatologists or pediatric neurologists can be expected to have entirely different perspectives when studying the issue of causation unless more effort is exerted to improve communication between them. Some pediatricians, for example, are prone to suggest an intrapartum cause of cerebral palsy if there was a simple "abnormality" of the EFM tracing no matter how minor the "abnormality." An obstetrician might find the "abnormality" trivial. The pediatrician thus may arrive at a wrong etiologic conclusion based on faulty obstetric information. Similarly, obstetricians are prone to lump all kinds of cerebral palsy as well as other neurologic abnormalities into one disparate group of "neuromotor dysfunctions." It is altogether likely that the various types of cerebral palsy have different etiologies (some, for example, may be due to prolonged prenatal asphyxia while others are not), and an experienced obstetrician who has little knowledge of pediatric neurology may insist there is no relationship between intrapartum asphyxia and the waste basket diagnosis of cerebral palsy when a more refined neurologic diagnosis might reveal a causal relationship between the asphyxia and one particular kind of neurologic disease.

I thus conclude, even before I get to my topic, that we do *not* know the precise cause of cerebral palsy in most individual patients and can therefore not hope to know with precision whether our obstetric intervention for intrauterine growth retardation (IUGR) really has had any effect or not in that individual patient. I am, however, not quite as pessimistic as I sound. I believe that we may be able to conclude, by studying groups of patients rather than individual patients, that it is possible or even likely that what we do may reduce the likelihood of neuromotor dysfunction, even if that reduction is more modest than our egos would like.

What Is the Cause of Cerebral Palsy?

What do we presently know about the "cause" of cerebral palsy and is IUGR likely to be one of the causes? I think there is now a widespread belief that the intrapartum period can be dismissed as the sole time-frame when neurologic damage occurred in the majority of cases of cerebral palsy - perhaps the vast majority. There also seems to be almost universal agreement that few cases of cerebral palsy are caused by events after birth. Thus, by a process of elimination, events during the prenatal period probably account for, or at least contribute to, most cases of cerebral palsy. One such "event" during the prenatal period is IUGR. Is IUGR a major cause of cerebral palsy? The evidence is conflicting on the issue. Hagberg and Hagberg (1984) find that it is; Stanley and Blair (1986, personal communication) find it is not. The possibility exists that modern methods of diagnosing and perhaps treating IUGR may have already had an impact on long-term morbidity. The proof for such an assumption is lacking, but at least one major investigator in the field thinks this may be so. Ounsted (1986, personal communication), using data collected prospectively at Oxford, has noted no relationship between the presence of IUGR and subsequent cerebral palsy. She thinks this lack of relationship is possibly due to the fact that her data were collected on children born in the 1970s rather than on earlier births which were the basis primarily for the contradictingreports. She points out that obstetric intervention in the 1950s and 1960s occurred only in extremis and that it was still the practice to starve low-weight babies for at least the first 24 h. Thus, while the proposition that the presumed deleterious neuromotor effects of IUGR may have been largely eliminated by modern perinatal care is unproved and may not even be true, I think we should continue to postulate that obstetric intervention for IUGR *may* reduce the risk of neuromotor disability, at least until we have positive proof that this is not so. Caution dictates, however, that we also consider the possibility that obstetric intervention may actually increase the risk of such damage. It is apparent that there is a very real need for randomized trials of many of our cherished obstetric treatments.

Types of IUGR

At this point we must also remind ourselves that IUGR is not all one piece, that there are two types of IUGR with differing etiologies. Type I IUGR, also called symmetrical growth retardation, apparently arises early in pregnancy with limitation of growth of all, or most, organs. The etiology is likely to be intrauterine infection, a toxin, or possibly very poor economic circumstances of the mother which lead to early stunting of fetal development, notably including the brain. Since this type of IUGR seems unlikely to be affected by obstetric intervention, this essay will dwell primarily on type II IUGR, also called assymetrical growth retardation. With this disease, fetal growth is normal until about the third trimester when interference with factors which affect placental support of the fetus develops. Clinically, such infants show smaller abdominal viscera and a lack of subcutaneous fat, but a normally sized head and brain. Since this type of IUGR can be potentially affected by obstetric intervention, this essay will emphasize this syndrome rather than symmetrical IUGR.

An earlier paper in this volume (Pontonnier) discussed the recognition and identification of IUGR and subsequent papers (Visser) will evaluate the specific usefulness of antenatal cardiotocography in the management of recognized IUGR. In discussing management, however, I must briefly refer to these issues.

It is easy to list possible causes of IUGR, poor obstetric history, poor pregnancy weight gain, obstetric events such as acute hypertensive disease and twins, medical complications such as chronic hypertension or cardiac or renal disease, but a substantial number of patients carrying an IUGR fetus will not have any of these causes operating. To make the diagnosis even more difficult, most patients with one or more of these predisposing causes will not display any IUGR at all. Accuracy of identification of the IUGR fetus is undoubtedly greater in a university hospital with a special interest in the problem than in a clinical care setting where routine antenatal care is offered. Thus Hall et al. (1980), in a routine antenatal clinic in Aberdeen offering, no doubt, a high level of antenatal care, detected only 44% of the 189 cases of IUGR defined as those whose birthweight fell below the 10th percentile. Several other studies have reported that accurate antenatal prediction of IUGR remains difficult. Rosenberg et al. (1982), using clinical tools alone, recognized only 50% of the small for gestational age (SGA) fetuses in their population. Hughey (1984) detected 23% of SGA infants when clinical means alone were used, while routine ultrasonic scanning increased the detection rate to 57%. There are similar studies which could be cited, but variations in the details of the studies make them difficult to compare.

Diagnosis of IUGR

Today, the diagnosis of IUGR is usually made or confirmed by ultrasound either in a patient thought to be at risk of IUGR or in one in whom routine ultrasound screening has been used during early pregnancy. The methods used for the ultrasonic diagnosis are the same as those used for monitoring growth of the fetus once the diagnosis has been established. Warsof et al. (1986) designed a prospective screening program of a large obstetric population to determine the effectiveness of ultrasonic biometry in diagnosing IUGR. Among 3616 pregnancies, ultrasound was used routinely before the 24th gestational week to date the pregnancy. Three ultrasonic parameters were measured: biparietal diameter (BPD), head circumference, and abdominal circumference. To maintain a high sensitivity, the authors considered ultrasonic measurements below the 25th percentile for gestational age to be abnormal. The predictive value of a positive test using this criterion ranged from 0.25 to 0.55 depending on the week of gestation in which the scan was performed. Abdominal circumference measurements were more predictive of IUGR than either fetal head circumference or BPD, or a combination of these parameters. They concluded that 34 ± 1 weeks of gestation was the optimal time to screen patients routinely examined by ultrasound before the 24th week for IUGR. Other authors have used various other methods for determining abdominal size such as a transverse diameter of the abdomen, but it seems clear that measurement of the size of the abdomen by one method or another, either alone or in relation to the fetal head circumference, is more accurate in detecting IUGR than is measurement of the fetal head by itself.

A new and fascinating technique for the measurement of vascular resistance in the uterine artery or its branches and the umbilical artery has been recently introduced (Cohen-Overbeek et al. 1985). Good correlation between increased vascular resistance and the presence of IUGR has been reported (Cohen-Overbeek et al. 1985). The technique employs a continuous wave Doppler ultrasound system and the investigating scientists seem certain that the hardware used will soon be sufficiently simple and inexpensive to allow widespread usage among clinicians. Briefly, arterial velocity waveforms are recorded and a calculation of the peak systolic/diastolic ratio is made, a reflection of vascular resistance distal to the point of measurement. Fleischer et al. (1985) studied 189 women at high risk for IUGR with umbilical artery velocity waveforms. Using a centile birthweight of less than 25% as the end point, these investigators reported a sensitivity of 78% and a specificity of 83% for the diagnosis of IUGR in the entire population. The predictive value of a positive test was 49% but rose to 66% when maternal hypertension was present. Similar results were reported by Trudinger et al. (1985) with measurement of arterial flow velocity waveforms in branches of the uterine artery. Among 91 complicated pregnancies, 25 delivered an IUGR infant. In 15 of these a high vascular resistance was recognized, reflecting probable reduced uterine artery perfusion. In ten of the 25 IUGR cases, normal uterine artery waveforms were present suggesting to the authors the probability that the IUGR in these cases was of fetal cause.

Management of IUGR

Management, of course, implies that a diagnosis of the condition to be managed has been made. In the case of IUGR, the diagnosis will have been made as precisely as possible on the basis of early gestational dating by all possible means, a high degree of suspicion for possible predisposing factors, careful physical examination of the gravida taking into account the wide variation of "normal" in the measurement of fundal height, and the appropirate use of ultrasound whether this is ultimately decided to be best used routinely or selectively. The use of arterial blood flow velocity waveforms may be important for this purpose in the near future. What then needs to be done, or can be done, to "manage" the growth-retarded fetus thus recognized? Possibly, we can increase the growth of the fetus in utero. If we recognize deterioration of the condition of the fetus, we can decide between continued in utero care or neonatal care depending on which we think is more appropirate. We should prevent or minimize the risk of intrapartum asphyxia if labor is allowed. Lastly, and perhaps primarily, we should treat any underlying maternal disease which may be aggravating the IUGR.

What can be done to increase the growth rate of the fetus thought to be suffering IUGR? Several possibilites come to mind although many of these are scientifically unproven. There will be very little disagreement that avoidance or cessation of maternal cigarette smoking, maternal alcohol ingestion, and maternal recreational drug use have the potential for increasing fetal growth potential. Little more needs to be said of these habits since there are many reasons other than the possibility of alleviation of IUGR for encouraging mothers to stop these deleterious practices.

Less certain is the impact of improved maternal nutrition on IUGR. There is ample evidence that low prepregnancy weight and low maternal weight gain reduce the size of the fetus (Niswander et al. 1969). Data confirming the attractive hypothesis that improved maternal nutrition will increase the size of the fetus and reduce the ill effects of IUGR are, however, lacking or, at best, conflicting. This is a reasonable assumption to make on the matter, however, and few would argue that better maternal nutrition is likely to exert a negative influence on the fetus. Stein et al. (1978), in a review of eight controlled studies of prenatal nutrition supplementation concluded that: (a) prenatal dietary supplements can lead to a moderate increase in birthweight; (b) a high protein diet is no more effective than is a balanced high calorie diet in raising birthweight. Hyperalimentation is a recent innovation in clinical medicine and can be accomplished by either enteral or intravenous means in the pregnant patient. Published experience with this method of increasing nutrition during pregnancy is scanty, and the method cannot at present be recommended except for serious maternal gastrointestinal disease. Further clinical experience may broaden the indications for this method of nutrition.

Bed rest has been widely prescribed to improve fetal growth with IUGR and is thought to be effective through a reduction of catecholamine release, a decrease in uterine activity, and an increase in uteroplacental blood flow. Scientific proof for the effectiveness of bed rest in reducing the risk of such poor outcomes as an SGA infant or newborn mortality and morbidity from this cause is lacking. Prevention of preterm delivery with twin pregnancy by the use of bed rest has been of special interest to investigators. Since IUGR is so common in twin pregnancies, these studies are of importance to us. Several investigators have concluded that bed rest in twin pregnancy may prolong that pregnancy and increase infant weight (Persson et al. 1979). Weekes et al. (1977), however, in a randomized clinical trial failed to demonstrate any difference in birthweight or gestational age among three groups of patients with twin pregnancy: those who received no special treatment, those managed with bed rest, and those treated with cervical cerclage. Thus, as with many other forms of therapy, we must fall back on clinical experience, and I think most of us would recommend bed rest, at least to some extent, in a gravida carrying an IUGR fetus.

The usefulness of bed rest in the treatment of serious medical complications in the gravida also needs review. A recent study of 157 hypertensive pregnant women showed that most of the 21 perinatal deaths occurred in infants with birthweights below the 50th percentile and an additional 22% of the total group of infants were SGA (Lin et al. 1982). Three categories of hypertensive patients had significantly higher incidences of SGA infants, those with glomerulonephritis, multiparous patients with pre-eclampsia without preceding chronic hypertension, and patients with chronic hypertension with superimposed pre-eclampsia. While bed rest for at least 2 h a day is advised for these patients, proof that such treatment reduces the risk of development of IUGR or its effects is lacking. There is a similar lack of data on the effectiveness of bed rest in reducing the IUGR found with severe renal disease of pregnancy and severe cardiac disease in pregnancy, but most would nevertheless empirically recommend such treatment.

Pharmacologic agents which might promote human fetal growth have also been suggested as possible therapeutic agents, but at the present time these must be considered experimental and are not recommended for routine clinical use. Various beta-adrenergic agonists, because of their peripheral vasodilator effects, significantly increase uterine blood flow during the third trimester of pregnancy. These agents have cardiovascular and metabolic side effects and must be used with care even for the accepted treatment of premature labor. Katz et al. (1982) reported an increase in the weights of various fetal organs in rabbits when maternal terbutaline was used. Whether this effect will be seen in the human and whether it will prove to be clinically useful remains to be seen.

An inherent part of prenatal management of IUGR is monitoring fetal growth, monitoring fetal condition, especially with regard to developing asphyxia, and monitoring maturation of the fetus which, when sufficient, will allow a good chance of survival outside of the uterus. When IUGR is recognized, the clinician must walk the fine line between allowing the fetus to remain in utero for additional growth and maturity and thus risk death in utero and delivery of the fetus with the possibility of resulting neonatal death or damage. Certain tools will help the clinician with this decision, but the tools do not always permit a satisfactory outcome. Still, the clinician hopes to maximize the number of infants with a good outcome by astutely balancing the risks between the two choices.

Delivery of the IUGR Fetus

When should the clinician deliver the growth-retarded fetus? With severe growth retardation, the fetal mortality is universally recognized to be high, and delivery, as soon as there is sufficient maturity of the fetus to promise likely neonatal survival, is usually the best course of action. With less severe IUGR, placental function tests which indicate continuing good fetal health will permit the clinician to allow the pregnancy to continue, sometimes until "term." The major dilemma occurs when severe IUGR with nonreassuring placental function tests is found to coexist with obvious fetal immaturity. Maturity of the fetus (really, maturity of the fetal lungs) is best documented by analysis of amniotic fluid for a lecithin/sphingomyelin (L/S) ratio of 2.0 or greater and the presence of phosphatidylglycerol (PG). In this instance, it is usually better to deliver the fetus since continued in utero care is probably more likely to result in death than is nursery care. Data are insufficient to predict whether delivery of such a fetus also reduces the likelihood of a neuromotor dysfunction or not.

There seems to be no universal agreement on which of the various placental function tests currently available is best. Indeed, randomized clinical trials have suggested that utilization of the nonstress test (NST) may not lower perinatal mortality or morbidity (Grant and Mohide 1982). Similarly, a randomized clinical trial on the use of plasma estrogens for management of high-risk pregnancies failed to show any improvement in fetal-neonatal outcome when estrogen levels were available to the clinician (Duenholter 1976). Nevertheless, in the absence of better tests of placental function, and with due regard that future developments may very well make my remarks passe, I do recommend the use of the NST and/or the contraction stress test (CST), and some would also recommend urinary or serum estrogen determinations. Fetal movement counts may provide useful information on fetal condition, but their use as the sole criterion for diagnosis of a condition as potentially serious as IUGR cannot at present be recommended.

The NST, CST, and estrogen levels as measures of placental function each have adherents. Perhaps the most prevalent view at present is that the NST should be the initial screening test. A reactive NST is reassuring, and weekly (or biweekly?) repetitions are presumed adequate to assure continuing good fetal health. A non-reassuring NST should be followed by a CST (now commonly accomplished with breast stimulation rather than oxytocin infusion). A negative CST (i.e., no late decelerations seen), expecially if the fetal heart rate (FHR) also shows reactivity, is reassuring of good fetal health and should be repeated 1 week later. A positive CST requires consideration of very early delivery of the fetus accomplished either by induction of labor with careful continuous EFM or by cesarean section. Induction or section ideally should be preceded by an amniocentesis to determine adequate fetal maturity. A positive CST in a severely growth-retarded fetus in the absence of fetal maturity is an especially distressing clinical problem, but such a fetus probably does better in the nursery than in the uterus.

If the clinician has been fortunate enough to carry an IUGR fetus to term, or, indeed, if induction of labor has been elected even before term, very careful assessment of fetal condition during labor should be undertaken. It is likely that an IUGR fetus tolerates labor less well than a normal fetus, and the clinician should have a higher index of suspicion of intrapartum asphyxia in such a fetus. Recognizing the many shortcomings of continuous EFM, the high false-positive rate, the variability of interpretation by even highly competent experts in reading tracings, and the lack of proof that intervention with an EFM pattern thought to indicate asphyxia will reduce the risk of subsequent neuromotor dysfunction, the clinician caring for a severely growth-retarded fetus should probably err on the side of overdiagnosis of fetal asphyxia (Sykes et al. 1982). This admonition, however, is made with full recognition that the cause of neuromotor dysfunction in an IUGR fetus with asphyxia during labor is obscure. It is possible that the neurologic dysfunction was caused by factors associated with the IUGR and existed prior to, or even caused, the intrapartum asphyxia. Also possible is that the cause is multifactorial both from the known factor of IUGR and/or intrapartum asphyxia and from other unknown or unrecognized factors. In short, we should exercise the best current medical knowledge and use the clinical tools we have for reducing the risk of asphyxia or other embarrassments to the fetus, but we should not exaggerate the likelihood that such skill will reduce or eliminate poor fetal outcome pending better data that might establish such cause and effect.

There is no doubt that the presence of IUGR seriously complicates obstetric care. An increase in the perinatal death rate is a well-known result. Less certain is the degree to which IUGR contributes to neuromotor dysfunction in the surviving child. We need not wait for reliable data on that issue, however, before aggressively trying to improve the accuracy of our diagnostic tools for recognizing IUGR and for maintaining the health of the IUGR fetus. While unproved, a happy by-product of these efforts may be a reduction in the risk of neuromotor dysfunctions. At least that is a reasonable hope.

References

Cohen-Overbeek T et al. (1985) The antenatal assessment of uteroplacental and fetoplacental blood flow using Doppler ultrasound. Ultrasound Med Biol 11: 329

Duenholter J (1976) An analysis of the utility of plasma immunoreactive estrogen measurements in determining delivery time of gravidas with a fetus considered at high risk. Am J Obstet Gynecol 125: 889

Fleischer A et al. (1985) Umbilical artery velocity waveforms and intrauterine growth retardation. Am J Obstet Gynecol 151: 502-505

Grant A, Mohide P (1982) Screening and diagnostic tests in antenatal care. In: Enkin M, Chalmers I (eds) Effectiveness and satisfaction in antenatal care. Spastics International Medical Publications, London

Hagberg B, Hagberg G (1984) Prenatal and perinatal risk factors in a survey of 681 Swedish cases. In: Stanley F, Alberman E (eds) The epidemiology of the cerebral palsies. Spastics International Medical Publications, Oxford

Hall M et al. (1980) Is routine antenatal care worth while? Lancet 2: 78-80

Hughey M (1984) Routine ultrasound for the detection and management of the small for gestational age fetus. Obstet Gynecol 64: 101-107

Katz M et al. (1982) Fetal organ weight changes after intravenous terbutaline administration in the rabbit (Abstr 10). 29th Annual Meeting of the Society for Gynecologic Investigations, Dallas

Lin C et al. (1982) Fetal outcome and hypertensive disorders of pregnancy. Am J Obstet Gynecol 142: 255

Niswander K et al. (1969) Weight gain during pregnancy and prepregnancy weight: Association with birth weight of term gestation. Obstet Gynecol 33: 482

Persson P et al. (1979) On improved outcome of twin pregnancies. Acta Obstet Gynecol Scand 58: 3

Rosenberg et al. (1982) Antenatal detection of growth retardation: Actual practice in a large maternity hospital. Br J Obstet Gynecol 89: 12-15

Stein Z et al. (1978) Prenatal nutrition and birth weight: Experiments and quasiexperiments in the past decade. J Reprod Med 21: 287
Sykes G et al. (1982) Do Apgar scores indicate asphyxia? Lancet 1
Trudinger B et al. (1985) Uteroplacental blood flow velocity-time waveforms in normal and complicated pregnancy. Br J Obstet Gynecol 92: 32
Warsof S et al. (1986) Routine ultrasound screening for antenatal detection of intrauterine growth retardation. Obstet Gynecol 67: 33-39
Weekes A et al. (1977) The relative efficacy of bedrest, cervical suture, and no treatment in the management of twin pregnancy. Br J Obstet Gynecol 84: 161

Abnormal Antepartum Cardiotocogram and Neuromotor Dysfunction in Term and Preterm Babies

U. LORENZ and F. KUBLI

Modern obstetricians pay more and more attention to the prevention not only of intrauterine fetal death (Hamilton et al. 1978; Kubli and Rüttgers 1974; Parer 1979) but also of chronic brain damage which can be caused by prolonged intrauterine hypoxia. In this connection, the evaluation of antepartum pathological cardiotocograms (CTGs) becomes more and more important (Freeman et al. 1982). Since the development of brain damage is a multifactorial process influenced not only by hypoxia and its duration (Flynn and Kelly 1979; Fricker et al. 1983; Hill and Volpe 1982; Schneider 1978) but also by other etiological noxae, a procedure has to be found by means of which other factors influencing brain development can be kept fairly constant. This paper tries to make a contribution to the role of pathological antepartum CTGs as a prognostic factor for the further development of term and preterm children.

Matched Pairs

Of the 5674 infants born during a 4-year period at the Department of Obstrics and Gynecology in Heidelberg, 219 infants had abnormal antepartum CTG recordings (4%). Fourteen infants died during the peri- or neonatal period. The mothers (205) of 210 infants were sent questionnaires on the neuromotor development of the children. We finally received 133 answers.

To establish a control group, we used the "matched pairs" method, i.e., we tried to find matched partners with *normal* antepartum CTG recordings in whom the following match criteria corresponded to one of the cases with *pathological* antepartum CTG:

1. Intrauterine growth retardation (< 10th percentile)
2. Gestational age at delivery
3. Complications and diseases of the mother during pregnancy
4. Time of delivery (± 6 weeks)

We based our considerations on the assumption that certain complications and conditions, in addition to fetal hypoxia manifested in CTG, influence the later neuromotor development of the child to a varying degree (match criteria 1 and 3) and that only children of roughly the same age can be compared with each other (match criterion 4).

Pilot Project - Pathological Antepartum CTG and Neuromotor Development of the Child

Results

Intrauterine growth retardation, gestational age at the time of delivery as well as the frequency and types of complications during pregnancy were identical in both groups. Only the incidence of maternal, non-pregnancy-related diseases was somewhat higher in the group with pathological antepartum CTG (for more details see Lorenz et al. 1986).

The comparison of pathological situations during delivery - not a match condition - reveals no significant differences between the group with pathological antepartum CTG and the control group. Only fever during delivery was seen more frequently in the target group.

There were clear differences in the mode of birth between both groups: the frequency of cesarean sections was 44% in the group with pathological antepartum CTG as compared to 12.6% in the group with normal antepartum CTG (Table 1).

As expected, there was also a high rate of infants with pathological CTG patterns during first and second stage of labor: pathological *intrapartum* CTGs were approximately four times more frequent in the group with pathological antepartum CTG than in the control group (Table 2).

The number of severely depressed neonates, which is indicated by an Apgar score ≤ at 5 and 10 min, was significantly increased after pathological antepartum CTG, as was the rate of severe and mild acidoses (Tables 3 and 4). A markedly increased resuscitation frequency could also be seen. Transfer to the neonatal intensive care unit was also required twice as often (Table 5).

The rate of complicated courses during the neonatal period in premature babies, where additional complications such as pneumonia, respiratory distress syndrome, and others occur, was slighly higher in the target group. Other diseases of the neonates not associated with premature delivery were also more frequent and led to a markedly higher transfer rate of the infants from this group.

Table 1. Mode of delivery in cases with and without pathological antepartum CTG (matched pairs)

	Pathological antepartum CTG ($n=118$)		Control group ($n=119$)	
	(n)	(%)	*(n)*	(%)
Cesarean section Total	52*	44.0	15	2.6
Primary	33**	28.0	8	6.7
Secondary	19**	16.0	7	5.9
Vaginally operative	11	9.3	12	10.1
Vaginally spontaneous	55*	46.7	92	77.3

* $p<0.001$; ** $p<0.01$

Table 2. Frequency of abnormal *intrapartum* CTG in cases with and without pathological antepartum CTG (matched pairs)

	Pathological antepartum CTG (n=123)		Control group (n=123)	
	(n)	(%)	*(n)*	(%)
Number of children reaching first stage of labor	87		115	
With pathological CTG in first stage of labor	60*	69	21	18.3
Number of children reaching second stage of labor	67		108	
With pathological CTG in second stage of labor	55*	82	30	27.8

* $p<0.001$

Table 3. Neonatal depression in cases with and without abnormal antepartum CTG (matched pairs)

Apgar score	Pathological antepartum CTG (n=123)		Control group (n=123)	
	(n)	(%)	*(n)*	(%)
1-min value ≤ 5	21	17.0	5	4.1
5-min value ≤ 7	13 (+4)*	10.6/13.8	5	4.1
10-min value ≤ 7	4 (+4)**	3.2/6.5	1	0.8

* $p\leq 0.01$; ** $p\leq 0.05$

Table 4. Acidosis (pH_{ua}) in cases with and without abnormal antepartum CTG (matched pairs)

pH_{ua}	Pathological antepartum CTG (n=123)		Control group (n=123)	
	(n)	(%)	*(n)*	(%)
≤ 7.10	7*	5.7	-	
$>7.10 \leq 7.20$	28**	22.8	11	8.9
>7.20	88***	71.5	112	91.1

* $p<0.05$; ** $p<0.01$; *** $p<0.001$

Table 5. Need for resuscitation and transferal rates to NICU in cases with and without abnormal antepartum CTG (matched pairs)

	Pathological antepartum CTG ($n=123$)		Control group ($n=123$)	
	(*n*)	(%)	(*n*)	(%)
Intubation/resuscitation	37*	26	6	4.9
Transferral rate	43	35	23	18.7

* $p<0.01$

Table 6. Neuromotor abnormalities in children following *abnormal* antepartum CTG and in the corresponding matched partners with *normal* CTG

Case No.	Pathological antepartum CTG group (13 reversible, one irreversible disorder)	Matched partner (normal CTG)
1	Minimal brain damage	–
2	Developmental retardation	–
3	Developmental retardation	–
4	Minimal brain damage and developmental retardation	–
5	Neuromotor dysfunction	–
6	Developmental retardation	–
7	Neuromotor dysfunction and developmental retardation	–
8	Developmental retardation and generalized seizures	–
9	Irreversible cerebral palsy (spastic diplegia)	–
10	Developmental retardation	Neuromotor dysfunction
11	Developmental retardation	–
12	Hypotonicity and developmental retardation	–
13	Developmental retardation	–
14	Developmental retardation	–

Evaluation of Questionnaires

The evaluation of the questionnaires reveals 14 cases with neuromotor abnormalities in the group with pathological antepartum CTG. These were reversible in 13 cases by adequate physiotherapy, but in one case, an irreversible spastic diplegia (case No. 9) developed (Table 6). Among the corresponding matched partners, there was only one case showing a reversible neuromotor dysfunction.

In the control group with normal antepartum CTG, there were six children with abnormal neuromotor findings. All disorders seen in these children were reversible. Among the corresponding matched partners with pathological CTG, one case with a reversible neuromotor disorder was found (Table 7). Thus, the frequency of neuromotor abnormalities is more than twice as high after pathological antepartum CTG than after normal antepartum CTG.

Despite the considerable variation in the number of random samples, several significant differences between these two groups can be found: higher incidence of pathological pregnancies (in particular, preeclampsia) in cases with later neu-

Table 7. Neuromotor abnormalities in children following *normal* antepartum CTG and in the corresponding matched partners with *pathological* antepartum CTG

Case No.	Control group (six reversible disorders)	Matched partner (with pathological antepartum CTG)
1	Minimal brain damage	-
2	Neuromotor dysfunction and seizures	-
3	Neuromotor dysfunction	Developmental retardation
4	Developmental retardation	-
5	Neuromotor dysfunction	-
6	Neuromotor dysfunction	-

Table 8. Pre- and perinatal conditions of children with and without neuromotor abnormalities following pathological antepartum CTG

	Children *with* neuromotor disorders ($n=14$)		Children *without* neuromotor disorders ($n=109$)	
Normal pregnancy course	3*		65	
EPH gestosis	7*		14	
Premature labor/tocolysis	2		8	
Gestational age at birth $\leq 37+0$	7*		18	
Percentile <10	5		24	
Birthweight <1500 g	4*	10	4	28
1500-2500 g	6		24	
Primary section	7	8	26	44
Secondary section	1		18	
Apgarscore 1 min ≤ 5	8*		13	
5 min ≤ 7	5*		12	
10 min ≤ 7	4*		4	
$pH_{ua} \leq 7.20 > 7.10$	5	6	23	29
≤ 7.10	1		6	
Resuscitation/intubation	11*		32	
Transfer to NICU	11		34	
Intrapartal CTG				
Pathological in first stage	5/7		55/83	
Pathological in second stage	6/6		49/65	

* $p<0.05$

romotor disorders; higher incidence of premature delivery prior to a gestational age of 37 weeks; higher incidence of newborn infants with a very low birthweight; higher incidence of low Apgar scores after 1, 5, and 10 min; higher incidence of resuscitation (Table 8). Full details of the matched pairs study have been recently published (Lorenz et al. 1986).

Infants with Low Birthweight

Since we found a predominance of children with low birthweight in the group of cases with later neuromotor dysfunction, our second attempt to elucidate the problem was a target group of infants with a birthweight ≤2000 g born at the Department of Obstetrics and Gynecology in Heidelberg. By evaluating this high-risk population we tried to find out whether there is a sort of cut-off point beyond which we have to interfere, i.e., to terminate pregnancy even if a rather immature child has to be expected.

There were originally 417 children with a birthweight ≤2000 g in the study, of whom 189 had to be excluded due to reasons such as intrauterine fetal death, no CTG tracing available, no followup of the children, or the need to exclude one of two twins. Finally, 239 infants remained in the study, of whom 41 died within the first 6 months postnatally. The distribution of the times of death of these 41 children is shown in Table 9.

Finally, 198 children were available for followup, i.e., regular examinations of the neuromotor development were performed by the neurodevelopmental team of the University Children's Department at Heidelberg. In accordance with the neuropediatricians, we subgrouped the neurodevelopmental findings into three categories:

1. Infants with normal or retarded development
2. Infants with mild or severe but transient neuromotor abnormalities
3. Infants with minimal brain damage and with cerebral palsy

The distribution of the 198 surviving children weighing 2000 g or less at birth in the three neurodevelopmental groups was as follows: 70 were in group 1 (29.3%), 123 belonged to group 2 with mild or severe but transient neuromotor abnormalities (51.5%), and five children (2.1%) developed either minimal cerebral dysfunction ($n=3$) or irreversible cerebral palsy ($n=2$). During the postpartum period of up to 6 months after birth, a total of 41 children died (Table 10).

Table 9. Incidence of perinatal, early, and late neonatal death in children weighing ≤2000 g at birth

	(n)	(%)
Intrapartum death	1	0.42
Neonatal death 1st-7th day	24	10.04
Death 8th-28th day	10	4.18
Death 29th day-6th month	6	2.51
Survivors	198	82.85
Total	239	100.00

Table 10. Allocation of children weighing ≤2000 g at birth to the neuromotor developmental groups 1-3 and group 4 (children dying within the first 6 months after birth)

	(n)	(%)
Normal/retarded	70	29.29
Transient unspecific neurologic abnormality	123	51.46
Minimal brain damage and cerebral palsy	5	2.09
Death within 6 months after birth	41	17.15
Survivors	198	82.85
Total	239	100.00

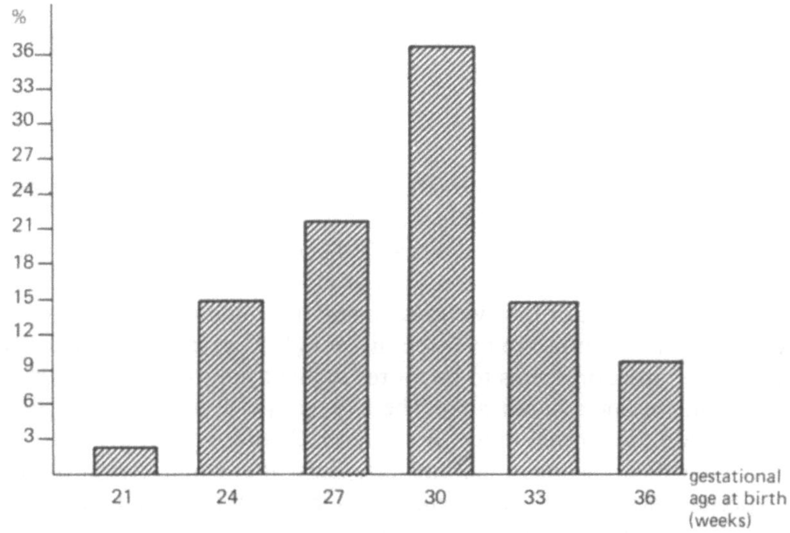

Fig. 1. Postpartum mortality of children weighing ≤2000 g at birth: relative frequency according to gestational age at birth

Results

Pregnancy and perinatal parameters as well as the neonatal course of events were evaluated and correlated to the later neuromotor development of the children. The majority of children who died during the first 6 months after birth ($n=41$) were born at 30 weeks of gestation or less, as expected (Fig. 1). The majority of these

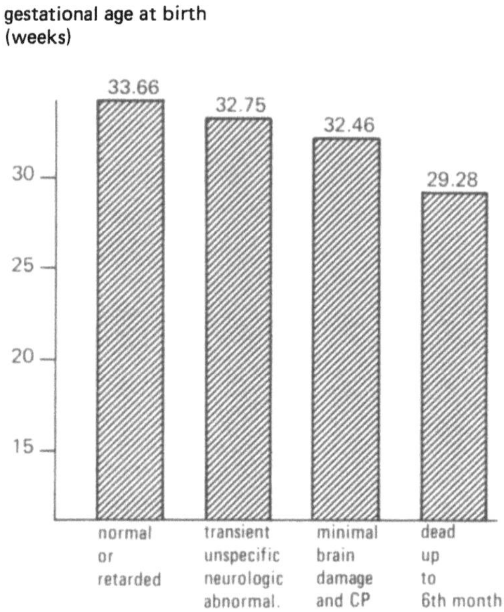

Fig. 2. Mean gestational age at birth of children weighing ≤2000 g compared to later neuromotor findings and infants' death

children died during the immediate neonatal period, i.e., in the perinatal period up to the 7th day of life (Table 9).

The mean gestational age, classified according to neurodevelopmental groups, dropped steadily from 33.6 weeks in group 1 to 29.3 weeks in group 4 (Fig. 2). The distribution of mean birthweights shows the same trend: the lowest birthweights (1254 g) were seen in group 4, the highest (1697 g) in group 1 (Fig. 3). Intrauterine growth retardation seems to be more frequent in group 3 (survivors with minor or major neuromotor handicaps). The average percentile is low in this group (9.00) and within the normal range in groups 1, 2, and 4 (16.9, 21.6, 30.5) (Fig. 4). From the immediate neonatal parameters, only the 1-min Apgar score showed the expected decline in the four neurodevelopmental groups: it was highest in group 1 (6.59) and lowest in group 4 (3.89), i.e., in children who died later. After 5 and 10 min, the same trend could be seen, but somewhat weaker, probably influenced by resuscitation procedures which are often necessary in these infants of low birthweight. Obviously, Apgar scores after 5 and 10 min do not show greater differences in the groups 1-3 (survivors), but a remarkably lower value in those children who died later on (Fig. 5).

Apgar scores are of some prognostic value regarding survival or impending death but cannot be of much help in discriminating children with or without later disturbance of neuromotor development.

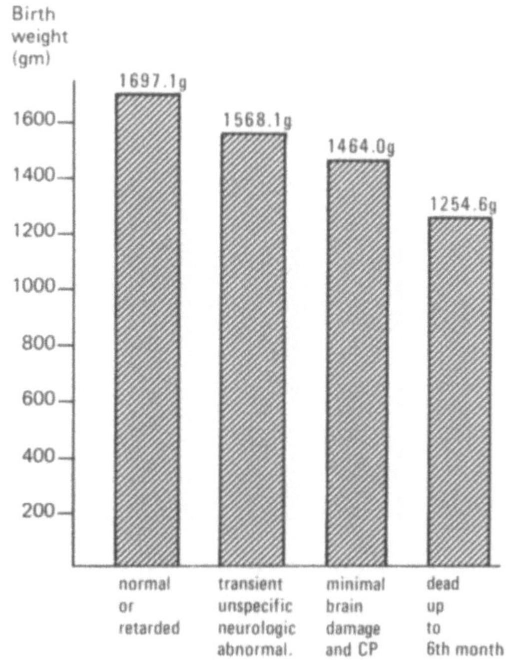

Fig. 3. Mean birthweight of children (≤2000 g) compared to later neuromotor findings and infants' death

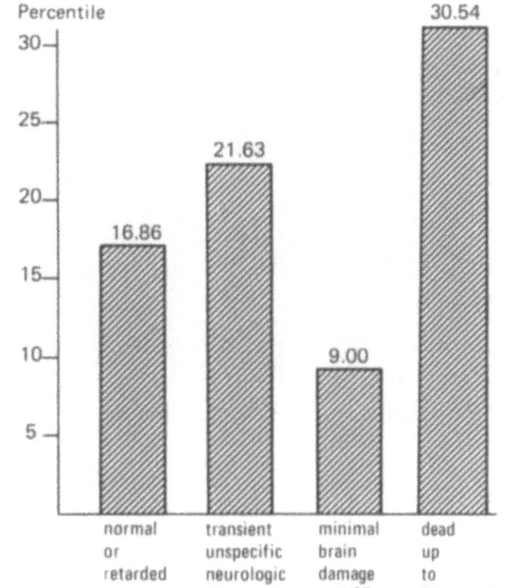

Fig. 4. Average values of percentile of birthweight in the three groups of different neuromotor development and cases dying within 6 months after birth

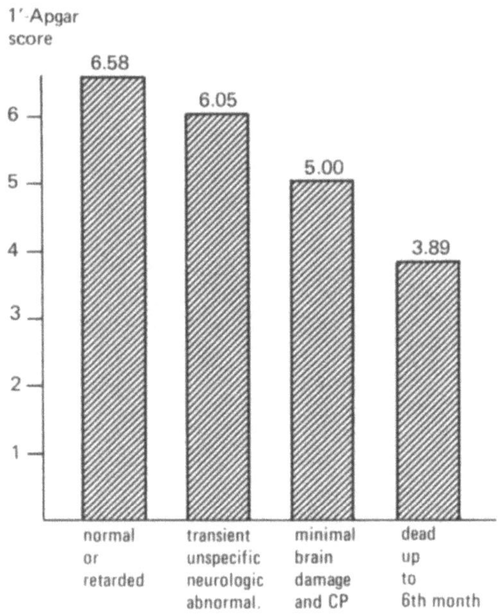
1'-Apgar score
6.58
6.05
5.00
3.89
6
5
4
3
2
1
normal or retarded
transient unspecific neurologic abnormal.
minimal brain damage and CP
dead up to 6th month

a

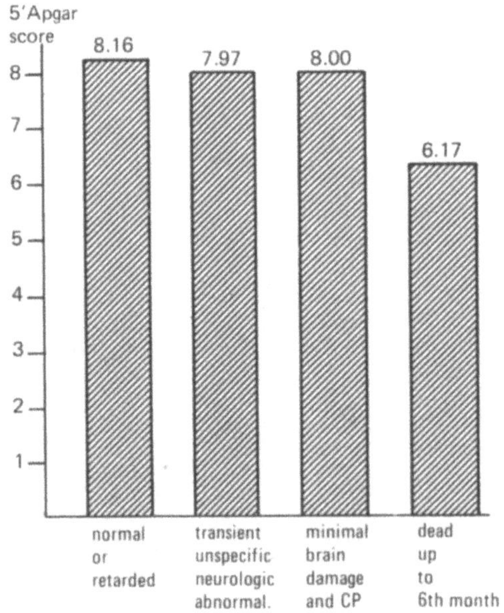
5'Apgar score
8.16
7.97
8.00
6.17
8
7
6
5
4
3
2
1
normal or retarded
transient unspecific neurologic abnormal.
minimal brain damage and CP
dead up to 6th month

b

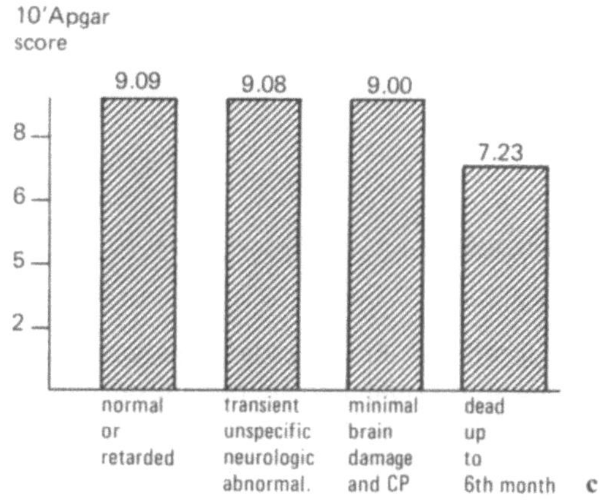

Fig. 5a–c. Mean Apgar scores after 1 (**a**), 5 (**b**), and 10 min (**c**) of children weighing ≤2000 g at birth. Distribution of values according to neurodevelopmental groups and infants dying within 6 months after birth

Table 11. Mean CTG values in the various groups of neuromotor development of surviving children with birthweights ≤2000 g and children dying within the first 6 months after birth. CTG values are compiled for various time intervals prior to delivery

Mean CTG scores prior to birth	Neurodevelopmental groups				Significance		
	1	2	3	4			
	Healthy and retarded	Transient unspecific neurological abnormalities	Minimal brain damage and cerebral palsy	Death within 6 months		Kruskal-Wallis test	Spearman test
-4 h	4.86	5.17	4.66	4.49	NS	$p=0.2144$	$p=0.5457$
-8 h	5.05	5.29	4.66	4.62	NS	$p=0.2029$	$p=0.3790$
-12 h	5.10	5.33	4.63	4.58	NS	$p=0.1205$	$p=0.2593$
-24 h	5.30	5.39	4.69	4.66	NS	$p=0.1132$	$p=0.0913$
-48 h	5.50	5.45	4.93	4.82	NS	$p=0.1716$	$p=0.0571$
-1 week	5.84	5.65	4.91	4.86	S	$p=0.0217$	$p=0.0056$
-2 weeks	5.90	5.67	4.91	4.94	S	$p=0.0260$	$p=0.0051$
-3 weeks	5.93	5.69	4.91	5.03	S	$p=0.0290$	$p=0.0055$
-7 weeks	5.96	5.69	4.94	5.02	S	$p=0.0216$	$p=0.0037$

CTG Evaluation

For short periods of CTG evaluation (evaluations up to 4, 8, 12, 24, 48 h prior to delivery), a correlation between CTG pathology and the neurodevelopmental state of the child could not be shown. However, a compilation of all CTG data during the last and the last but one week of pregnancy showed a correlation between antepartum CTG pathology and later outcome: irreversible brain dysfunction (in five cases) or early or later neonatal death (in 41 cases) are associated with low CTG scores (Table 11). The comparison of mean score values in groups 1 and 2 as well as groups 3 and 4 shows remarkable differences between more or less undisturbed children who survive and those who die or survive with handicaps (Table 11).

Comment

The results of our investigations can be summarized as follows: in a case-controlled study (matched pairs method), children with pathological antepartum cardiotocograms showed a two-fold higher incidence of later neuromotor abnormality (one irreversible, 13 reversible dysfunctions) compared to children with normal antepartum CTG. Pathological antepartum cardiotocograms lead to higher rates of pathological intrapartum CTGs, higher cesarean section rates, more cases of neonatal depression, and more frequently to severe and mild acidosis in the umbilical artery.

Comparison of cases with and without neuromotor dysfunction following pathological antepartum CTG reveals higher rates of pregnancy-related complications, more premature births (<37 weeks), more infants of low (<2500 g) and very low (<1500 g) birthweight. Thus - and this can be confirmed by the second part of our study - the combination of pathological antepartum CTG and immaturity leads to a more unfavorable prognosis for the neonates; a substantial part of the children with a birthweight ≤2000 g will die of immaturity (17% in our study population); 2.5% will develop irreversible brain damage, whereas 80% will survive with either no serious complications except for retarded somatic development as expected after premature birth (29%), or with transient prematurity-associated neuromotor dysfunctions.

The compiled mean scores of antepartum CTG during the last weeks of pregnancy show substantially lower values associated with later unfavorable outcome for the child (irreversible brain damage or death within the first 6 months of life). In cases with imminent premature delivery and antepartum CTG pathology, the decision in favor of earlier intervention (i.e., earlier delivery) has to be based on the duration of CTG pathology.

In agreement with other authors (Hensleigh et al. 1986), we could confirm that prematurity and asphyxia are definitely associated with cerebral palsy. However, there must be other causes for cerebral palsy than those mentioned above, since in a considerable number of cases, no documented depression occurred at birth (Paneth and Staris 1983). Since antepartum CTG is a more or less crude cardiovascular parameter detecting established fetal hypoxia, other parameters are needed to elucidate earlier changes in fetal blood flow, especially impairment of blood flow in the fetal brain. First results show impairment or even a loss of flow in the umbilical artery and fetal aorta days before a suspicious or even pathological antepartum CTG can be registered (Arabin et al. unpublished).

Fortunately, irreversible brain damage is a rare event, therefore larger studies of fetal blood flow and CTG events have to be designed to bring us nearer to the solution of the problem of whether there is a more definite cut-off point up to which we could wait and postpone delivery, or beyond which we have to intervene, i.e., to induce delivery, even if we expect infants of very low birthweight.

References

Flynn AM, Kelly J (1979) Unstressed antepartum cardiotocography in the management of the fetus suspected of growth retardation. Br J Obstet Gynaecol 86: 106-110

Freeman RK, Anderson G, Dorchester W (1982) A prospective multi-institutional study of antepartum fetal heart rate monitoring. Am J Obstet Gynecol 143: 771-777

Fricker HS, Sauter M, Buchs B (1983) Antepartale hypoxische Hirnschädigung (antepartale CTG und postpartale CT-Veränderungen). Z Geburtshife Periantol 187: 50-53

Hamilton LA, Gottschalk W, Vidyasagar D, Horn C, Wynn RM (1978) Effect of monitoring high-risk pregnancies and intrapartum FHR monitoring on neonates. Int J Gynaecol Obstet 15: 483-490

Hensleigh PA, Fainstat T, Spencer R (1986) Perinatal events and cerebral palsy. Am J Obstet Gynecol 154: 978-981

Hill A, Volpe JJ (1982) Hypoxic-ischemic brain injury in the newborn. Semin Perinatol 6: 25-41

Kubli F, Rüttgers H (1974) Probleme und Bedeutung der kardiotokographischen Überwachung des Fetus. Geburtshilfe Frauenheilkd 34: 1-20

Lorenz U, Fischer R, Kubli F (1986) Pathologisches antepartales CTG als prognostischer Faktor für die weitere Entwicklung des Kindes. Z Geburtshilfe Perinatol 190: 114-122

Paneth N, Staris RI (1983) Cerebral palsy and mental retardation in relation to indicators of perinatal asphyxia. Am J Obstet Gynecol 147: 960-966

Parer JT (1979) Fetal heart rate monitoring. Lancet 22: 632-633

Schneider R (1978) Hirnfunktionsstörungen im Kindesalter. Enke, Stuttgart, pp 2-11

Antepartum Fetal Heart Rate and Movement Pattern in Relation to Oxygenation and Neonatal Neurological Morbidity

G. H. A. VISSER

Introduction

Antepartum fetal heart rate monitoring is widely used to evaluate the fetal condition in utero, as is, to a lesser degree, the monitoring of fetal movements. Knowledge about the etiological backgrounds of abnormal patterns, especially with respect to fetal oxygenation, is essential when relating antepartum heart rate and/or movements to neonatal neurological morbidity.

Abnormal patterns of both diagnostic indices have been found in relation to various pregnancy complications, such as congenital malformations, infections, Rh disease, maternal drug administration, and, last but not least, fetal intrauterine growth retardation. In this paper only data on growth-retarded fetuses are presented for reasons of simplicity. First, data on the changes in heart rate and movement patterns with progressive deterioration of the fetal condition in utero are presented and related to the status of fetal oxygenation. Secondly, the relationship between the presence of antepartum late heart rate decelerations with neonatal neurological outcome is considered.

Heart Rate and Movement Patterns in Growth-Retarded Fetuses

Murata et al. (1982) found that with progressive deterioration in the fetal condition of the rhesus monkey, late decelerations appeared first. This condition was associated with fetal hypoxemia. With a gradual decline in the pH the incidence of accelerations (and of movements?) decreased (Fig. 1). In growth-retarded fetal sheep, a low arterial pO_2 also precedes acidemia (Robinson et al. 1985). In the latter, chronic hypoxemia (and hypoglycemia) was sometimes present for weeks before acidemia and finally intrauterine death occurred.

There is evidence that changes in heart rate (and movement) patterns in the growth-retarded human fetus follow more or less the same patterns as those found in the rhesus monkey. A possible rank ordering at which these changes occur with progressive deterioration of the fetal condition is shown in Fig. 2. The occurrence of late heart rate decelerations is centrally placed in this figure. The suggested rank ordering is based on the data presented below.

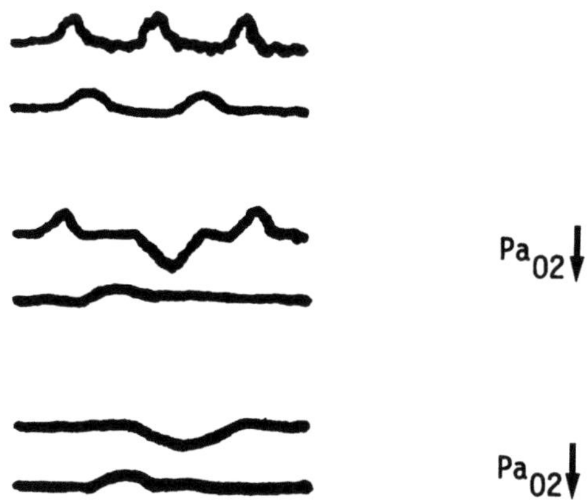

Fig. 1. Changes in fetal heart rate pattern and oxygenation in rhesus monkeys, with progressive deterioration of the fetal condition. These data are based on the study of Murata et al. (1982)

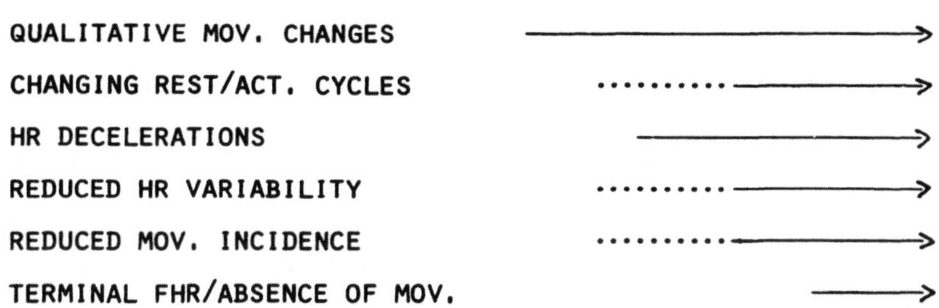

Fig. 2. Suggested rank ordering at which movement *(MOV)* and heart rate *(HR)* changes occur in growth-retarded human fetuses with progressive deterioration of the fetal condition *ACT.*, active

In intrauterine growth-retarded fetuses, a low long-term heart rate variation is usually found during both "reactive" and "nonreactive" episodes. In the absence of late decelerations, however, this variation is nearly always within the normal range (Visser 1984). It has, on the other hand, recently been found that in the presence of late decelerations, heart rate variation was reduced in 23 of 26 cases (88%; Bekedam and Visser 1984; Bekedam et al. 1987). This implies that the heart rate variation pattern of growth-retarded fetuses cannot be distinguished from that of normal ones before late decelerations appear, and, consequently, that a reduction of long-term heart rate variation has to be considered as a rather late sign of fetal compromise. It is, as yet, uncertain if short-term ("beat-to-beat") variation drops below the norm at an earlier stage.

The data are almost identical, with respect to fetal body movements (as observed by real-time ultrasound), to those found for long-term heart rate variation. In the absence of late decelerations, movements dropped below the norm ($\cong$5% of recording time) in only one out of ten cases, whereas in the presence of decelerations this incidence was reduced in 18 of the 27 cases (Bekedam et al. 1987). It is also known from subjective fetal movement records kept by the pregnant women that before the sudden decline in movement occurs, usually indicat-

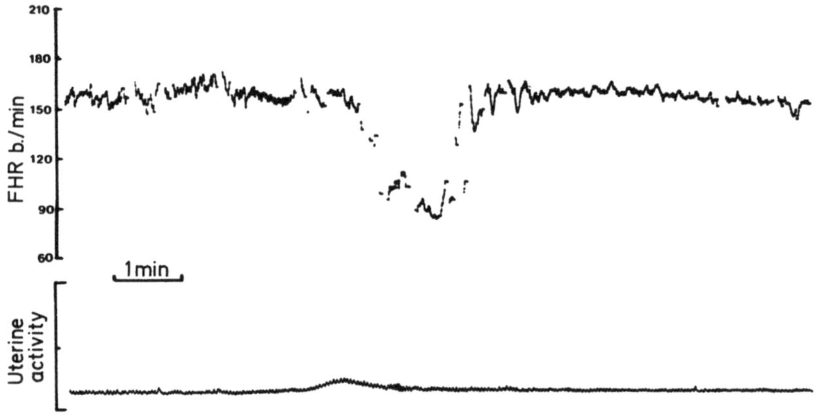

Fig. 3. Example of a "decelerative" fetal heart rate *(FHR)* pattern

ing impending fetal death, the movement incidence is still within the normal range (Sadovski et al. 1974; Pearson and Weaver 1976). A decline in the incidence of fetal movements must, therefore, also be considered as a late sign of fetal impairment.

Recently, we studied the relationship between antepartum heart rate decelerations and fetal blood gases obtained at elective cesarean section (Bekedam et al. 1987). With a decelerative cardiotocogram, as shown in Fig. 3, a normal pH was, generally, found in both the umbilical artery and vein, when compared to a control group. The pO_2 was, however, significantly reduced (mean pO_2 1.61 and 2.81 kPa, respectively). In a group of growth-retarded fetuses with a normal heart rate pattern, the pO_2 was usually in the lower normal range. This indicates that antepartum late heart rate decelerations - and a decrease in heart rate variation and movement incidence - coincide with the occurrence of fetal hypoxemia. A causal relationship is suggested as oxygen administration to the mother results in an increase of both heart rate variation and movements (Bekedam et al. 1986). Henson et al. (1983) also showed that the initial reduction in heart rate variation occurs before acidemia develops.

With further deterioration of the fetal condition fetal movements are usually absent and the fetal heart rate shows a "terminal pattern," namely, flat with shallow late decelerations. This condition is strongly associated with fetal acidemia and at elective cesarean section a pH in the umbilical artery (pH_{ua}) of less than 7.15 has been found in 70% of the cases (Visser et al. 1980).

Fetal heart rate and movement changes that precede the occurrence of late decelerations are, in general, more difficult to quantify. It is known, from subjective records kept by the women, that an increase in the percentage of weak movements occurs, with a decrease of strong and "rolling" movements sometimes weeks before movements decline (Sadovski et al. 1979). Using real-time ultrasound, slow monotonous movements of small amplitude can be observed. Although techniques for quantification have been developed, objective assessment of these changes remains difficult. For the ultrasonographist familiar with normal fetal motility these changes are, however, usually evident and in a series in which this has been previously been investigated a high interobserver agreement was found (Bekedam et al. 1985). Manning et al. (1981), who developed a biophysical profile score, assess this aspect by observing limb movements. A high score is given when a movement from a position of flexion to extension with a rapid return to flexion is observed. A low "fetal tone" exists when the fetus is in a position of semi- or full-limb extension with no return to flexion after the movements.

A disturbance in the development of fetal behavioral states also precedes the occurrence of late decelerations. From 36-38 weeks the normal fetus exhibits well-regulated fetal behavioral states with simultaneous changes in heart rate, eye movement, and gross body movement patterns. Van Vliet et al. (1985) found that in term growth-retarded fetuses the transition from one state to another was disturbed. It is, as yet, uncertain if changes in the distribution of rest/activity cycles and behavioral states, resulting in an increase in the percentage of time of non-reactive ("flat") heart rate episodes, precede the occurrence of heart rate decelerations.

It can be concluded from the data presented that in intrauterine growth-retarded fetuses, changes in heart rate and motility are relatively late signs of impairment. In general, a growth-retarded fetus will be found to have a normal heart rate and motility pattern. It is not growth retardation that is detected with these assessment techniques but presumably, in the first instance, hypoxemia. Earlier signs of impairment may be detected by other techniques such as recordings of umbilical artery velocity wave forms.

Antepartum Heart Rate Decelerations and Neonatal Neurological Morbidity

The relationship between antepartum fetal heart rate patterns and neonatal neurological morbidity was investigated in 23 small-for-date (SFD) term infants and in 33 SFD infants delivered before 37 weeks. All the subjects were selected from the data base of the Groningen Perinatal Project, containing pre- and perinatal data on 3162 children from consecutive singleton pregnancies, all surviving the neonatal period. Details as to the obstetrical-neonatal neurological relationship of the total study population have been published previously (Jurgens-van der Zee et al. 1979; Huisjes et al. 1980). The selection criterion for the current study in SFD infants was the availibility of umbilical blood gas values at birth. A standardized neonatal neurological examination (Prechtl 1977) was performed during the newborn period; infants born prematurely were examined at term age. The results were expressed in a neurological classification (normal, suspect, abnormal) and in a neonatal neurological optimality score (NNOS, range 0-60; Touwen et al. 1980).

Details of this study have yet to be published (Dijxhoorn et al., in preparation). The results, with respect to the relationship between the presence or absence of heart rate decelerations and neonatal brain function, are summarized in Table 1. There was a strong correlation between heart rate decelerations (of which 80%

Table 1. Neonatal neurological outcome in relation to antepartum fetal heart rate (FHR) patterns in small-for-date (SFD) term and preterm fetuses

	n	CS	pH_{ua} (mean)	Neonatal neurological diagnostic category			NNOS (median)
				Normal	Suspect	Abnormal	
SFD term							
Normal FHR	9	9	7.25	8	1	-	56
Decelerations	14	14	7.14	3	7	4	51.6
Total	23						
SFD preterm							
Normal FHR	12	-	7.18	7	5	-	53
Decelerative FHR	14	11	7.16	4	6	4	50.5
Terminal FHR	7	7	6.99	-	3	4	48.5
Total	33						

CS, cesarean section; NNOS, neonatal neurological optimality score

occurred antenatally and the remainder in early labor) and neonatal neurological morbidity. Neurologically "abnormal" infants were restricted to the group with decelerations, with the poorest outcome in the subgroup with a "terminal" fetal heart rate pattern antepartum. There was also a good correlation between the pH_{ua} and neurological morbidity. No relationship between pH and morbidity was, however, found within the term group with decelerations. This suggests the presence of two separate study populations, of which one had decelerations, a lower pH_{ua}, and more severe growth retardation (Dijxhoorn et al., in preparation), as opposed to a direct relationship between neurological morbidity and the pH at birth. All eight neonatal neurologically abnormal infants of the preterm group had an abnormal fetal heart rate pattern of which this was already present antepartum in seven of the cases. Four of these infants had a more or less normal pH_{ua} at birth (>7.15). These data indicate that the occurrence of antepartum decelerations is more important with respect to neurological outcome than the actual pH value at birth.

The strong relationship between antepartum late decelerations and neurological morbidity stresses the impact of prenatal hypoxemia on brain development. As hypoxemia in growth-retarded fetuses is probably associated with chronic hypoglycemia and deprivation of other nutritients, brain damage in the growth-retarded fetuses is more likely to be due to chronic malnutrition (including hypoxemia) rather than simply to hypoxemia.

Management with Respect to The Prevention of Nervous System Impairment

The data presented suggest that growth-retarded fetuses should be delivered before antepartum signs of hypoxemia occur. Fetuses at risk for the development of antepartum heart rate decelerations might be detected by studying velocity wave forms in the umbilical artery or fetal aorta, as there is increasing evidence that, in growth-retarded fetuses, changes in these usually precede the occurrence of decelerations (Hernandez et al. 1984; Trudinger et al. 1986). In eight of ten growth-retarded fetuses that we followed longitudinally, abnormal wave forms were present for more than 3 weeks before decelerations occurred (Visser et al. 1986a). However, to date there is inadequate knowledge concerning false-positive abnormal wave forms, whereas preterm delivery at an earlier age might increase other (neonatal) risks. At present, the best option to prevent neurological handicap is to prevent growth retardation. In pregnancy-induced hypertension, leading to intrauterine death or delivery before 34 weeks, the recurrence rate during a subsequent pregnancy is nearly 50% (Visser et al. 1986b). Antiplatelet therapy seems promising in preventing growth retardation in these cases (Beaufils et al. 1985; Wallenburg et al. 1986).

Conclusions

1. In growth-retarded fetuses, antepartum changes in heart rate and movement patterns are relatively late signs of impairment
2. Antepartum heart rate decelerations are usually the first abnormalities detected and are associated with fetal hypoxemia
3. In growth-retarded fetuses there is a close association between antepartum heart rate decelerations and neonatal neurological morbidity
4. Prolonged nutritional deprivation, especially if associated with early signs of hypoxemia, seems to be more important with respect to neonatal neurological outcome than indicators of "asphyxia" determined at birth

References

Beaufils M, Uzan S, Donsimoni R, Colau JC (1985) Prevention of pre-eclampsia by early antiplatelet therapy. Lancet 1: 840–842

Bekedam DJ, Visser GHA (1984) Heart rate variation and movement incidence in growth-retarded fetuses with decelerative heart rate patterns. Correlations with fetal acid-base status. Eur J Obstet Gynecol Reprod Biol 18: 236–237

Bekedam DJ, Visser GHA, de Vries JJ, Prechtl HFR (1985) Motor behaviour in the growth retarded fetus. Early Hum Dev 12: 155–165

Bekedam DJ, Visser GHA, Kamstra A, Mulder EJH (1986) Effects of maternal hypoxia on fetal breathing movements, body movements and heart rate variation; a study in growth retarded human fetuses (Abstr) 13th Conference of the Society for the Study of Fetal Physiology, Bauff, Canada

Bekedam DJ, Visser GHA, Mulder EJH, Poelmann-Weesjes G (1987) Heart rate variation and movement incidence in growth retarded fetuses. Am J Obstet Gynecol (in press)

Henson GL, Dawes GS, Redman CWG (1983) Antenatal fetal heart-rate variability in relation to fetal acid-base status at Caesarean section. Br J Obstet Gynaecol 90: 516–521

Hernandez CE, Cohen-Overbeek TE, Campbell S, Pearce JMF (1984) A comparison of fetal aorta flow velocity waveforms with cardiotocography and biophysical profiles in the antenatal assessment of fetal wellbeing (Abstr). 11th Annual Meeting of the Society for the Study of Fetal Physiology, Oxford

Huisjes HJ, Touwen BCL, Hoekstra J, van Woerden-Blanksma JT, Bierman-van Eendenburg MEC, Jurgens-van der Zee AD, Fidler V, Olinga AA (1980) Obstetrical-neonatal neurological relationships. A replication study. Eur J Obstet Gynecol Reprod Biol 10: 247-256

Jurgens-van der Zee AD, Bierman-van Eendenburg MEC, Fidler V, et al. (1979) Preterm birth, growth retardation and acidemia in relation to neurological abnormality of the newborn. Early Hum Dev 3: 141-154

Manning FA, Baskett TF, Morrison I, Lange I (1981) Fetal biophysical profile scoring: a prospective study in 1184 high-risk patients. Am J Obstet Gynecol 140: 289-294

Murata Y, Martin CB, Ikenone T, et al. (1982) Fetal heart rate accelerations and late decelerations during the course of intra-uterine death in chronically catheterized rhesus monkeys. Am J Obstet Gynecol 144: 218-223

Pearson JF, Weaver JB (1976) Fetal activity and fetal wellbeing: an evaluation. Br Med J 1: 1305

Prechtl HFR (1977) The neurological examination of the full term newborn infant. Clin Dev Med 63: 1-65

Robinson JS, Falconer J, Owens JA (1985) Influence of growth retardation on functional capacity of fetal organ systems. In: Beard RW, Sharp F (eds) Preterm labour and its consequences. The Royal College of Obstetricians and Gynaecologists, London, pp 39-52

Sadovsky E, Yaffe H, Polishuk WZ (1974) Fetal movement monitoring in normal and pathologic pregnancy. Int J Gynaecol Obstet 12: 75

Sadovsky E, Laufer N, Allen JW (1979) The incidence of different types of fetal movements during pregnancy. Br J Obstet Gynaecol 86: 10-14

Touwen BCL, Huisjes HJ, Jurgens-van der Zee AD, Bierman-van Eendenburg MEC, Smrkovsky M, Olinga AA (1980) Obstetrical condition and neonatal neurological condition. An analysis with the help of the optimality concept. Early Hum Dev 4 (3): 207-228

Trudinger BJ, Cook CM, Jones L, Giles WB (1986) A comparison of fetal heart rate monitoring and umbilical artery waveforms in the recognition of fetal compromise. Br J Obstet Gynaecol 93: 171-175

Van Vliet MAT, Martin CB, Nijhuis JG, Prechtl HFR (1985) Behavioural states in the growth retarded human fetus. Early Hum Dev 12: 183-198

Visser GHA (1984) Antenatal cardiotocography in the evaluation of fetal well-being. Aust NZ J Obstet Gynecol 24: 80-85

Visser GHA, Redman CWG, Huisjes HJ, Turnbull AC (1980) Nonstressed antepartum heart rate monitoring: implications of decelerations after spontaneous contractions. Am J Obstet Gynecol 138: 429-435

Visser GHA, Poelmann-Weesjes G, Bekedam DJ (1986a) Umbilical artery velocity wave forms in growth retarded fetuses; a comparison with heart rate and movement patterns (Abstr). 24th British Congress of Obstetrics and Gynaecology, Cardiff

Visser GHA, Huisman A, Saathof PWF, Sinnige HAM (1986b) Early fetal growth retardation: obstetric background and recurrence rate. Obstet Gynecol 42: 40-43

Wallenburg HCS, Dekker GA, Makowitz JW, Rotmans P (1986) Low-dose aspirin prevents pregnancy-induced hypertension in angiotensin-sensitive primigravidae. Lancet 1: 1-3

Intrapartum Asphyxia and Birth Trauma

Intrapartum Events and Cerebral Palsy

K. B. Nelson and J. H. Ellenberg

"Difficult birth in itself in certain cases is merely a symptom of deeper effects that influenced the development of the fetus." Sigmund Freud (1897)

The medical literature contains many studies of high-risk newborns, most of these concerning infants who were very low in birthweight or who were seriously asphyxiated as newborns. These studies have contributed greatly to continuing improvements in the care of a sector of the newborn population that is at high individual risk. The need for such studies is beyond any question.

It is also true that very low birthweight and seriously asphyxiated infants are quite uncommon among all births. It is possible that many of the children who are later recognized as neurologically disabled, even excluding those injured by infection or trauma after the newborn period, were not members of any high-risk group before or near the time of birth. In fact, Scott and Masi (1979) have reported that "the majority of children who suffer from handicaps experience no identified perinatal complications."

Studies that follow only high-risk children obviously do not include children who are later disabled but were not members of perinatal high-risk groups. Therefore such studies of high-risk populations cannot provide information on what proportion of neurologic disability arises among children who were not recognized in the perinatal period to be at special risk. For an estimate of the degree to which disability has its origin in perinatal complications, it is necessary to turn to studies that strive to identify children in a population who have, and those who do not have, the suspected risk factors, and compare the rate of later disability among those with and those without the complications. This strategy permits recognition in disability arising among children who were not members of high-risk groups, as well as among those who were.

It has been the experience in other situations that high-risk groups may not account for a large proportion of a specific form of morbidity. For example, it is well known that older mothers are at high risk for having an infant with Down's syndrome. Yet most children with Down's syndrome are not born to women of relatively advanced age, since such women make up only a small part of the childbearing population.

Cerebral palsy is the form of long-term neurologic morbidity that has been linked most confidently with perinatal events. Most population studies of cerebral palsy (CP) that have offered an estimate of the contribution of prenatal and perinatal factors to the outcome have had to make fairly arbitrary guesses in assigning cause. In one major study, any child with CP who had had a 1-min Apgar score below 7 had his/her disability attributed to intrapartum asphyxia. But 99% of children with 1-min Apgar scores in that range did *not* have CP (Nelson and Ellenberg 1981); this measure is not a good discriminator of risk.

To our knowledge, only one population study has gathered and analyzed the data in order to identify the leading empirically recognizable predictors of CP, and then applied that information to the question of the proportion of CP that has been contributed by those same predictive factors. That study was the Collaborative Perinatal Project of the National Institute of Neurological and Communicative Disorders and Stroke, the NCPP. Analyses of the results of that study, which involved about 54000 pregnancies between 1959 and 1966 at 12 American teaching hospitals, have now been completed and form the subject of this report.

We began involvement with this study with the assumption that the results would indicate just which birth events were the important determinants of CP and were major contributors to childhood seizure disorders. The results have been something of a surprise: factors of labor and delivery appear to play a relatively small role in the etiology of CP, and an even smaller role for childhood seizure disorders.

This presentation will focus on perinatal, and especially on intrapartum, asphyxia and its relationship to CP, with discussion of three points:

1. Mild or brief intrapartum asphyxia does not produce lasting brain damage. Only severe and prolonged intrapartum asphyxia is associated with a substantial risk of CP. Such a degree and duration of asphyxia is very uncommon, and when it occurs, the usual outcome is death or clinically normal development. Only a small percentage of survivors of this uncommon and severe degree of asphyxia manifest clinically evident long-term neurologic handicap.
2. Indicators of intrapartum asphyxia may be misleading if interpreted to establish causation of lately-identified neurologic abnormality.
3. Maldevelopment appears to be an important factor in CP, and important also in childhood seizure disorders. In the one population for which such data are available, events of labor and delivery appeared to contribute to a lesser degree.

In the analyses discussed here, children with major brain malformations and those with postnatally acquired CP have been excluded.

Asphyxia

We all know that a sufficient dose of asphyxia can cause severe damage in the brain of a newborn and produce CP. Both clinical and experimental studies establish this very clearly. What is less often realized is that the *severity* and *duration* of the asphyxia required to produce such damage is extreme, and in the circumstances in which infants in developed countries are born, is very uncommon.

The clinical indicator of asphyxia employed was the Apgar score. In the NCPP, Apgar scores were recorded at 1 and 5 min for approximately

50000 infants born between 1959 and 1966. A specially trained independent observer, not responsible for patient care, performed the Apgar rating. Apgar scoring was continued at 10, 15, and 20 min for babies who did not achieve a score of 8 or higher at 5 min. During this period, resuscitative measures were undertaken as considered clinically appropriate.

Babies with very low Apgar scores, 0-3, were at increased risk of death. The longer the scores remained very low, the greater was the risk of death. Babies of low birthweight were more likely to die than babies of similar Apgar score who weighed more than 2500 g. In infants who survived, the risk of CP was related to the Apgar score, and especially to very low, very late low Apgar scores.

CP was observed in only 0.4% of children with Apgar scores of 4-6 at 1 min. Scores in that range are fairly common at 1 min. The risk of CP rose to 5% among infants whose 5-min Apgar score was 0-3. Fewer than 1% of surviving infants had 5-min scores that low, but of those who did, one on 20 later had handicapping CP. Continuing very low Apgar scores were even more uncommon and were associated with risks of CP that reached 162 times the risk of children whose scores were 7-10 at 5 min. Counting each very low-scoring child only once, at the latest time his/her Apgar score was 0-3, the risk of CP in term weight children jumped sharply in those infants whose very low Apgar scores persisted past 15 min. In infants over 2500 g with a 5-min Apgar score of 0-3, the observed rate of CP did not exceed 1% in those whose scores improved to 4 or better by 10 min. It required severe and prolonged asphyxia, 15 min or more postpartum, to produce a substantial risk of CP.

So children who developed CP after perinatal asphyxia were mostly term babies who had had lengthy asphyxia. The form of CP later seen in those babies was usually spastic quadriparesis, often with athetosis. These children were usually severely mentally retarded and half had seizure disorders.

Most low birthweight children with very low late scores died. Surviving infants who weighed more than 2500 g and whose Apgar scores were 3 or less at 20 min had a CP rate of 57%. The very low late Apgar score in the term infant is an extremely powerful predictor of CP.

Although at very high risk, these babies with very low Apgar scores at 20 min were in a rare and extreme situation; they constituted only a small fraction of 1% of surviving infants.

Perinatal asphyxia as measured by Apgar scores, then, if severe and prolonged, is a powerful risk factor for CP. But it accounted for little of the CP in the one population for which information is available. Almost three-quarters of children with CP in the NCPP had scores of 7-10 at 5-min.

What were children like who experienced this severe a degree of perinatal asphyxia, but survived without CP? Of 390 infants with Apgar scores of 0-3 at 10 min or later, 270 died before the first birthday. Of the 99 survivors, 12% had CP and, as noted, most of those 12% had multiple neurologic handicaps as well as the motor disability. In the severely asphyxiated group 87 children survived without CP. Of these, none was epileptic, none was blind, none was severely mentally retarded. The rate of mild retardation did not exceed the rate in the general population of the NCPP. Hyperactivity was not increased in frequency in this group. Three of these children were deaf and had defective speech, and three others had abnormal speech articulation without deafness. It warrants mention that some of the children who were normal by school age were neurologically symptomatic as newborns and in their early months of life. Some of these children may have sustained brain lesions that could have been revealed by currently available imaging techniques, but all were functioning as normal young citizens according to a variety of clinical measures. In all, 80% of survivors of Apgar scores of 0–3 at 10 min or later were neurologically normal at 7 years of age.

What emerges, then, is a surprising discontinuity: a degree of asphyxia sufficient to kill more than half the babies who experienced it, left three-quarters of survivors apparently neurologically healthy by early school age. There was very little middle ground. The NCPP was the largest study to document this phenomenon, but far from the only one.

Perinatal asphyxia, if severe and prolonged, is a powerful risk factor for CP. Such an extreme condition is rare, and only studies with large sample size are likely to contain more than a few such infants. Mild and brief asphyxia is not associated with heightened risk of long-term neurologic deficit. Most children who survived even extreme asphyxia were later apparently intact on clinical evaluation, and most children with CP probably did not reach that outcome via the route of perinatal asphyxia.

High Risk, Low Prevalence

CP is a relatively infrequent condition. There is a relationship between the power of a factor as a predictor of CP and the prevalence of the risk factor. On the y-axis of Fig. 1 are some of the factors with highest risk of CP. At the top, over the 50% mark, is an Apgar score of 3 or below at 20 min in a baby over 2500 g in birthweight. Another strong predictor is birthweight below 1500 g in a white infant. That birthweight level in a black infant is also associated with considerable risk of CP, although with a risk well below that for a white infant; the same very low birthweight level may be less extreme for a black than for a white baby.

So comparing the factors ranging up the y-axis gives a view of the magnitude of the risk of CP associated with some of the strongest predictors. Near the lower end of the y-axis, indicating low absolute risk of CP, are two clinical markers of intrapartum asphyxia: fetal heart rate of 60 beats per minute or less, as recorded by auscultation, and first cry delayed to 5 min or more. Less extreme degrees of bradycardia and delay in initial cry were not associated with significant increase in risk. So these markers had to be fairly extreme to be indicators of any increase in risk, and in absolute terms even fairly extreme abnormality was not associated with a level of risk that was high in absolute terms.

The other point Fig. 1 is intended to illustrate relates to the emptiness of the middle of the graph. The x-axis represents the percentage of the population that had the strongest risk factors for CP. All the powerful risk factors are huddled at the left extreme of the figure or near the baseline, indicating that all the predictors associated with relatively high levels of risk were rare factors. No risk factors were

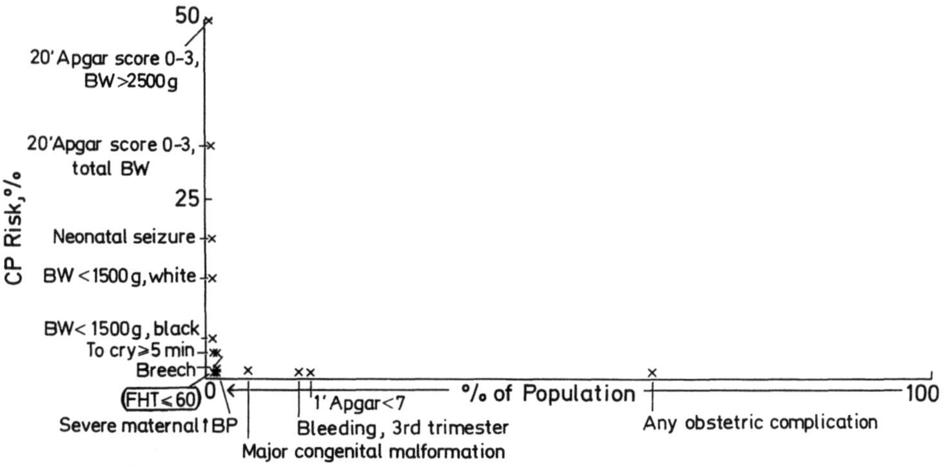

Fig. 1. The *y-axis* represents risk of CP, and the *x-axis* indicates the percentage of the population possessing certain risk factors. All the characteristics associated with considerable risk of CP were rare characteristics. *BW*, birthweight

both common and powerful. This is reasonable, since if there were predictors that were both powerful and common, CP would have to be much more frequent than it is.

What are the implications of this statement for other predictors? It is a real possibility that what holds true for the predictors examined here may apply also to other risk factors. For example, Sykes et al. (1982) criticized the Apgar score because it did not correlate well with pH measurements. But most of the Apgar scores, and most of the pH values under scrutiny, were in the range of common and mild depressions, which definitely for Apgar scores and probably for pH values do not predict outcome. The sample being relatively small, it did not include many severe and extreme depressions. In the range in which they (Apgar scores and pH values) do not matter for outcome, it would not seem to be of enormous importance if they are not closely correlated with one another. At the most extreme values examined by Sykes et al. (1982) agreement was better between Apgar scores and pH; and as indicated, it is only with respect to extreme values that Apgar scores have implications for outcome.

We would predict that for pH, for ominous fetal heart rate patterns, and for other potential predictors, only extreme and uncommon degrees of abnormality will be important predictors of outcome. The sample size required to test the relationships of these predictors with long-term status will therefore be large and research design difficult. However, short-term outcomes will be of uncertain value as measures of outcome, since none that has yet been widely tested is a strong predictor of long-term neurologic status.

Birth Complications and CP

We examined 14 late pregnancy birth conditions, selected because they might be associated with perinatal asphyxia, for their association with CP. Late pregnancy and birth complications were common: one or more of the 14 complications studied was present in 62% of 51 285 singleton pregnancies.

Among infants below 2500 g born by breech delivery, the CP rate was almost one in 20; this was the only complication for which the risk of CP was statistically significantly higher than among uncomplicated births. For babies over 2500 g, the CP rate did not exceed 2% for any of the complications and for many of the conditions was not higher than for uncomplicated births.

When complications were examined in babies over 2500 g in the light of the infants' condition in the first minutes of life, as evaluated by 5-min Apgar score, it was observed that the Apgar score could discriminate those infants at special risk: the CP rate was highest among a small subgroup of infants who, following a birth complication, had a 5-min Apgar score of 3 or less. Most babies over 2500 g born following each complication achieved 5-min scores of 7 or higher, and for them the risk of CP was not significantly greater than for babies born of uncomplicated deliveries.

Infants with very low 5-min Apgar scores who had not had birth complications were not at much increase in risk of CP. Presumably the mothers of many of this group had received larger than optimal doses of analgesic medication, or the infants had secretions in the upper airway, so in both situations there was probably a fairly prompt response to resuscitation.

So it required *both* a complication *and* evidence in the early moments of life of neurologic symptomatology (that symptomatology, in this instance, on the first measure of neonatal neurologic status, the Apgar score) to mark an infant at significantly heightened risk of CP. And most cases of CP came from the large group not at increased risk by virtue of obstetric or immediate neonatal condition.

It is know that brain-injuring events, related to severe drops in maternal blood pressure, for example, can occur long enough before delivery to allow the infant to "pink up" and be asymptomatic in the early minutes of his/her life. There is no known way, at present, to estimate the frequency of such events, nor the proportion of later neurologic morbidity they might contribute.

Seizure disorders in children who did not also have CP were not significantly associated either with birth complications evaluated, or with Apgar scores. Broman (1979) reported that low Apgar scores and other measures of birth asphyxia were not important antecedents of mental retardation in children without other neurologic abnormality, and we have observed that children who survived very low Apgar scores without developing CP did not demonstrate an excess of mental retardation (Nelson and Ellenberg 1981). Unless they occur in the same individual, childhood seizure disorders and mental retardation cannot be assumed to have the same antecedents as CP.

Prelabor Versus Labor/Delivery Factors as Contributors to CP

The NCPP contained more than 400 variables describing the family, the mother, the pregnancy, labor and delivery, and newborn period. We examined these characteristics through a number of stages, including univariate correlations and multivariate regression procedures, to select major predictors and reduce these to a number feasible for entry into multiple logistic regression analyses.

In the analyses of factors one at a time, it was observed that a number of factors often assumed to be important risk factors for CP could not be demonstrated to have a significant association with CP. For example, among factors ascertainable by the time of a first prenatal visit, maternal diabetes, extremes of maternal age, parity, smoking history, and socioeconomic status, were not significantly related to risk of CP. The leading prepregnancy factors among those examined were maternal mental retardation as clinically recognized, hyperthyroidism, or seizure disorders before pregnancy, and fetal loss in two or more prior pregnancies.

Among labor and delivery factors that were *not* significantly related with CP, when examined one factor at a time, were oxytocin administered either for induction or for augmentation of labor, nuchal cord, midforceps, or duration of labor. For some of these factors, the small subgroup of children whose births were complicated by these conditions and whose 5-min Apgar scores were very low were at heightened risk. By themselves, however, these conditions were not sufficiently strongly related to CP to demonstrate a significant relationship. We were startled by the observation that duration of labor was not in itself a significant risk factor; not first stage of labor and not second, not precipitate labor, nor prolonged labor. Dale and Stanley (1980) also did not observe a significant association between duration of labor and CP in a case-control study.

Factors that *were* major predictors ascertained during the labor and delivery period were gestational age below 32 weeks, lowest fetal heart rate 60 beats per minute or less, breech presentation, chorionitis, placental weight below 325 g, and placental complications (previa, abruption, or marginal sinus rupture). Of these, only breech presentation was a significant predictor among infants weighing over 2500 g. Breech presentation was the significant predictor, breech delivery was not.

On the final multivariate analysis, ten characteristics from before the onset of labor were the most important of the prelabor predictors of CP. (There were ten, not by arbitrary selection, but because the 11th strongest did not add additional predictive power to these ten.) The most powerful of these predictors present or absent by the moment before labor began were:

- Birthweight below 2001 g
- Major congenital malformations, noncerebral
- Maternal mental retardation
- Breech presentation

Breech *delivery* was not a major predictor. Congenital malformations were, next to low birthweight, the most powerful of predictors of CP. There were interactions between birthweight, congenital malformations, and breech presentations. The rate of major noncerebral congenital malformation in the NCPP was 6% among infants born weighing more than 2500 g, 11% in those 1500–2500 g, and 19% – three times the rate of normal-weight infants – in babies born weighing less than 1500 g.

Among infants with CP, 22% had at least one major congenital anomaly outside the central nervous system. Among infants with CP who were born weighing less than 2001 g, the malformation rate was 29%; among infants with CP who had had neonatal seizures, it was 30%; among infants with CP who had been breech presentation it was 33%; and among infants who had either a lowest fetal heart rate below 60 beats per minute or a 5-min Apgar score of 3 or less, or who required 5 min or more to cry, 35% had a major congenital malformation. To reiterate, of children with CP who had one or more clinical markers suggestive of intrapartum asphyxia, 35% had a major congenital malformation.

Of children with CP who had one or more markers of asphyxia, more than half had a birthweight below 2001 g, or microcephaly at birth, or major congenital malformation, or an alternate explanation for their CP, such as rubella syndrome.

Markers of asphyxia must be severe to be associated with substantially heightened risk of CP. And such markers may be misleading if used to imply causality, for it is not obvious that preventing asphyxia in these children would have prevented unfavorable neurologic outcome. The same is true for others of the major risk factors. For example, Braun et al. (1975) state that 50% of infants with the Prader-Willi syndrome and 40% of those with fetal alcohol syndrome present in the breech. Delivery by well-timed cesarean section of these infants would have produced, just as would vaginal delivery, a child with Prader-Willi syndrome or with fetal alcohol syndrome. While we cannot state what proportion of all infants presenting in the breech have such intrinsic defects, we can report that a third of children with CP who were breech presentations had major congenital malformations. To jump to the conclusion, with respect to a neurologically abnormal child who was a breech delivery, that abdominal delivery would have prevented the outcome, may not always be warranted.

Prediction of CP

The best test of whether we understand the causation of an outcome is whether or not we can predict the occurrence of that outcome. To consider the predictability of CP, we were fortunate to be able to use a program used in the National Heart, Lung, and Blood Institute to examine the predictability of heart attacks. Heart attacks are the number one cause of death in the United States, and a great deal of effort has gone into identifying the risk factors for, and judging the contribution of those risk factors to, the occurrence of heart attacks.

Considering the top ten predictors of CP that were present or absent by the moment before labor began, we found that 5% of the NCPP population at highest predicted risk contributed 34% of the CP. Clearly this *was* a high-risk sector of the population, since it contained almost a seven-fold excess of CP cases. However, two-thirds of the CP in this population did not come from this high-risk sector.

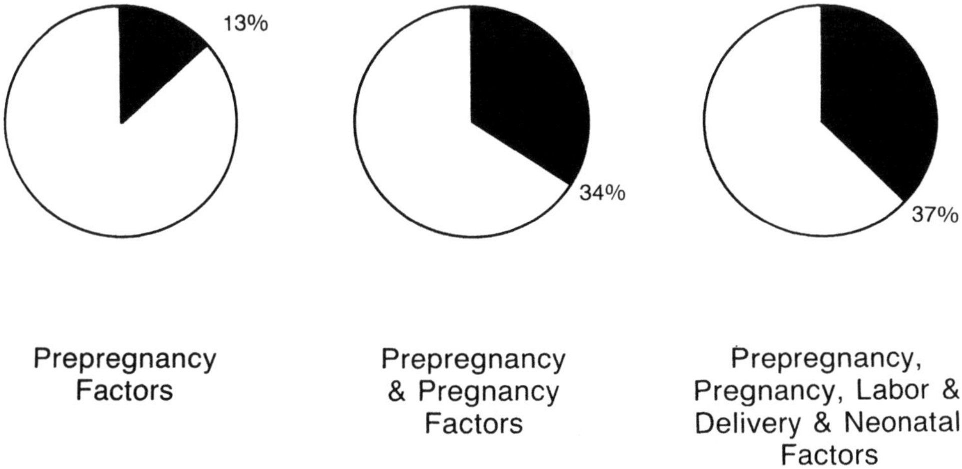

Fig. 2. Considering the 5% of the population at highest predicted risk, factors from before pregnancy contributed 13% of the CP. Counting congenital malformations, gestational age and birthweight, and breech presentation among characteristics determined by the moment before labor began, prepregnancy and pregnancy stage factors contributed 34% of the CP. The addition of information from labor, delivery, and the neonatal period led to a negligible increase in predictive ability

And worse, this level of prediction included a very high false-positive rate: more than 97% of children identified as within the high-risk group did not turn out to have CP. Our ability to predict CP based upon prelabor characteristics was not very good.

When the chief predictors of CP from labor, delivery, and the nursery period were added to the prelabor factors, the top 5% of the population by risk contributed 37% of the CP (Fig. 2). So with addition of data on birth and the newborn period, there was a negligible increase in the power to predict CP.

We conclude, then, that much less is known about the etiology of CP than has been supposed. And these data seem to indicate that of processes identified that might be causal of CP, maldevelopment seems to be more prominent than events of labor and delivery.

It will be obvious that the data described here, concerning births between 1959 and 1966 in North American university hospitals, cannot be assumed to apply to births in other circumstances or at other times, before or since. It should also be obvious that the relatively small contribution of factors of labor and delivery to long-term neurologic disability observed in this study does not make that contribution unimportant; some of that component may be further reducible. It is likely that the achievement of this level of noncontribution to long-term neurologic morbidity represents the success of almost-modern obstetric care, and it is possible that further advances have been made since the time of births into the NCPP.

The contribution of modern obstetrics and modern neonatal care should probably not be judged by their relationship to the rate of CP in the population, but rather by the rate of maternal and birthweight-specific infant mortality, and the rates of certain forms of neonatal morbidity; the likelihood is great that long-term neurologic outcome is, in developed countries, chiefly related to other factors, many of them still unknown. Assuring that obstetric and neonatal care are not limiting factors in healthy survival should be a goal sought with great urgency for developing nations as well.

References

Braun FHT, Jones KL, Smith DW (1975) Breech presentation as an indicator of fetal abnormality. J Pediatr 86: 419-421

Broman SH (1979) Perinatal anoxia and cognitive development in early childhood. In: Field TF (ed) Infants born at risk. SP Medical and Scientific Books, New York, pp 29-52

Dale A, Stanley FJ (1980) An epidemiological study of cerebral plasy in Western Australia, 1956-1975. II. Spastic cerebral palsy and perinatal factors. Dev Med Child Neurol 22: 13-25

Freud S (1897) Die Infantile Cerebrallähmung. In: Nothnagel H (ed) Specielle Pathologie und Therapie. Holder, Vienna, pp 1-327

Nelson KB, Ellenberg JH (1981) Apgar scores as predictors of chronic neurologic disability. Pediatrics 68: 34-44

Nelson KB, Ellenberg JH (1984) Obstetric complications as risk factors for cerebral palsy or seizure disorder. JAMA 251: 1843-1848

Nelson KB, Ellenberg JH (1986) Antecedents of cerebral palsy, multivariate analysis of risk. N Engl J Med, 315: 81-86

Scott KG, Masi W (1979) The outcome from and utility of registers of risk. In: Field TI (ed) Infants born at risk. SP Medical and Scientific Books. New York, pp 485-496

Sykes GS, Molloy PM, Johnson P, Gu W, Ashworth F, Stirratt GM, Turnbull AC (1982) Do Apgar scores indicate asphyxia? Lancet 1: 494-496

The Relationship Between Obstetrically Preventable Intrapartum Asphyxia, Abnormal Neonatal Neurological Signs and Subsequent Motor Impairment in Babies Born at or after Term

A. GRANT

Introduction

In the comprehensive review *Prenatal and Perinatal Factors Associated with Brain Disorders* recently published by the National Institutes of Health, the editor, Freeman (1985), commented that "many of our assumptions about factors associated with brain disorders, such as cerebral palsy, mental retardation and epilepsy, remain rooted in outdated 'knowledge'". Yet, as Freeman implies, these assumptions still dominate public and professional beliefs about physical and mental handicap. Hey (1985), a British paediatrician, has described the situation in the United Kingdom: the House of Commons' Social Services Committee's "bold statement (1980) that at least 5000 children in England and Wales are surviving each year with handicap that could have been prevented by better obstetric care neatly encapsulates the current climate of expectation – a climate fostered by expert (medical) witnesses to that Committee and further enhanced by those of our (medical) colleagues who tell mothers, 'If you don't do as I say you may damage your baby'". He later continues "the profession's ideas about the obstetric antecedents of cerebral palsy are, at present, dangerously simplistic; those of the general public are even more so".

The aim of this paper is to explore the relationship between obstetrically – preventable intrapartum asphyxia and long-term motor impairment. Motor impairment has been singled out because it is this form of cerebral handicap which is most plausibly related to intrapartum events. As is reviewed elsewhere in this volume, there is little evidence that isolated mental retardation has any link with birth and the minority of cases of severe mental retardation attributed to perinatal events almost always have physical disabilities, particularly cerebral palsy (CP). Furthermore, the epidemiology of mental retardation associated with CP seems to be similar to that of the CP, and mental retardation in this context appears to be a concomitant of the neurological impairment of CP (Susser et al. 1985). Other forms of neurodevelopmental disability such as "global delay", motor delay, speech delay and behaviour disorder also appear to be unrelated to events during labour and delivery (Taylor et al. 1985). Nevertheless, it should be recognised that uncertainty still remains about the relationship between intrapartum asphyxia and these and other forms of neurodevelopmental dysfunction in childhood such as perceptual problems and learning difficulties (Dennis 1985).

Long-term Motor Impairment and Intrapartum Asphyxia

Although the majority of cases of cerebral palsy appear to be unrelated to labour and delivery there is an association between "poor condition at birth" and subsequent CP. The association is not strong and most babies in poor condition at birth (variously defined) either survive apparently intact or die. The striking feature of all such follow-up studies is that in the minority who survive with sequelae, the "handicap is usually severe and almost always involves the motor system" (Paneth and Stark 1983). Quadriplegia in conjunction with severe mental retardation has been singled out in this context (Susser et al. 1985). The challenge is to gauge the extent to which these latter cases reflect "intrapartum asphyxia" rather than problems which existed prior to the onset of labour, or the consequences of neonatal events or paediatric management.

The last 20 years have been marked by the introduction of increasingly intensive intrapartum surveillance aimed at reducing the effects of intrapartum asphyxia. One justification for the widespread introduction of continuous fetal heart rate monitoring during labour was the claim that more intensive monitoring could reduce perinatal morbidity by 50% (Quilligan and Paul 1975). Yet geographically based surveys of long-term impairment in children born during this time period provide little evidence of a similar trend to support this contention. Indeed, the most recently reported data suggest that, if anything, there may have been an increase in the prevalence of CP in normal birthweight babies during the years when continuous electronic fetal heart rate monitoring was being rapidly introduced into routine clinical practice (Jarvis et al. 1985; Hagberg et al. 1984).

Only one study has systematically examined the relationship between the quality of intrapartum care and perinatal outcome (Niswander et al. 1984). This study is currently being replicated in the northern region of England. Niswander et al. (1984) found no evidence of an association between suboptimal care during labour and CP. Failure to respond appropriately to an abnormal fetal heart rate trace may plausibly be considered as a surrogate measure of obstetrically preventable intrapartum asphyxia. Yet, in none of the 34 cases of CP reviewed in this study was it judged that such a failure had occurred.

What Constitutes Intrapartum Asphyxia?

Clearly, even for CP the relationship with intrapartum asphyxia is far from straightforward. The situation is further confused, however, by the vagueness of the term "asphyxia". It is rarely defined. When it is defined, it has attracted a wide variety of meanings. Obstetrical accidents such as cord prolapse or abruptio placentae have been judged by some to signify severe asphyxia. (In the context of this discussion it is questionable whether such "asphyxia" is, anyway, obstetrically preventable, or indeed whether asphyxia is the fundamental problem in these cases). Asphyxia has also been inferred on the basis of intrapartum observations such as fetal heart rate abnormalities, low fetal scalp blood pH and meconium staining of the liquor amnii. None of these is strongly predictive of the clinical status of the baby at birth and their relationships to long-term status are unknown. "Asphyxia" is most commonly defined on the basis of poor condition at birth. The common practice of basing the diagnosis on clinical indices such as the Apgar score, the time to spontaneous respiration or the need for resuscitation has been criticised because these may all reflect factors other than intrapartum asphyxia. The attraction of the Apgar score is that its (albeit weak) relationship with long-term disability has been well described (Nelson and Ellenberg 1981). The same does not, at the moment, apply to the measurement of acid base status at birth (which is poorly correlated with the Apgar score, Lumley and Wood 1969; Sykes et al. 1982). A variety of cord blood parameters is now in clinical use, the strictest definitions of "asphyxia" requiring a combination of hypoxia, hypercarbia and acidosis (Steer 1985). Neonatal seizures have also been suggested as indicators of intrapartum asphyxia and are known to be potent predictors of long-term neurological status (Brann 1985). Less severely abnormal neonatal neurological signs have also been attributed to preventable events during labour (Amiel-Tison 1985).

Experimental Evidence that Neonatal Seizures Are a Valid Epidemiological Indicator of Obstetrically Preventable Intrapartum Asphyxia

Until recently the validity of these various putative indicators of birth asphyxia had not been assessed using a controlled experiment involving human fetuses and neonates. The Dublin randomised controlled trial of intrapartum fetal heart rate monitoring (MacDonald et al. 1985) provided an opportunity to do this (Table 1). Strong support was given to the hypothesis that neonatal seizures reflect intrapartum asphyxia: a statistically significant halving of the risk of neonatal seizures occurred in the more intensively monitored group. In contrast, the experiment yielded no good evidence to support claims that the other variables mentioned above are valid indicators of intrapartum asphyxia: there were no substantial differences between the two experimental groups in respect of other abnormal neonatal neurological signs, depressed Apgar score, low umbilical cord venous pH, apnoea at birth or endotracheal intubation. This experimentally derived evidence is consistent with that contributed by earlier smaller trials (Chalmers 1979). The summary odds ratio (Yusuf et al. 1985) for neonatal seizures among infants born following the more intensive methods of intrapartum fetal monitoring studied in the relevant trials (Renou et al. 1976; Haverkamp et al. 1979; MacDonald et al. 1985) is 0.4 with 95% confidence intervals of 0.2 to 0.7.

This contrasting experience of the trials' two experimental groups may reflect differences in fetal trauma, or in fetal asphyxia, or both; but of these two possible aetiological factors, asphyxia seems likely to have been dominant. In the largest trial (MacDonald et al. 1985) trauma of various kinds was documented somewhat *more* frequently in the group which had received more intensive intrapartum fetal

Table 1. Frequency of putative indices of birth asphyxia in two groups of babies, one randomly allocated to a policy of continuous electronic fetal heart rate monitoring (EFM), the other randomly allocated to a policy of intermittent auscultation of the fetal heart rate (IA) (MacDonald et al. 1985)

	EFM		IA		
	(n)	(%)	*(n)*	(%)	
Neonatal seizures	12/6530	1.8	27/6554	4.1	$p<0.025$
Other abnormal neonatal neurological signs	67/5035	13.3	67/5058	13.2	
Apgar score <3					
-At 1 min	57/6530	8.7	62/6554	9.5	
-At 5 min	10/6530	1.5	5/6554	0.8	
Umbilical venous pH					
<7.05	2/540	3.7	2/535	3.7	
7.05-7.10	3/540	5.5	6/535	11.2	
7.10-7.20	41/540	75.9	40/535	74.8	

monitoring and which experienced the lower incidence of seizures. Nevertheless, it is important to acknowledge that neonatal seizures may result from several causes besides birth asphyxia (Brann 1985), some of which will not declare themselves until long after the perinatal period (Dennis 1978). Although the situation is changing with the advent of modern imaging techniques (Levene and Trounce 1986), it has usually been difficult and is still often impossible to make specific aetiological diagnoses in individual cases of neonatal seizures.

Are Subcategories of Neonatal Seizures a Better Index of Obstetrically Preventable Intrapartum Asphyxia?

As noted by Brann (1985), several investigations have suggested that the day on which seizures begin may be a clue to aetiology. Dennis (1978), for example, noted that those cases of neonatal seizures which (after prolonged follow up) she ultimately assigned to a "perinatal" aetiology had almost all experienced their first seizure within 48 h of birth and that over three-quarters of those babies who experienced seizures within 48 h and who were born at term were ultimately assigned to a "perinatal cause" category. It was against this background that Dennis and Chalmers (1982) hypothesised that seizures occurring within 48 h of birth in babies born at term were more likely to reflect intrapartum asphyxia than other categories of seizures. This hypothesis was supported by the results of the Dublin intrapartum monitoring trial in that the relative risk (RR) between the two trial groups for this subcategory of seizures was more extreme (0.35; 95% confidence

Table 2. Frequency of three putative indices of birth asphyxia based on neonatal seizures in two groups of babies, one randomly allocated to a policy of continuous electronic fetal heart rate monitoring (EFM), the other randomly allocated to a policy of intermittent auscultation of the fetal heart rate (IA)

	EFM $n=6530$	IA $n=6554$	RP (95% CI)
All neonatal seizure cases	12	27	0.45 (0.23-0.86)
Very early onset neonatal seizures in infants at or after term	7	20	0.35 (0.15-0.80)
Neonatal seizures within one week of birth + Apgar score <5 at 1 or 5 min *or* apnoea at birth *or* endotracheal intubation[a]	6	12	0.50 (0.19-1.31)

[a] Adapted from Finer et al. (1981, 1983)

interval 0.15-0.80) than that for neonatal seizures overall (RR 0.45; 95% confidence interval 0.23-0.86) (Table 2).

Case control studies (Niswander et al. 1984; Derham et al. 1985) have provided further support for the claim that very early neonatal seizures in babies born at or after term reflect intrapartum asphyxia. Niswander et al. (1984) for example, reported an RR for very early neonatal seizures of 6.6 associated with suboptional reaction to fetal distress. Even within this group of babies, however, it is clear that not all are suffering from intrapartum asphyxia. Other aetiological factors are known to manifest themselves in this way (Dennis 1978; Ohtahara 1978, 1984; Dennis and Chalmers 1982; Clarke et al. 1987), and it will often be impossible to implicate asphyxia or other specific perinatal factors in individual cases. Clearly it is desirable that indicators of "birth asphyxia" based on neurologically abnormal neonates should be refined further so that aetiologically more specific syndromes can be identified. Finer et al. (1981, 1983; Robertson and Finer 1985) have proposed that birth asphyxia (hypoxic-ischaemic encephalopathy) should only be diagnosed if abnormal neurological signs evident within 1 week of birth have been associated with either an abnormal fetal heart rate, or a 1- or 5-min Apgar score of less than 5, or the need for immediate resuscitation or intubation. Abnormal fetal heart rate could not be used as a refining criterion for the Dublin monitoring trial data because the basis of the trial was that these abnormalities would be recognised more often in the intensively monitored group. Applying Finer's other criteria to the seizures cases in the Dublin trial, however, did not increase the contrast in seizure rates in the two experimental groups (RR 0.50; 95% confidence interval 0.19-1.31) (Table 2).

The results of the randomised controlled trials, taken together with other evidence, lead one to conclude that when the incidence of early onset seizures in babies born at or after term is relatively high (over three per 1000 live births) a relatively large proportion of cases is likely to be a manifestation of obstetrically preventable intrapartum asphyxia. Seizures in some other cases may reflect trauma.

The remaining cases seem likely to reflect causes which are less amendable to prevention by clinical action. These include asphyxia due to unpredicted catastrophes like sudden, massive intrapartum placental abruption and pre-existing fundamental abnormalities whose aetiology may be obscure. These latter, less preventable causes of early-onset seizures are likely to predominate when the overall incidence of this class of neonatal seizures is relatively low (less than one case per 1000 live births).

Other Abnormal Neurological Signs in the Neonatal Period

It is possible that more minor degrees of abnormal neurological behaviour in the neonatal period may signal less profound degrees of intrapartum asphyxia. Sheridan-Pereira, the paediatric neurologist in the Dublin intrapartum monitoring trial, identified a syndrome seen within 48 h of birth of distal hypertonia, abnormal movements and altered neurobehaviour, signs which are qualitatively similar to the premonitory signs of very early neonatal seizures. Babies with these signs, in contrast to babies with isolated hypotonia alone, tended to have relatively low cord venous pH values at delivery; in a series of 18 such babies the venous pH was always below the population mean. Furthermore, these cases also had epidemiological characteristics such as associations with primiparity, prolonged labour, oxytocin use in labour and instrumental delivery which have been described for cases of very early neonatal seizures (MacDonald et al. 1985; Minchom et al. 1987). However, applying Sheridan-Pereira's criteria to babies with abnormal neurological signs other than seizures in the Dublin trial of intrapartum fetal heart rate monitoring failed to show any clear difference in frequency between the two trial groups (Grant 1986).

In summary, the results of recent research suggest first, that the incidence of early onset seizures in term babies does indeed reflect the quality of perinatal, particularly intrapartum, care (as proposed by Dennis and Chalmers 1982); and second, that this subgroup of seizure cases is currently the most rigorously validated of all putative neonatal indicators of intrapartum asphyxia.

The Relationship Between Early-Onset Seizures and Long-term Motor Impairment

Other recently published evidence (Finer et al. 1981; Derham et al. 1985) has also confirmed earlier research (Harris and Tizard 1966; Brown et al. 1972; Combes et al. 1975; Dennis 1978) demonstrating that early-onset seizures, like neonatal seizures in general (Brann 1985), are strongly predictive of later death and disability. So it is easy to understand why the National Institutes of Health report (Freeman 1985) concluded that "neonatal seizures appear to be the best evidence of

Table 3. Outcome at 1 year of age of infants who experienced neonatal seizures in the Dublin randomised controlled trial of intrapartum fetal heart rate monitoring. (From MacDonald et al. 1985)

	EFM $n=6530$	IA $n=6554$
All cases of neonatal seizures	12	27
Survival following neonatal seizures	9	21
Severe disability at 1 year of age	3	3

asphyxia and the best predictor of later damage". Although both elements of this statement are true, however, it encourages an assumption that those babies who experience seizures attributable to perinatal asphyxia are the same babies who go on to manifest "later damage". Even in the class of neonatal seizures which seems most likely to reflect perinatal asphyxia - those of early onset in babies born at or after term - however, the neurological dysfunction of some of the infants, as discussed above, is certainly a reflection of other, less tractable aetiological factors (Dennis and Chalmers 1982). This is particularly important because cases of early-onset seizures in which the aetiology was almost certainly not asphyxia appear to be far more likely to manifest some serious disability in later childhood (Dennis 1978; Ohtahara 1978; Clarke et al. 1987). What remains unclear, therefore, is the extent to which the two epidemiological characteristics of neonatal seizures noted in the National Institutes of Health report are mediated by the same individual babies. In other words, to what extent do cases of disability among survivors of neonatal seizures reflect not preventable perinatal asphyxia, but other aetiological factors?

Two recently published analyses have brought this question into sharp focus. The first is the large randomised trial referred to above (MacDonald et al. 1985). Although babies born following random allocation to the more intensive method of intrapartum fetal monitoring experienced less than half the rate of early-onset neonatal seizures than that experienced by babies born following the less intensive method, follow up of these two cohorts of seizure cases at 1 year of age revealed equal numbers (three) of CP in each group (MacDonald et al. 1985; Table 3). Clearly this picture may change if additional, less severe cases of CP are diagnosed as the survivors of neonatal seizures grow older - a review at 4 years of age is currently underway. But the case-control study conducted by Niswander et al. (1984) has raised similar questions. As mentioned earlier, suboptimal care was found to be associated with an increased risk of early onset seizures in babies born at or after term, but not with an increased risk of CP.

The majority of babies who experience very early neonatal seizures either die or survive apparently intact. In the minority who survive with impairment the disability is usually severe and includes CP. Does this latter group reflect an intermediate degree of intrapartum asphyxia (a balance which has proved very hard to accomplish in animal studies) or do they in fact have a distinct aetiology, as suggested by the two human studies mentioned above?

Are Babies Whose Seizures Are Followed by Disability in Childhood Less Likely to Have Experienced Perinatal Asphyxia than Those Who Die or Develop Normally?

To explore the possibility that babies whose seizures are followed by disability in childhood are less likely to have experienced perinatal asphyxia than those who died or developed normally, two case series of babies born at or after term who experienced very early onset seizures - one from Dublin and one from Cardiff - have been studied. The smaller series from Dublin comprises the babies in the Dublin intrapartum monitoring trial. The larger Cardiff series was identified from the Cardiff Births Survey, a geographical population-based survey (Andrews et al. 1986). The derivation of this study group and a description of the antecedents of early neonatal seizures in this population have been described in detail elsewhere (Minchom et al. 1987). For both case series the frequencies of "adverse" perinatal

Table 4. Comparison of perinatal factors for two cohorts of infants born at or after term who experienced early-onset seizures and who either died within 28 days of birth, or had a handicap diagnosed or who were apparently well at follow up (3 years in Cardiff; 1 year in Dublin)

	Seizures cases, by outcome											
	Neonatal death				Disability diagnosed				No disability diagnosed			
	Cardiff ($n=5$)		Dublin ($n=4$)		Cardiff ($n=11$)		Dublin ($n=4$)		Cardiff (n=38)		Dublin (n=19)	
	(n)	(%)	*(n)*	(%)	*(n)*	(%)	*(n)*	(%)	*(n)*	(%)	*(n)*	(%)
Gestation 41 weeks+	2	40.0	1	25.0	3	27.3	0	0.0	21	55.3	8	42.1
Mother primiparous	3	60.0	2	50.0	5	45.5	3	75.0	28	73.7	11	57.9
Oxytocin augmentation	2	20.0	4	100.0	4	36.4	3	75.0	13	34.2	13	68.4
Fetal distress	5[b]	80.0	1[d]	25.0	7[b]	63.6	1[d]	25.0	24[b]	63.2	4[d]	21.1
Prolonged fetal heart abnormality[a]	0/2	0.0			2/7	28.6			5/21	23.8		
Emergency Caesarean section	1	20.0	0	0.0	1	9.1	0	0.0	10	26.3	6	31.6
Labour >5 h		NA	3	75.0		NA	2	50.0		NA	14	73.7
Second stage 2 h+	0	0.0[c]		NA	1	9.1[c]		NA	2	5.3[c]		NA
Assisted vaginal delivery	3	60.0	2	50.0	4	36.4	1	25.0	15	39.5	1	5/3
Apgar 0-3 at 1 min	4	80.0	4	100.0	4	36.4	2	50.0	12	31.6	7	36.8

[a] For cases born between 1975 and 1979 only.
[b] Fetal heart rate persistently outside the range 120-160 beats per minute and/or meconium staining.
[c] Vaginal deliveries only.
[d] Operative delivery prompted by fetal distress.

characteristics were compared in three subgroups of seizure cases categorised by outcome: survivors of early seizures who died in the neonatal period, those who manifested a disability at follow up (3 years of age in Cardiff and 1 year of age in Dublin), and those who showed no evidence of disability at follow up (Table 4). The "adverse factors" examined were those found to have a statistically significant association with (all) early-onset seizures in previous analyses of the Cardiff and Dublin data sets. These factors are listed on the left side of Table 4. Cases in which a disability had been diagnosed were less likely to have prolonged pregnancies (more than 41 weeks, pooled odds ratio: 0.24, 95% confidence interval 0.07-0.92) and less likely to have had emergency Caesarean deliveries (pooled odds ratio: 0.20, 95% confidence interval 0.03-1.45). Otherwise no pattern emerges. This was the case, for example, for oxytocin use and length of labour, both of which appear to be related to the preventability of neonatal seizures as judged by the results of the Dublin trial. However, this may be due to the fact that, although numbers of cases have been increased by amalgamating the results of the two studies, they are nevertheless small for cross-tabulation. A clearer picture may emerge if others tabulate data on the outcome of early neonatal seizures against perinatal risk factors in babies born at term or after term in a similar way to that presented in Table 4.

New Developments in Neonatal Diagnosis

Perhaps the greatest hope for earlier and more precise identification of the individual babies who comprise the three broad aetiological categories (preventable asphyxia, trauma and other pathology) lies in the use of recently introduced methods of neonatal brain imaging (Fitzhardinge et al. 1981; Cady et al. 1983; Levene and Trounce, 1986) combined with neonatal electroencephalographic studies (Eyre et al. 1983a, b; Aziz et al. 1986). If it becomes possible to make more precise diagnoses for babies who exhibit abnormal neonatal neurological signs (some of whom are undoubtedly suffering from preventable asphyxia and trauma) then it should be possible to make more confident statements than are possible at present both about the effects of particular modes of obstetrical practice and about the relationship between obstetrically preventable asphyxia, birth trauma and long-term disability.

Acknowledgements. I am extremely grateful to Iain Chalmers for his generous help with this paper; to Lesley Mierh and Myrna Holmes for typing the manuscript; and to the Department of Health and Social Security for its support of the National Perinatal Epidemiology Unit.

References

Amiel-Tison C (1985) Outcome and long term follow up. In: Clinch J, Mathews T (eds) Perinatal medicine. MTP Press, Lancaster, pp 109-114

Aziz SS, Wallace SJ, Murphy JF, Sainsbury CPQ, Gray OP (1986) Cotside EEG monitoring using compressed spectral analysis. Arch Dis Child 61: 242-246

Brann AW (1985) Factors during neonatal life that influence brain disorders. In: Freeman JM (ed) Prenatal and perinatal factors associated with brain disorders. National Institutes of Health, Bethesda, pp 263-358

Brown JK, Cockburn F, Forfar JO (1972) Clinical and chemical correlates and convulsions in the newborn. Lancet 1: 135-139

Cady EB, Costello AM de L, Dawson MJ, Delpy DT, Hope PL, Reynolds EOR, Tofts PS, Wilkie DR (1983) Non-invasive investigation of cerebral metabolism in newborn infants by phosphorous nuclear magnetic resonance spectroscopy. Lancet 1: 1059-1062

Chalmers I (1979) Randomized controlled trials of fetal monitoring 1973-1977. In: Thalhammer O, Baumgarten K, Pollak A, (eds) Perinatal medicine. Thieme, Stuttgart, pp 260-265

Clarke M, Gill J, Noronha M, McKinlay I (1987) Early infantile epileptic encephalopathy with suppression burst: Ohtahara syndrome. Dev Med Child Neurol, (in press)

Combes J, Rufo M, Vallade MJ, Pinsard N, Bernard R (1975) Les convulsions néonatales: circonstances d'apparition et critères de pronostic. Pediatrie 30: 477-492

Dennis J (1978) Neonatal convulsions: aetiology, late neonatal status and long term outcome. Dev Med Child Neurol 20: 143-153

Dennis J (1985) The long-term effects of intrapartum cerebral damage. In: Crawford JW (ed) Risks of labour. Wiley and Sons, Chichester, pp 157-188

Dennis J, Chalmers I (1982) Very early neonatal seizure rate: a possible epidemiological indicator of the quality of perinatal care. Br J Obstet Gynaecol 89: 418-426

Derham RJ, Matthews TG, Clarke TA (1985) Early seizures indicate quality of perinatal care. Arch Dis Child 60: 809-813

Eyre JA, Oozeer RC, Wilkinson AR (1983a) Continuous electroencephalographic recording to detect seizures in paralysed newborn babies. Br Med J 286: 1017-1018

Eyre JA, Oozeer RC, Wilkinson AR (1983b) Diagnosis of neonatal seizure by continuous recording and rapid analysis of the electroencephalogram. Arch Dis Child 58: 785-790

Finer NN, Robertson CM, Richards RT, Rinnell LE, Peters KL (1981) Hypoxic-ischemic encephalopathy in term infants: perinatal factors and outcome. Pediatrics 98: 112-117

Finer NN, Robertson CM, Peters KL, Coward JH (1983) Factors affecting outcome in hypoxic-ischaemic encephalopathy in term infants. Am J Dis Children 137: 21-25

Fitzhardinge PM, Flodmark O Fitz CR, Ashby S (1981) The prognostic value of computed tomography as an adjunct to assessment of the term infant with post asphyxial encephalopathy. Pediatr 99: 777-781

Freeman JM (ed) (1985) Prenatal and perinatal factors associated with brain disorders. National Institutes of Health, Bethesda, p. 447

Grant A (1986) The Dublin randomised controlled trial of intrapartum fetal heart rate monitoring. Thesis, University of Oxford

Hagberg B, Hagberg G, Olow I (1984) The changing panorama of cerebral palsy in Sweden. IV. Epidemiological trends 1959-78. Acta Paediatr Scand 73: 433-440

Harris R, Tizard JPM (1966) The electroencephalogram in neonatal convulsions. J Pediatrics 137: 245-250

Haverkamp AD, Orleans M, Langendoerfer S, McFee J, Murphy J, Thompson HE (1979) A controlled trial of the differential effects of intrapartum fetal monitoring. Am J Obstet Gynecol 134: 399-408

Hey E (1985) Fetal hypoxia and subsequent handicap: the problem of establishing a causal link. In: Chamberlain GVP, Orr CJB, Sharp F (eds) Litigation and obstetrics and gynaecology. Royal College of Obstetricians and Gynaecologists, London, pp 233-242

Jarvis SN, Holloway JS, Hey E (1985) Increase in cerebral palsy in normal birthweight babies. Arch Dis Child 60: 1113-1121

Levene MI, Trounce JQ (1986) Cause of neonatal convulsions: towards more precise diagnosis. Arch Dis Child 61: 78-87

Lumley J, Wood C (1969) Fetal acidosis. Aust NZ J Obstet Gynaecol 9: 145-151

MacDonald D, Grant A, Sheridan-Pereira M, Boylan P, Chalmers I (1985) The Dublin randomized controlled trial of intrapartum fetal heart rate monitoring. Am J Obstet Gynecol 152: 524-539

Minchom P, Niswander K, Chalmers I, Dauncey M, Newcombe R, Elbourne D, Mutch L, Andrews J, Williams G (1987) Antecedents and outcome of very early neonatal seizures in infants born at or after term. Br J Obstet Gynaecol 94: 431-439

Nelson KB, Ellenberg JH (1981) Apgar scores as predictors of chronic neurologic disability. Pediatrics 6: 31-44

Niswander K, Henson G, Elbourne D, Chalmers I, Redman C, Macfarlane JA, Tizard P (1984) Adverse outcome of pregnancy and the quality of obstetric care. Lancet 2: 827-831

Ohtahara S (1978) Clinico-electrical delineation of epileptic encephalopathies in childhood. Asian Med J 21: 499

Ohtahara S (1984) Seizure disorders in infancy and childhood. Brain Dev 6: 509-519

Paneth N, Stark RI (1983) Cerebral palsy and mental retardation in relation to indicators of perinatal asphyxia. Am J Obstet Gynecol 147: 960-966

Quilligan EJ, Paul RH (1975) Fetal monitoring: is it worth it? Obstet Gynecol 45: 96-100

Renou P, Chang A, Anderson I, Wood C (1976) Controlled trial of fetal intensive care. Am J Obstet Gynecol 126: 470-476

Robertson C, Finer N (1985) Term infants with hypoxic-ischemic encephalopathy: outcome at 3.5 years. Dev Med Child Neurol 27: 473-484

Social Services Committee (1980) Report on perinatal and neonatal mortality. HMSO, London

Steer PJ (1985) Fetal distress. In: Crawford JW (ed) Risks of labour. Wiley and Sons, Chichester, pp 11-31

Susser M, Hauser WA, Kiely JL, Paneth N, Stein Z (1985) Quantitative estimates of prenatal and perinatal risk factors for perinatal mortality, cerebral palsy, mental retardation and epilepsy. In: Freeman JM (ed) Prenatal and perinatal factors associated with brain disorders. National Institutes of Health, Bethesda, pp 359-439

Sykes GS, Molloy PM, Johnson P, Gu W, Ashworth F, Stirratt GM, Turnbull AC (1982) Do Apgar scores indicate asphyxia? Lancet 1: 494-496

Taylor DJ, Howie PW, Davidson J, Davidson D, Drillien CM (1985) Do pregnancy complications contribute to neurodevelopmental disability? Lancet 1: 713-716

Yusuf S, Peto R, Lewis T, Collins R, Sleight P (1985) Beta blockade during and after myocardial infarction: an overview of the randomised trials. Prog Cardiovasc Dis 27: 336-371

Available Evidence Relating Abnormal Intrapartum Fetal Acid Base Balance (pH) to Neuromotor Dysfunction and Mental Handicap

E. HOCHULI and H. P. VOGT

Causes of Brain Injury

The pathophysiological mechanism by which asphyxia causes the brain injury associated with cerebral palsy is not totally clear. Myers et al. 1981 think that the damage to neuronal tissues is caused by a critically high level of lactic acid, an end product of anaerobic metabolism which the tissues employ for energy in the absence of oxygen. Animal work confirms the clinical observation that severe fetal hypoxia results in brain injury. It also suggests an explanation for the confusing clinical observation that most fetal hypoxia does not result in brain injury.

It is apparent that a precise definition of the severity and the type of the acidotic state in the human fetus must be evaluated before any prediction of the likelihood of the development of brain injury in an individual fetus can be assessed.

Long-term Morbidity After Acidosis

Present figures in relation to the yearly birth rate (n=75000) for Switzerland (Table 1) show that 3.5%–5% of school-age children are afflicted with a severe mental handicap (IQ <50) while seven out of 1000 schoolchildren suffer from a moderate mental handicap (IQ 50–70). One-third of the severely handicapped cases are due to trisomy 21. Malformations of the central nervous system (anencephaly, meningomyelocele, etc.), as well as cerebral palsy occur at about the same rate.

Reported Studies

Only a few studies have been reported in which newborns asphyxiated by various causes were examined for neurological intactness months or years after the intrapartum asphyxial episode. Low et al. (1978) first studied 42 children at the ages of 6 and 12 months who had suffered asphyxia (umbilical artery buffer base

Table 1. Main neuropediatric handicaps (per 1000 and in the 75000 annual live births in Switzerland (Data from Kamillo Eisner-Stiftung, Switzerland)

	1000	75000
Severe mental retardation (IQ <50)	3.5–5	262.5–375
Trisomy 21 Age of mother: 25 years: 1:1000 35 years: 1: 365 44 years: 1: 44	1.4	105
Anencephaly	1	75
Meningomyelocele	1.2–2.5	90–187.5
Cerebral palsy	1.0–2.5	75–187.5
Congenital hypothyroidism	0.3	22.5
Phenylketonuria	1:20000	

<34.0 mEq/per liter) at birth and compared them to a group of 69 children born without asphyxia (umbilical artery buffer base >36.1 mEq/per liter). They used the intrapartum buffer base values described by Saling (1966).

Low's two groups were not significantly different in respect to maternal characteristics, maternal medical complications, parity, past obstetrical history, obstetrical complications in the present pregnancy, or labor and delivery characteristics. There were no differences in mental or physical development at the ages of 6 and 12 months or neurological examination at the age of 12 months in the control and study group children. In a follow-up study (Low et al. 1983) between 1 and 6 years of age there was also no significant difference in the pattern of physical growth and the incidence of motor and cognitive handicap or developmental delay, language developmental delay, and tests of vision and hearing in the children of the hypoxia group and the children of the control group.

Influence of the Apgar Score

The data available on the predictive value of low Apgar scores and neurological damage is at variance and there is a notable lack of correlation between Apgar scores and acidosis in the newborn. Sykes et al. (1982) found that only 21% of babies with a low 1-min Apgar score and 19% of babies with a low 5-min Apgar score had severe acidosis at birth. Similarly, 73% of babies with severe acidosis had a 1-min Apgar score of 7 or more, and 86% had a similar 5-min score.

Influence of Chronic Acidosis

There is some evidence that chronic asphyxia or repeated acute episodes superimposed on chronic asphyxia may be the culprit in "causing" brain injury. Dweck et al. (1974) observed no increased risk of brain damage in a group of severely asphyxiated newborns compared to nonasphyxiated infants unless the former had also suffered intrauterine growth retardation.

In our unit, we have carried out pH evaluation in the umbilical cord in all babies born since 1973. The rate of severe and advanced acidosis (ph <7.10) has decreased from about 24‰ to an average 8‰–9‰ over the past 10 years (Fig. 1). Our results were compared with results obtained from other Swiss centers (Figs. 2

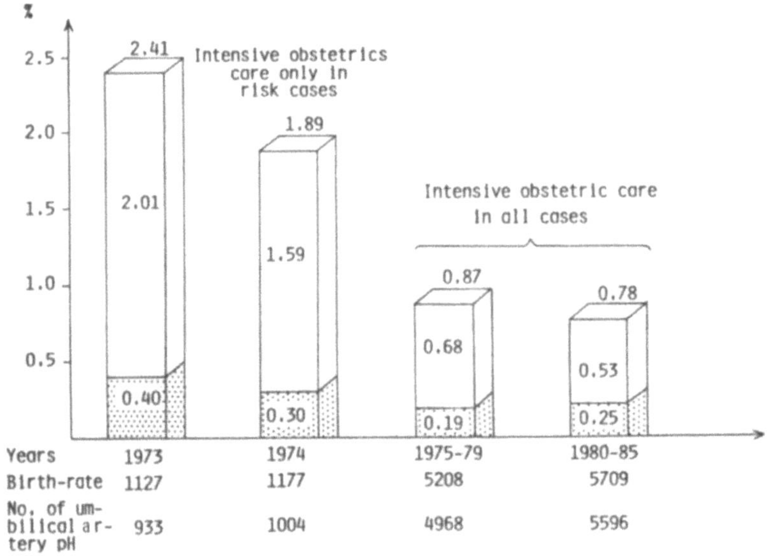

Fig. 1. Frequency of advanced and severe acidosis, in the umbilical, artery. □ pH 7.0–7.9; ▦ pH <7.0

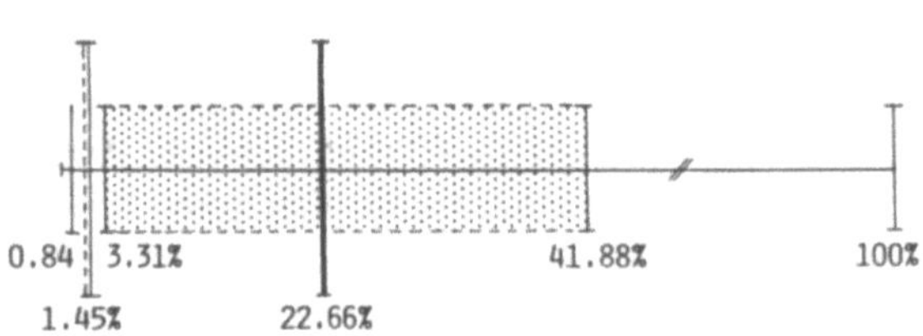

Fig. 2. pH measurements, not taken in the umbilical artery. Extract from the Swiss multicenter data bank. Range of pH values comparing the statistical profile of a single clinic (Kantonsspital Münsterlingen average I) to the Swiss average (I). The 25–75% range ▦ marks the middle field between the lowest (p<25%) and the highest (p>75%) noticeable part. It allows the placement of any clinic and the evaluation of results outside the normal range

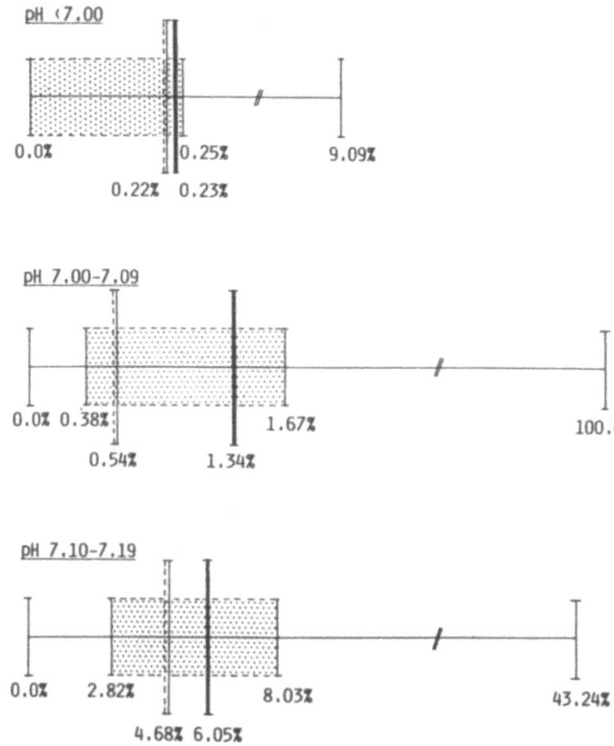

Fig. 3. These graphs show several ranges of pH values comparing the clinic of Münsterlingen (I) to the Swiss average (I). ▒ 25%-75% range

and 3). There has been a concomitant reduction in the perinatal deaths when compared to multi-centers in Switzerland (Table 2).

Analyzing the follow-up examinations of 84 newborns with acidosis (pH < 7.10 in the umbilical artery) and correlating the perinatal acidosis with later neuropediatric handicaps our findings are as follows. Of the cases with acidosis over a period of 11 years (1967-1977: 112 acidosis cases), 25 foreign children in the study group and three in the control group could no longer be reached (they had left the country).

The age range of the 84 children who had acidosis at birth is as shown in Table 3. These 84 children were divided into two groups (Fig. 5). Group I ($n=63$) comprised those for whom exact intrapartum records could be traced, with the acidosis presumably due to the birth process itself (for example, in cases of uterine inertia, difficult delivery, umbilical cord complications). Group II ($n=21$) consisted of all newborns with one or more additional risks, such as prematurity, small for date, and postnatal respiratory distress syndrome. Subgroups were differentiated as to cases with advanced acidosis (pH 7.09-7.00) and severe acidosis (pH <7.00) (Fig. 4).

Table 2. Extract from the Swiss multicenter data bank. Rate of perinatal mortality 1983–1985 comparing a single clinic (Kantonsspital Münsterlingen – KSM) to the Swiss average (according to WHO)

	KSM		Switzerland	
	(n)	(%)	*(n)*	(%)
Fetal death rate before admission to the clinic	7	0.25	353	0.40
Fetal death rate after admission to the clinic	0	0.00	77	0.09
Fetal death rate during labor before admission to the clinic	0	0.00	22	0.02
Fetal death rate during labor after admission to the clinic	2	0.07	76	0.09
Neonatal death rate (including the first 7 days of life)	7	0.25	281	0.32
Total	16	0.57	809	0.92

Table 3. Neuropediatric examination of children ($n = 84$). (Data from Hochuli 1980)

	(n)
Infants	3
Toddlers of age 2–6 years	61
Schoolchildren of age 7–10 years	20

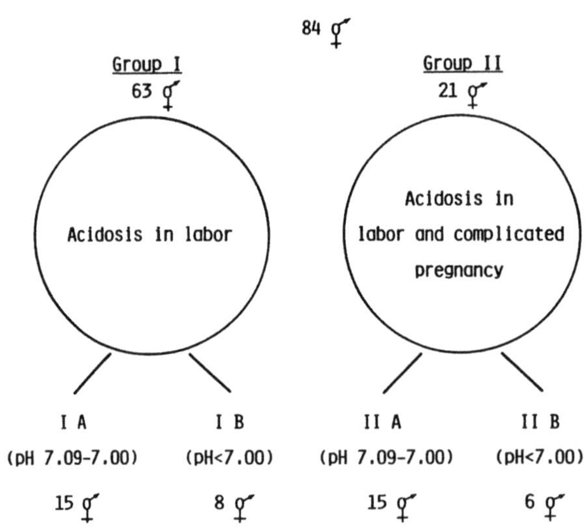

Fig. 4. Follow-up data on controlled children. (Data from Hochuli 1980)

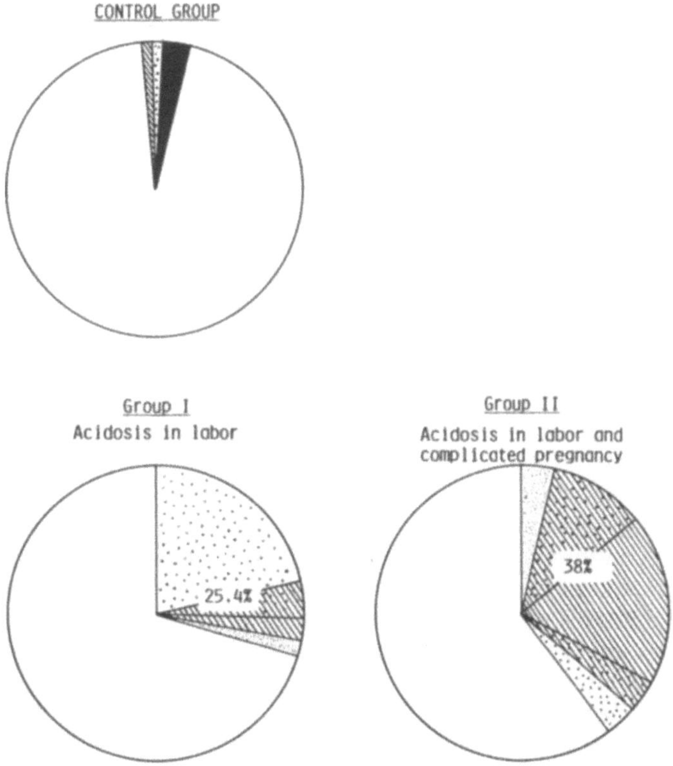

Fig. 5. Graphs of the distribution of disturbances in a control group compared with groups I and II. Distribution of disturbances in the early childhood per 1000 births = 2%-(3%?) (Hagberg 1975). Cerebral palsy; retardation; minimal brain disorders; other factors; mixed factors; healthy.
(Data from Hochuli 1980)

Definitions

The children were neuropediatrically examined according to the following definitions and in accordance with Barnett and Einhorn (1972):

- Cerebral palsy (CP) - different symptoms affecting the brain functions which show themselves in disability of the motor functions
- Minimal brain disorders (slight infantile brain injury) - no feeble-mindedness and no dementia, no gross neurological deficiency, no epilepsy or malformation of the CNS, but school problems, behavioral disorders, enuresis, encopresis, disciplinary problems, developmental problems, nervoussness, speech deficiencies
- Retardation - definition = smiling > 2 months, grasping > 5 months, sitting > 12 months, standing > 12 months, walking > 18 months, first words > 18 months, first sentences (with 2-3 words) > 36 months

Broad Outlines of Our Results

Since the disorders partly overlap, influence one another and are sometimes hardly or not at all separable from one another, they are classified into separate groups according to the importance of the apparent symptoms. In view of the difficulty in attributing the neuro-psychomotor handicaps to the individual obstetrical episodes we are only able to give the broad outlines of our results (Fig. 5).

Differences appear if we compare the results with our postacidosis figures with the distribution of the "main neuropediatric handicaps" according to Hagberg (1975). We are surprised by the number of handicaps (especially minimal brain disorders) present in our postacidosis cohort, particularly when further risk factors are added. Even when taking into account the fact that the follow up of controls was performed at different ages these results at least show trends which are of interest.

These figures certainly cannot stand up to critical examination. They represent neither a randomized cohort nor a prospective study. The numbers are too small to consider, for example, maternal factors such as parity, age, and pregnancy complications, etc. If we want to make firm statements, the only possibility we can think of is randomized, prospective, multicentric, and comprehensive studies taking into account all factors, something which should be feasible with the widespreach use of computer technology all over the world.

There is no comparison possible with other work in this field, neither as to the type nor to the quality of the follow up examinations (= standardization) because of the differences not only in examination methods but also in age groups.

Given that our figures relating to newborn acidosis have stabilized at a very low level during the past 10 years and assuming that, in purely arithmetical terms, the neonatal problems due to acidosis have also been reduced, the results are, however, similar to those obtained by Ingemarsson et al. (1981).

In conclusion, we think that there is a very strong correlation between neuropediatric handicaps and acidosis, but we do not know the exact critical level of acidosis nor the critical duration needed for permanent neurological sequelae.

References

Barnett HL, Einhorn AH (1972) Pediatrics, 15th edn. Appleton Century Crofts, New York

Dweck H, Huggings W, Dorman L et al. (1974) Development sequelae in infants having suffered severe perinatal asphyxia. Am J Obstet Gynecol 119: 811

Hagberg B (1975) Pre-, peri- and postnatal prevention of major neuropediatric handicaps. Neuropediatrics 6: 331

Ingemarsson E, Ingemarsson I, Niels W (1981) Impact of routine fetal monitoring during labor on fetal outcome with long-term follow-up. Am J Obstet Gynecol 141: 29-38

Low J, Galbraith R, Muir D et al. (1978) Intrapartum fetal asphyxia: a preliminary report in regard to longterm morbidity. Am J Obstet Gynecol 130: 525

Low J, Galbraith R, Muir D et al. (1983) Intrapartum fetal hypoxia: a study of long-term morbidity. Am J Obstet Gynecol 145: 129

Myers RE, Wagner KR, de Courten GM (1981) Lactic acid accumulation in tissues as cause of brain injury and death in cardiogenic shock from asphyxia. In: Lauerser NH, Hochberg HM (eds) Perinatal biochemical monitoring. William and Wilkins, Baltimore
Saling E (1966) Das Kind im Bereich der Geburtshilfe. Thieme, Stuttgart
Sykes G, Johnson P, Ashworth E et al. (1982) Do Apgar scores indicate asphyxia? Lancet 1: 494

Intrapartum Cardiotocogram, Apgar Score and Acidaemia at Birth: Relationship to Neonatal Neurological Morbidity

G. H. A. VISSER and M. J. DIJXHOORN

Measuring the fetal condition during the perinatal period must be continued, but we should not fool ourselves by insisting that we can avoid most brain damage by avoiding perinatal asphyxia. (Niswander 1981)

Up until now there have been no studies relating intrapartum fetal heart rate (FHR) patterns to the neurological condition of the newborn infant. Intrapartum FHR is, however, related to the direct neonatal outcome as measured by the Apgar scoring system or by the blood gases obtained from the umbilical vessels. So indirectly a relationship between intrapartum FHR and neurological outcome can be made.

Studies showing a relation between in intrapartum FHR patterns and direct neonatal outcome are numerous (e.g. Kubli et al. 1969; Bissonnette 1975; Tejani et al. 1975; Chik et al. 1976; Zanini et al. 1980). They all report, however, a wide variation in outcome with particular FHR patterns. This might be due to the fact that many variables influence intrapartum FHR. Also the initial reserve capacity of the individual fetus is likely to play a role. In the controlled trials on intrapartum FHR monitoring a beneficial effect - e.g. reduction of acidaemia at birth or of neonatal morbidity - was only found when FHR monitoring was combined with intrapartum fetal acid-base assessment when indicated (MacDonald et al. 1985). There appears to be a general agreement that intrapartum FHR monitoring and additional fetal scalp pH measurements should identify fetuses at risk for intrapartum acidaemia and/or a low Apgar score at birth. This brings us to the importance of preventing 'asphyxia' during labour, e.g. to the relationship between 'birth asphyxia' and neurological outcome. In this context data of the Groningen Perinatal Project will be summarized and discussed in relation to other investigations.

Apgar-score and Acidaemia at Birth in Relation to Neonatal Neurological Morbidity

In 1975 the Groningen Perinatal Project was started with the aim of studying the relationship between pre- and perinatal events and the development of the nervous system. Over 3000 singleton infants, consecutively born in the course of 3 years, underwent a standardized neonatal neurological examination (Prechtl 1977). Term infants were examined on the 4th or 5th postnatal day. Infants born

Table 1. Groningen Perinatal Project. Number and percentages of neonatal neurologically abnormal infants in the various study groups (for details see Jurgens-Van de Zee et al., 1979; Huisjes et al., 1980)

	Total *(n)*	Neurologically *(n)*	abnormal (%)
AFD term	2658	104	3.9
SFD term	333	31	9.3
Preterm	171	26	15.2
Total	3162	161	5.1

prematurily were also studied at term age. The neonatal neurological condition was classified using a qualitative and quantitative approach. The qualitative approach entailed assigning each infant to one of three diagnostic categories: normal, suspect, abnormal. An infant was considered abnormal if one or more of the following neurological symptoms were present; hyper- or hypokinesia, hyper- or hypotonia, hemisyndrome, apathy syndrome, hyperexcitability syndrome. An infant was classified as suspect if only isolated symptoms were present, but no defined syndromes. A detailed description of this classification has been published elsewhere (Jurgens-van der Zee et al. 1979). Another manner of quantifying the neurological findings was the optimality concept as described by Prechtl. This entailed defining an optimal range for 60 representative neurological items. Each infant obtained a neonatal neurological optimality score (NNOS), consisting of the number of items falling within the optimal range (Touwen et al. 1980).

From all cases the 1- and 3-min Apgar scores were noted. In approximately one-third complete neonatal (umbilical vein and artery) and maternal blood gas analyses were also available.

Not surprisingly it was found that the incidence of neonatal neurological abnormality was increased in the growth retarded and in the preterm infants (9% and 15% respectively) as compared to the appropriate-for-dates (AFD) term infants (4%). Because of the large size of the latter group the majority of neonatally abnormal infants were, however, born at term and were AFD (69%; Table 1).

Appropriate-For-Dates Term Infants

In the AFD term infants only a marginal effect of 'acidaemia at birth' on neonatal neurological morbidity was found (Dijxhoorn et al. 1985). This relationship was only present for (minor) neurological symptoms (suspect infants) and for the NNOS. However, the percentages of variance in NNOS explained by the blood gas variables were very low ($<1\%$). Neonatal neurological abnormality was not at all related to pH_{ua} or to $\Delta pH_{m\text{-}ua}$ and was equally distributed over the pH ranges (Fig. 1). Apparently, acidaemia at birth in this group of infants was only related to neurological symptoms, not to syndromes. Even though according to normal crite-

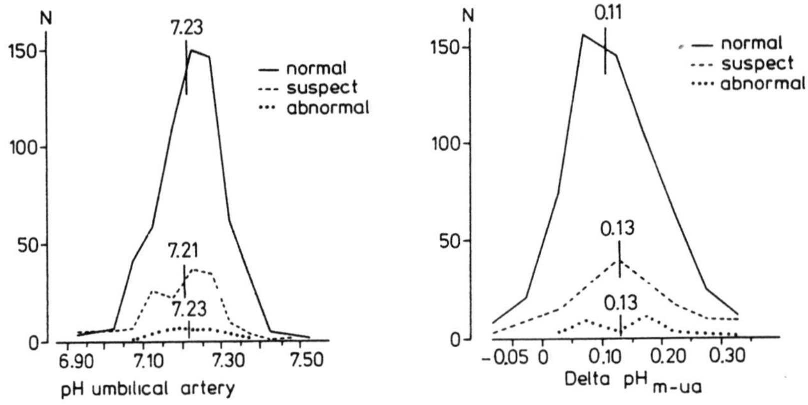

Fig. 1. Appropriate-for-dates term infants ($n=805$). Distribution and median values of umbilical arterial pH and of maternal vein pH and umbilical arterial pH differences (ΔpH_{m-ua}) in the three neonatal neurological diagnostic subgroups (from Dijxhoorn et al. 1985)

Table 2. Percentage of explained variance (squared multiple correlation coefficient) by the combined 'asphyxia' variables (Apgar score; pH, ΔpH, BE; meconium) in neonatal neurological optimality score (NNOS), in the different subpopulations (*$p<0.05$)

Population	Total (*n*)	Explained variance in NNOS (%)
Term infants		
AFD	805	2.0*
SFD vaginal born	224	7.1*
(<2.3 centile	46	22.1)
SFD caesarean section	23	93.0*
Preterm infants		
AFD	93	18.3
SFD	33	54.3*

ria a considerable number of infants were born acidaemic, severe acidaemia at birth ($pH_{ua}<7.00$) was present in only a few cases ($n=9$). Although none of these nine infants was abnormal, assessment of the effect of severe acidaemia at birth could not be made. On the other hand, in a recent follow-up study of 56 AFD term infants who were born extremely acidaemic ($pH_{ua}<7.00$), no differences could be found at the age of 2.5–9 years as compared to matched controls (Aarnoudse et al. 1985).

In the AFD term infants the 1- and 3-min Apgar scores were related to neonatal neurological morbidity, but the variance explained in NNOS was - again - very low (<1%) (Dijxhoorn et al. 1986). A combination of the Apgar score with one of the pH variables increased this percentage to 1.5 and with all 'asphyxia variables' to 2.0 (Table 2). The highest incidence of neurologically suspect and abnormal infants, as well as the lowest median NNOS values, were found in infants with a low 1-min Apgar score but with a normal pH. This unexpected finding suggests that factors other than hypoxia are involved and also that a low Apgar score is more a marker of defective reactions as a result of various other insults than an indicator of hypoxia. This suggestion was also made on the basis of the follow-up study of the 1970 British Birth Survey (Peters et al. 1984).

Thus in this population of AFD term infants asphyxia at birth was not responsible for evident neonatal neurological abnormalities. This implies that the causes could not be identified for the majority of neurologically abnormal infants (see Table 1). These data seem to contradict earlier reports on the relationship between asphyxia at birth and neurological handicap. However, the infants discussed before were all carefully selected as being AFD and born at term. In other studies often different population were combined. Moreover, it may well be that with modern management, including intensive monitoring during labour and intensive neonatal treatment of hypoxia at birth - facilities available at our hospital - the incidence of prolonged hypoxia during labour as well as after birth is low. Others also found that mature AFD infants will not exhibit an increased incidence of neurological sequelae following intrapartum hypoxia of short duration (Low et al. 1983). With a persisting low Apgar score, which may indicate on the one hand a severe birth hypoxia and on the other inadequate resuscitation, it has been shown that the incidence of neurological sequelae increases strikingly (Nelson and Ellenberg 1981). Finally it may be that many infants born with a low Apgar score or otherwise being thought to be 'asphyxiated' during labour were already abnormal before birth. Recent literature (Sims et al. 1985; Paul et al. 1986; Mann 1986) indicates that central nervous system injuries occurring prior to the labour process are not rare. Up until now many of these infants have probably been left with the diagnosis 'birth asphyxia'.

Small-For-Dates Infants

In small-for-dates (SFD) term infants ($n = 224$) the predictive value of the indicators of asphyxia was higher than in the AFD term group (percentage of explained variance in NNOS: 7; Dijxhoorn et al. 1987). This percentage was three times higher in the severely SFD infants (birthweight <2.3 centile; Table 2). Although these figures are higher than in AFD term infants, they still only indicate a small contribution of intrapartum asphyxia to neonatal neurological morbidity. In the 23 SFD term infants delivered abdominally, the combination of measured asphyxia variables explained 93% of the variance in NNOS. On the other hand, poor neurological outcome in the latter group was restricted to those in whom late fetal heart rate decelerations had been present. It is suggested that these signs of fetal hypoxaemia, which were mostly present antenatally (80%), are more important with respect to neurological outcome than the commonly used indicators of asphyxia at birth. Similar data were obtained in the SFD infants born prematurily. In this group heart rate decelerations (present in 80% of cases antenatally) also correlated better with neurological outcome than the Apgar score and/or pH variables at birth. Impaired neurological functioning in these infants is therefore more likely to be due to 'chronic' antepartum hypoxaemia (and malnutrition) than to 'acute' asphyxia at birth. This reasoning is to a large extent supported by morphological findings in human growth-retarded infants (Dobbing 1974) and in animal studies (Bedi 1984), where a smaller brain size, fewer cells etc. are found, rather than distinct lesions as is often the case after acute asphyxia (Kreusser and Volpe 1984). These data suggest that growth-retarded fetuses should preferably be delivered before antepartum signs of hypoxaemia occur. The benefits of prevenient intervention must, however, be weighed against the risks of premature delivery, and the methods for early identification of fetuses at risk for intra-uterine hypoxaemia still have to be validated (see the chapter by Visser, this book).

Appropriate-For-Dates Preterm Infants

In the AFD preterm infants the relationship between 'asphyxia' variables and neonatal neurological morbidity was evident, although less pronounced than in the SFD preterm group (Table 2). As there is no reason to presume that chronic malnutrition/asphyxia had been present in the former group, it is suggested that the effect on the neonatal neurological condition is mainly the result of more-or-less acute 'asphyxia' during labour. Westgren et al. (1984) also observed in acidotic (fetal scalp pH less than 7.25), premature, mostly AFD infants significantly more neurological abnormalities in the neonatal period and a higher rate of neurodevelopmental disabilities at follow-up than in nonacidotic infants of the same gestational age.

In a combined group of 303 high-risk preterm and term newborn infants, Low et al. (1985) observed newborn encephalopathy in 92 cases (30%). A significant association was found with severe intrapartum fetal hypoxia, newborn respiratory complications and major infections. According to the data of Low et al. (1985), prevention of intrapartum hypoxia would only reduce the incidence of moderate newborn encephalopathy by approximately 5% and of severe encephalopathy by 15%. In a subsequent study (Low et al. 1986) of 220 infants, of whom two-third were born prematurely, little evidence was found that fetal hypoxia contributed to newborn intracranial haemorrhage. In infants born before 34 weeks of gestation Beverley et al. (1984) also found no relation between umbilical pH and intraventricular haemorrhage. In infants with a birthweight of less than 1500 g Strauss et al. (1985) did find, however, a correlation between abnormal antepartum FHR and intraventricular haemorrhage. Shennan et al. (1985) studied the perinatal data and follow-up of the survivors (till 1 year) of 383 live-born infants delivered between 26 and 30 weeks of gestation. The initial condition of the infants, as measured by the Apgar scores, umbilical venous pH and base deficit, appeared to be correlated with neonatal death, but not to subsequent handicaps.

These data indicate that, even in infants born prematurely, birth asphyxia is not the major causative factor for subsequent handicap; prevention of 'asphyxia' at birth will only slightly reduce the incidence of handicaps. Preterm birth itself is the most important cause of handicap in these infants and all efforts should be directed into preventing early delivery.

Conclusions

From these data it can be concluded that:

1. The majority of neonatal neurologically abnormal infants are appropriate-for-dates and born at term
2. With modern management in a teaching hospital 'asphyxia at birth' is not a main causative factor of neurological abnormality in appropriate-for-dates term infants
3. In growth-retarded infants chronic malnutrition (including chronic hypoxaemia) appears to be more important with respect to neurological outcome than the actual condition at birth
4. 'Asphyxia at birth' is related to neurological impairment in preterm appropriate-for-dates infants; however, even in these infants it plays only a relatively minor role

References

Aarnoudse JG, Yspeert-Gerards J, Touwen BCL et al. (1985) Severe fetal hypoxia (umbilical arterial pH $\leqq$7.00) in preterm and growth retarded infants. A neurological follow-up study (Abstract). International workshop on dev neurol fetus preterm infant, Groningen, Holland

Bedi KS (1984) Effects of undernutrition on brain morphology: a critical review of methods and results. In: Current topics in research on synapses, vol 2, Liss Inc, New York, pp 93-163

Beverley DW, Chance GW, Coates CF (1984) Intraventricular haemorrhage-timing of occurrence and relationship to perinatal events. Br J Obstet Gynaecol 91: 1007-1013

Bissonnette JM (1975) Relationship between continuous fetal heart rate patterns and Apgar score in the newborn. Br J Obstet Gynaecol 82: 24-28

Chik L, Sokol RJ, Rosen MG (1976) Prediction of the one-minute Apgar score from fetal heart rate data. Obstet Gynecol 48: 452-455

Dijxhoorn MJ, Visser GHA, Huisjes HJ et al. (1985) The relation between umbilical pH values and neonatal neurological morbidity in full-term AFD infants. Early Hum Dev 11: 33-42

Dijxhoorn MJ, Visser GHA, Fidler V et al. (1986) Apgar score, meconium and acidaemia at birth in relation to neonatal neurological morbidity in term infants. Br J Obstet Gynaecol 93: 217-222

Dijxhoorn MJ, Visser GHA, Touwen BCL et al. (1987) Apgar score, meconium and acidaemia at birth in small-for-dates term infants and their relation to neonatal neurological morbidity. Br J Obstet Gynaecol (in press)

Dobbing J (1974) The later development of the brain and its vulnerability. In: Davis JA, Dobbing J (eds) Scientific foundations of paediatrics. Heinemann, London, p 565

Huisjes HJ, Touwen BCL, Hoekstra JJ et al. (1980) Obstetrical-neonatal neurological relationship. A replication study. Eur J Obstet Gynaecol Reprod Biol 10: 247-256

Jurgens-van de Zee AD, Biermann-van Eendenburg MEC, Fidler JV et al. (1979) Preterm birth, growth retardation and acidaemia in relation to neurological abnormality of the newborn. Early Hum Dev 3: 141-154

Kreusser KL, Volpe JJ (1984) The neurological outcome of perinatal asphyxia. In: Almli CR, Finger S (eds) Early brain damage, vol 1, Academic, Orlando, pp 151-168

Kubli FW, Hon EH, Khazin AF et al. (1969) Observations on heart rate and pH in the human fetus during labor. Am J Obstet Gynecol 104: 1190-1206

Low JA, Galbraith RS, Muir DW et al. (1983) Intrapartum fetal hypoxia: a study of long-term morbidity. Am J Obstet Gynecol 145: 129-134

Low JA, Galbraith RS, Muir DW et al. (1985) The relationship between perinatal hypoxia and newborn encephalopathy. Am J Obstet Gynecol 152: 256-260

Low JA, Galbraith RS, Sauerbrei EE et al. (1986) Maternal, fetal, and newborn complications associated with newborn intracranial hemorrhage. Am J Obstet Gynecol 154: 345-351

Mann LI (1986) Pregnancy events and brain damage. Am J Obstet Gynecol 155: 6

MacDonald D, Grant A, Sheridan-Pereira M et al. (1985) The Dublin randomized controlled trial of intrapartum fetal heart rate monitoring. Am J Obstet Gynecol 152: 524-509

Nelson KB, Ellenberg JH (1981) Apgar scores as predictors of chronic neurologic disability. Pediatrics 68: 36-44

Niswander KR (1981) In: Clapp JF, Mann LL, Peress NS, Szeto HH: Neuropathology in the chronic fetal lamb preparation: structurefunction correlates under different environmental conditions (Discussion). Am J Obstet Gynecol 142: 984-985

Paul RH, Yonekura ML, Cantrell CJ et al. (1986) Fetal injury prior to labor: does it happen? Am J Obstet Gynecol 154: 1187-1193

Peters TJ, Golding J, Lawrence CJ et al. (1984) Delayed onset of regular respiration and subsequent development. Early Hum Dev 9: 225-239

Prechtl HFR (1977) The neurological examination of the fullterm newborn infant. In: Clinics in developmental medicine, no 63, 2nd edn. Spastics International Medical Publications, Heinemann, London

Prechtl HFR (1980) The optimally concept. Editorial Early Hum Dev 4: 201-205

Shennan AT, Milligan JE, Hoskins EM (1985) Perinatal factors associated with death or handicap in very preterm infants. Am J Obstet Gynecol 151: 231-238

Sims ME, Beckwitt Turkel S, Halterman G et al. (1985) Brain injury and intrauterine death. Am J Obstet Gynecol 151: 721-723

Strauss A, Kirz D, Modanlou HD et al. (1985) Perinatal events and intraventricular/subependymal hemorrhage in the very low-birth weight infant. Am J Obstet Gynecol 151: 1022-1027

Tejani N, Mann LI, Bhakthavathsalan A et al. (1975) Correlation of fetal heart rate uterine-contraction patterns with fetal scalp blood pH. Obstet Gynecol 46: 392-396

Touwen BCL, Huisjes HJ, Jurgens-van de Zee AD et al. (1980) Obstetrical condition and neonatal neurological morbidity. An analysis with the help of the optimality concept. Early Hum Dev 4: 207-228

Westgren M, Holmquist P, Ingemarsson I et al. (1984) Intrapartum fetal acidosis in preterm infants: fetal monitoring and long-term morbidity. Obstet Gynecol 63: 355-359

Zanini B, Paul RH, Huey JR (1980) Intrapartum fetal heart rate: correlation with scalp pH in the preterm fetus. Am J Obstet Gynecol 136: 43-47

Neurological Morbidity of Term Infants as an Indicator of Safe Obstetrical Practice

C. AMIEL-TISON

Introduction

The Stresses of a "Normal" Delivery Have Been a Long-standing Source of Anxiety Among Obstetricians. Lacomme wrote in 1960: "I do not know what a 'normal delivery' is; I only know of an 'optimal' labor, i.e. labor where minimal stress is exerted on the fetus." Later on, with fetal heart rate (FHR) monitoring and acid base balance measurements during labor, the definition of an "optimal labor" was refined by taking into account: mechanical forces related to uterine contractions, hemodynamic changes associated with uterine contractions, and secondary fetal changes, as reviewed in 1974 by Sureau. However, the obstetrical anxiety not only persisted but increased with each new method of evaluating the risk of fetal asphyxia. In 1973, Valkeakari offered the first echoencephalographic demonstration of changes in the fetal brain as the result of a normal cephalic delivery. These changes were midline shifts depending on the fetal position during the vaginal delivery (significant with p less than 0.05 from 6 to 12 h postnatally) which were probably related to cerebral edema (normal up to 3 h and back to normal at 24 h). At the same time, it appeared clinically (Amiel-Tison et al. 1977a) that mild signs of cerebral dysfunction linked with the birth process were often observed in the absence of overt fetal distress and therefore with Apgar scores of 8 or more at 1 and 5 min, particularly in occipito posterior presentations.

Confidence Came with the Improving Results of Modern Obstetrics, Anesthesiology and Immediate Pediatric Care. After an obstetrical difficulty of short duration and/or a cesarean section, perinatal care prevents most of the deleterious consequences of an asphyxic or a traumatic birth on the neonatal brain; this result can be evaluated precisely in optimal neurosensorial behavior (Amiel-Tison et al. 1982). Mechanical difficulties in the course of the cesarean section, such as encountered in repeat cesarean sections or an already engaged head, are rare. This safety in surgical techniques resulted in an increased reluctance to perform dangerous obstetrical maneuvers.

Temptation to Extend Cesarean Section Indications Was Therefore Resisted Less and Less. Pressure from parents and lawyers reinforced this trend, resulting in rapidly rising rates of cesarean sections (Bottoms et al. 1980).

Reaction Came: Nature Is Wise, Physiologists Say. The benefits for the newborn of the stress of labor which promote adaptation through increasing fetal catecholamine levels have recently been reviewed (Lagercrantz and Slotkin 1986): high catecholamine levels have a favorable effect on breathing, distribution of blood flow, metabolic adaptation, and even parent-infant bonding. The question then becomes: what is the optimal cesarean section rate, and how does one define this optimal rate?

Neurological Evaluation of the Newborn is a Starting Point in Finding the Answer. Immediately after birth, the preceding definitions of fetal risk, gestational or obstetrical, have to be replaced by the neurosensorial evaluation of the newborn. The recent advances in the assessment of these capacities, or competences, are such that a normal newborn can be defined as normal (Amiel-Tison and Grenier 1986; Brazelton 1984; Touwen 1976) and confirmed as normal by repeated evaluations within the 1st week or 1st month. Certainly, the number of data have to be increased for the following statement to become an indisputable finding: a normal newborn will become a normal child, neurologically speaking (which does not exclude unfavorable effects of a low sociocultural status on school performances), no matter how dreadful the pregnancy or delivery was.

Elaboration of Clinical Methodology to Evaluate Neurological Status in the Neonatal Period

No Single Specific Sign Characterizes Hypoxic Ischemic Encephalopathy. Severe neurological signs present in the first hours of life after overt birth asphyxia have been well described: coma and repeated seizures are recognized and associated with severe EEG abnormalities. Therefore, in this category, everybody is talking about the same condition, the severe type of ischemic-hypoxic encephalopathy.

Beside this condition, a cluster of signs of CNS depression are also easily recognizable involving defects in three areas: consciousness, tone, and primary reflexes. There is little spontaneous activity and crying is rare; the tone is globally deficient; the primary reflexes are either totally absent or difficult to obtain. In particular, deficient sucking and swallowing can make feeding dangerous or impossible. In my first study (Amiel-Tison 1969), the 41 full-term newborn subjects belonged to two groups: status epilepticus and/or CNS depression. Later on, it became clear that milder signs and symptoms could represent the clinical expression of a milder degree of birth trauma and/or birth asphyxia.

A Classification of Signs and Symptoms into Three Grades. This was proposed in 1977 (Amiel-Tison et al. 1977a) and has been used in our work since then. Signs and symptoms often change rapidly during the 1st week of life, thus a detailed daily observation is necessary. These data may be collected on a grid (Amiel-Tison 1979, s. Appendix p. 187-191). At the end of the 1st week, they can be summarized into one of three grades: mildly abnormal, moderately abnormal, and severely

Table 1. Classification of signs of cerebral dysfunction in the term newborn during the neonatal period (1st week of life)

Mild distress (Grade 1)	Abnormalities of tone + hyperexcitability (seizures excluded)
Moderate distress (Grade 2)	Signs of CNS depression ± signs of intracranial hypertension (isolated seizures included)
Severe distress (Grade 3)	Repeated seizures and overt CNS depression

abnormal (Table 1). A similar classification, including EEG, was described by Sarnat and Sarnat (1976). Echography and/or computerized tomography (CT) scan findings have not been added to the grades which remain purely clinical. However, early CT scans, before the age of 3 days, may offer considerable information when the mechanism and timing of hypoxic-ischemic encephalopathy is not clear, such as when there are changes indicative of damage preceding birth.

There Are Some Pitfalls in Defining the Milder Degree of Brain Dysfunction. On the one hand, it is necessary to eliminate the very transient signs which might be considered as within the normal limits in the first 3 days. This is why we only take into account signs which persist after 3 days. On the other hand, as the clinician becomes more interested in and more observant of neurological signs of symptoms, more attention is paid to the diagnosis of more moderate dysfunction. So in the absence of a scoring system, there is a tendency in research studies to classify a greater proportion of cases as "moderately affected."

Clinical Diagnosis of Intracranial Hypertension Is Interesting From a Pathophysiological Point of View. Clinical diagnosis can be made from a cluster of cranial and neurological signs (Amiel-Tison et al. 1977b; Amiel-Tison and Grenier 1986) which cannot be fully described here. Early recognition of this condition following birth asphyxia allows palliative treatment. We have shown that intracranial hypertension was clinically present in 40% of mild degree and 70% of moderate degree cerebral dysfunction following birth asphyxia (Amiel-Tison et al. 1977b). It is always present in severe degree cerebral dysfunction (Larroche 1976).

Identification of Intracranial Bleeding Needs Other Investigations. A lumbar puncture may demonstrate a moderate arachnoid hemorrhage, a common finding after birth asphyxia with no prognostic implication per se; the mechanism has to do with hypoxia or with moderate trauma. Echography can localize severe intracranial bleeding, intraventricular hemorrhage or intracerebral hematoma. Both localizations were indicators of poor prognosis in Fitzhandinge's study of 62 asphyxiated full-term newborns (Fitzhardinge et al. 1981).

Prediction of Outcome Is One of the Goals of Such a Classification.

- *Extremes of neurological outcome* can be predicted accurately; that is, the determination of those newborns who will have sequelae and the determination of

Table 2. Estimate of risk for late sequelae based on neonatal classification of neonatal signs

Neonatal signs	Handicap at school age (estimate) (%)	
Grade 1	10	Mild
Grade 2	20–30	Moderate to mild
Grade 3	50–70	Moderate to severe

those who will be normal (Amiel-Tison and Ellison 1986; Amiel-Tison and Grenier 1986). *Prediction of abnormal outcome* can be based on: (a) persistence of abnormal function after 7 days of life, particularly in association with brain stem abnormalities during that timespan; (b) intraventricular or intraparenchymal hemorrhage in the first 3 days; (c) extensive infarcted or ischemic areas within the first 2 weeks; (d) repetitive seizures which are difficult to control; (e) low amplitude wave V with BAEP; and (f) markedly abnormal EEG patterns within the first 3 days. On the other hand, *prediction of normal outcome* can be based on: (a) normal neurological assessment during the 1st week of life; (b) recovery from mild neurological signs within the 1st week of life; (c) normal EEG within the 1st week of life.

- *After moderate and mild but persisting neurological signs,* the prediction of later outcome is presently much less accurate (Amiel-Tison et al. 1983; Amiel-Tison and Grenier 1986); much more work needs to be done, and the prediction should be significantly improved with new developments in technology.

Based on our successive studies using the clinical grades described, a rough estimate of later risk of sequelae is shown Table 2 and may be provisionally used as a guideline. However, for a group evaluation aimed at assessing progress in obstetrical methods, these grades are satisfactory, as they carry prognostic implications.

No Single Specific Type of Neurological, Psychological or Behavioral Handicap Characterizes the Outcome After Birth Asphyxia. Any type of motor handicap, seizure disorder, mental retardation, or behavioral problem can be the consequence of a perinatal lesion or dysfunction ranging in severity from complete disaster to very mild dysfunction (Amiel-Tison and Ellison 1986). EEG or CT scan findings later in childhood will be no more specific than the clinical aspects of sequelae: generalized cortical atrophy, porencephaly, and hydrocephalus ex vacuo are not specific findings. This is why it is so important in the neonatal period to consider, with the obstetricians, the whole history to obtain a precise estimate of the perinatal insult as often as possible. After that, it is essential to follow up the child for several years to observe how the clinical aspects change as cerebral function progresses. Detecting each step in the cerebral handicap will provide a clue that no retrospective study will ever be able to offer.

Personal Data on the Incidence of Birth Asphyxia in Term Infants in Two University Maternity Centers

Clinical Methodology Became Stable in 1973. In the first two studies (Amiel-Tison 1969, 1973) all the severe cases and some of the moderate cases were included; mild cases were not properly identified. Since 1973, moderate and mild cases have been identified better and the grades described above have been applied in routine pediatric care. In the third study (Amiel-Tison et al. 1977a), every full-term newborn was included in a formal study where each infant was classified as having severe, moderate, or mild cerebral dysfunction, transient signs (<3 days), or normal. Later on, the same methodology was applied in routine clinical practice (Amiel-Tison et al. 1980; Lebrun et al. 1985).

Trends Observed over a Period of 20 Years. It can be seen from Table 3 that the incidence per 1000 live birth of grade 3 decreased very slowly, from 1.6 to 0.5 per 1000. The trend for grade 2 is completely different: ignored or not properly assessed in the first two studies, the incidence decreased dramatically between 1973-1975 and 1976-1978 from 9.5 to 1.4 per 1000, which is statistically significant with a p value below 0.001. Later on, the incidence of grade 2 continued to decrease, although at a slower rate, to reach the same very low figure as for grade 3. The mild degree, grade 1, also decreased dramatically between 1973-1975 and 1976-1978 and then remained stable around 2-3 per 1000.

As seen above, the borderline between grade 1 and transient signs or normal status is somewhat imprecise, which is not of great consequence since grade 1 has, in most cases, an excellent outcome, as shown Table 2. It is, however, useful to identify these cases for the significance that this situation carries for the obstetricians (warning without cost).

Interpretation of Data. Our conclusion was that FHR monitoring for every delivery and the permanent presence of experienced staff allowed a more active management when signs of fetal distress and/or dystocia occur. The almost complete eradication of grade 2 has been the major achievement of modern obstetrics. This is very important since formerly the incidence was nearly 1% and an unfavorable outcome was observed in about one-third of the cases (Table 2). Classical obstetrics, without FHR monitoring but with appropriate clinical care was already able to obtain a very low incidence of grade 3, to such an extent that it has been very difficult to make any further significant progress. As shown in Baudelocque Maternity Hospital in the last 5 years, safety can be guaranteed for the full-term birth.

Table 3. Cerebral dysfunction in the full-term newborn, according to a classification based on the signs and symptoms observed within the 1st week of life

Publications			Full-term live births (n)	Neurological signs and symptoms						Method for neurological assessment
Years studied	Maternity hospital	Reference		Severe		Moderate		Mild		
				(n)	(per 1000)	(n)	(per 1000)	(n)	(per 1000)	
1962–1964	Baudelocque	Amiel-Tison (1969)	6200	10	1.6	31	5	?		Unstable
1968–1969	Port-Royal	Amiel-Tison (1973)	3257	5	1.5					
						61			18	
1973–1975	Port-Royal	Amiel-Tison et al. (1977a)	1785	2	1.1	17	9.5] *	38	21] *	Stable
1976–1978	Port-Royal	Amiel-Tison et al. (1980)	5825	5	0.9	8	1.4	15	2.6	
1979–1980	Baudelocque	Unpublished	2880	2	0.7	?		?		
1981–1982	Baudelocque	Lebrun et al. (1985)	2364	0	0	1	0.4	5	2.1	
1983–1984			3170	2	0.6	2	0.6	7	2.2	
1985	Baudelocque	Unpublished	2022	1	0.5	1	0.5	7	3.5	

* $p < 0.001$

Comments on the Identification of Etiological Factors in Birth Asphyxia

The Classification of Etiological Factors is Difficult for the Following Reasons: concentrating on birth asphyxia in full-term newborns means firstly the separate classification of any other neurological problems related to fetopathies, prenatal infection, CNS malformation, metabolic diseases, or genetic syndromes. So by definition, cases in which the neurological signs and symptoms are considered a direct consequence of late pregnancy and/or the birth process will be included.

In some cases, the birth process alone is clearly responsible; one typical example is prolapse of the cord at the end of a perfectly normal pregnancy. Such a case will be classified in the group of obstetrical factors. In other cases, the acute accident is clearly related to an abnormal pregnancy, such as an abruptio placentae as a complication of maternal hypertension. Such a case will be classified in the group of gestational factors. In many cases, however, a compromised fetus (due to postmaturity, for example) will not tolerate normal labor well and will demonstrate signs of birth asphyxia. In this kind of situation, it may be difficult to separate the gestational from the obstetrical factors in identifying the etiology. It is why we must classify these cases under the categories of both gestational factors ± obstetrical factors. Using this type of simple classification, our data are shown Table 4.

Obstetrical Factors Were and Still Are Considered as the Only Cause of Birth Asphyxia in About 50% of Cases. A more detailed examination of these obstetrical factors, which have not been completely eradicated in modern obstetrics, enables us to group them into two categories.

- *The first category is an emergency situation,* such as prolapse of the cord, abruptio placentae, or severe bradycardia, in which the clinical indication for an emergency cesarean section is obvious, according to the stage of labor, but there is a delay in performing this cesarean section for technical or decisional reasons.
- *The second category is a situation in which there is more progressive evidence* that something is going wrong in the course of labor, such as organic or functional dystocia with fetal tolerance decreasing as time passes. In these cases, obstetrical decisions are dependent on the interpretation of the judgement on the

Table 4. Etiological factors observed in full-term newborns with signs of cerebral dysfunction

Publications		Obstetrical factors		Gestational ± obstetrical factors	Various or unknown	Total
Years studied	Reference	*(n)*	(%)	*(n)*	*(n)*	*(n)*
1962-1964	Amiel-Tison (1969)	19	46	15	7	41
1973-1975	Amiel-Tison et al. (1977a)	17	53	6	9	32
1976-1978	Amiel-Tison et al. (1980)	14	50	10	4	28
1981-1984	Lebrun et al. (1985)	12	70	5	0	17
1985	Unpublished	5	56	4	0	9

obstetrical situation, FHR, measurement of pH, results of therapeutic actions such as oxytocin and/or analgesia-anesthesia, and the personal experience and confidence of the obstetrician in performing a difficult vaginal delivery. The debate on midforceps delivery is still open and crucial, as discussed recently by Cyr et al. (1984) analyzing their obstetrical results over the last 20 years.

Gestational Factors Are More Difficult to Delineate and Various Biases Make Historical Comparisons More Difficult.

- *First example: displacement* from the "full-term" category to the "preterm" category. This effect is well demonstrated by the recent management of fetus with intrauterine growth retardation (IUGR); when the growth retardation is severe enough, it is diagnosed early in the pregnancy, and fetal risk evaluated precisely enough to indicate cesarean section long before 37 weeks. Therefore, most of these newborn infants are no longer classified in the full-term cohort.
- *Second example: eradication of a category of risk by the routine application of new technologies.* Postmaturity is not tolerated anymore; the echographic determination of gestational age, the determination of fetal wellbeing when term is reached, and the progress in the management of cervical maturation have made it possible to eradicate this cause of birth asphyxia without a significant rise in the cesarean section rate. This is a real advance in obstetrical care.
- *Third example: better evaluation of brain damage resulting in a better identification of gestational factors.* A better identification of prenatal brain lesions is now possible thanks to echography and CT scanning. In the past (in our first two studies, for instance), status epilepticus could be observed with no detected abnormality in gestation or delivery. When FHR was performed routinely in any low-risk labor, it became clear that this was compatible with a completely normal tracing. But the demonstration of the prenatal origin of such cases was only offered by early CT scans. In such cases, when the CT scan performed before day 3 shows well-organized cerebral infarction (Mannino and Trauner 1983; Ment et al. 1984; Voorhies et al. 1984), the prenatal origin can be confirmed (hypoxic-asphyxic cell damage needs 2–3 weeks to organize into residual lesions). More and more cases of this type are now being identified and published, allowing us to establish a provisional list of suggestive gestational

Table 5. Suggestive gestational events or findings compatible with an encephalopathy of fetal origin (infections and malformations excluded) with recent references

Twin pregnancy with one stillborn fetus	Yoshioka et al. (1979)
Carbon monoxide asphyxia	Gosseye et al. (1982)
Maternal hypotension	Erasmus et al. (1982)
Maternal phlebitis	Unpublished
Maternal trauma	Amiel-Tison and Grenier (1986)
Maternal cocaine use	Chasnoff et al. (1986)
Decreasing fetal movements with abnormal FHR pattern ("near-miss" in utero?)	Unpublished
Knots in the cord	Classical
Thrombopenia	Naidu et al. (1983)
Polycythemia	Koffler et al. (1974)

events or findings compatible with such an encephalopathy. A list of these situations is proposed in Table 5, together with recent references. However, the history is fairly often not contributive and cannot provide any clue as to the etiology of a perinatal cerebral infarction. However, the precise diagnosis of such a prenatal lesion is important for the obstetrical staff to show that it is not the consequence of an intrapartum event. Unfortunately, the pathogeny remains obscure and the absence of risk indicators in mother or fetus makes prevention impossible. Clinical evaluation alone is insufficient in establishing the prenatal origin in these cases, as signs and symptoms mimic the clinical picture produced by birth asphyxia. Due to these morphological investigations, a relative shift from intrapartum asphyxia to prenatal asphyxia is now generally observed.

Discussion on Prevention and Cesarean Section Rate

Prophylactic identification of high-risk vaginal deliveries is obviously the first step in preventing birth asphyxia. The careful detection of cephalopelvic disproportion (CPD), by clinical, radiological, and echographic evaluations, is one of the most important recent achievements. The active management in postterm pregnancies is another important step, the safety rules in breech presentation in multiple pregnancies; the detection of IUGR, and the treatment of hypertensive disorders have decreased the risk of abruptio placentae. It is not our aim to review the routine obstetrical practice in every risk situation identified, but to consider that nowadays there is the possibility of detecting and preventing most of the obstetrical complications, and that the end result is an increasing number of elective cesarean sections. In the recent literature, the proportion of elective cesarean sections is about two-thirds of the total number of cesarean sections, whatever the total may be.

Early detection of unexpected obstetrical difficulties in the low-risk full-term fetus is the second step in prevention of birth asphyxia. The circumstances commonly encountered are summarized in three sections in Table 6: umbilical cord problems (maternal and staff education has proven very efficient in preventing prolapse of the cord or minimizing its fetal consequences); first stage problems may find a retrospective explanation in a moderate and unsuspected CPD or may be considered as a functional dystocia. Fetal factors such as the maturation of sutures or the degree of ossification of the skull may add a deleterious influence to the mechanical difficulties due to pelvic dimensions or type of cephalic presentation. Second stage problems, for example, mid-pelvis dystocia or a narrow vulvovaginal outlet, are often unsuspected and may have severe consequences; a decision to perform a cesarean section so late in the course of delivery is not easy; however the consequences of a midforceps and/or a delay in extraction may be dramatic. Whatever the decision is, it is important not to stop FHR monitoring at this stage, both for the obstetrical management itself and for medico-legal reasons.

Sometimes a bacterial infection transmitted from mother to fetus, with or without premature rupture of membranes, may be responsible for fetal tachycardia and decelerations and requires rapid decisions. In a few cases, a severe brady-

Table 6. Unexpected obstetrical difficulties in the low-risk full-term fetus

	Mechanical difficulties	Adverse factors on fetal tolerance	Risk of fetal asphyxia and/or birth trauma
Umbilical cord problems	Prolapse		Severe bradycardia
	Coils around the neck or short umbilical cord	Individual variations in fetal tolerance to ischemic-anoxic insult (metabolic or hormonal factors?)	Decelerations (various patterns)
First stage problems	Unsuspected cephalo-pelvic disproportion	If *hard skull,* poor compliance of sutures, no molding	No engagement with risk of fetal asphyxia
		If *soft skull* (craniotabes) (large anterior fontanelles) excessive molding	Insufficient protection of the brain, risk of arachnoid hemorrhage and brain edema
	Uterine dysfunction		Risk of fetal asphyxia
Second stage problems	Difficult forceps with or without contraction of mid-pelvis		Risk of trauma (subdural hemorrhage, skull fracture)
	Protracted expulsion (hypocinesia, narrow vulvovaginal outlet)		Risk of asphyxia
Any time during labor	None	Unsuspected materno-fetal bacterial infection	Fetal tachycardia + decelerations
	None	None	Unexplained bradycardia

cardia remains totally unexplained, even after careful reappraisal of the whole history. The proportion of cesarean sections decided during labor in any of the situations described in Table 6 reaches about one-third of the total number.

Graded neurological morbidity used as an indicator for safe obstetrics is therefore interesting to study in parallel with the cesarean section rate (Table 7). In the last 5 years in the Baudelocque Maternity Hospital, the safety of full-term birth has been nearly perfect and the cesarean section rate has been between 15% and 20% (Lebrun et al. 1985). An effort has been made by the whole staff to decrease as much as possible the cesarean section rate of 20% which had been reached in 1981-1982; the results show that about the same level of safety was maintained for the newborn by a cesarean section rate of 15%-17%. This means that for the population in this particular university hospital, the cesarean section rate of 15%-17% is compatible with safe obstetrics. Taking into account the maternal risk of an increased cesarean section rate, it is known from experience that an elective cesarean section is safer for the mother than an emergency cesarean section. As recently calculated (Feldman and Freiman 1985), any effort to increase the proportion of elective and decrease the proportion of emergency cesarean sections, the total rate

Table 7. Neurological morbidity in the full-term newborn and cesarean section rate in the last 5 years at the Baudelocque Maternity Hospital (Lebrun et al. 1985)

Full-term live births		Cerebral dysfunction (in full-term births only)						Cesarean section rate (in total population) (%)
Years	*(n)*	Severe		Moderate		Total		
		(n)	(per 1000)	*(n)*	(per 1000)	*(n)*	(per 1000)	
1981-1982	2364	0	0	1	0.4	1	0.4	20.3
1983-1984	3170	2	0.6	2	0.6	4	1.3	14.8
1985	2022	1	0.5	1	0.5	2	1	17.2

remaining unchanged, will be beneficial to the mother. Conversely, if one wants to decrease the total cesarean section rate, it is necessary to attempt vaginal delivery in circumstances such as minimal CPD or previous uterine surgery, even when there is no certainty of success.

Conclusions

Our data show that nearly total safety is obtainable for the full-term bith in level 3 obstetrical centers; this safety is obtained by a combination of careful evaluation of the fetus throughout pregnancy and during delivery. Modern obstetrics has markers which detect the risk of fetal distress early enough to extract a fetus not yet compromised, as long as the decision and execution are fast enough.

The price for this safety is a fairly high rate of cesarean sections. In our experience, rare cases are still unavoidable: intrapartum asphyxia for purely obstetrical reasons is becoming an exception; most prepartum damage is still out of our reach.

References

Amiel-Tison C (1969) Cerebral damage in full-term newborn. Aetiological factors, neonatal status and long term follow-up. Biol Neonate 14: 234-250

Amiel-Tison C (1973) The follow-up of infants presenting neurological abnormalities in the first days of life. In: Brossart H, Cruz JM, Huber A, Prod'hom LS, Sistek J (eds) Perinatal medecine. Huber, Bern, pp 207-218

Amiel-Tison C (1979) Birth injury as a cause of brain dysfunction in full-term newborns. In: Korobkin R, Guilleminault C (eds) Advances in perinatal neurology. Spectrum, New York, pp 57-83

Amiel-Tison C, Ellison P (1986) Birth asphyxia in the full-term newborn. Dev Med Child Neurol 28: 671-682

Amiel-Tison C, Grenier A (eds) (1986) Neurological assessment during the first year of life. Oxford University Press, New York

Amiel-Tison C, Henrion R, Esque-Vaucouloux MT, Goujard J, Firtion G, Tchobroutsky C, Varangot J (1977a) La souffrance cérébrale du nouveau-né à terme. J Gynecol Obstet Biol Reprod (Paris) 6: 971-989

Amiel-Tison C, Korobkin R, Esque-Vaucouloux MT (1977b) Neck extensor hypertonia: a clinical sign of insult to the central nervous system of the newborn. Early Hum Dev 1 (2): 181-190

Amiel-Tison C, Dalisson C, Henrion R (1980) Evolution de la pathologie cérébrale du nouveau-né à terme. Arch Fr Pediatr 37: 87-92

Amiel-Tison C, Barrier G, Shnider SM, Levinson G, Hughes SC, Stefani SJ (1982) A new neurologic and adaptive capacity scoring system for evaluating obstetric medications in full-term newborns. J Anesthesiol 56: 340-350

Amiel-Tison C, Dube R, Garel M, Jequier JC (1983) Outcome at age five years of full-term infants with transient neurologic abnormalities in the first year of life. In: Stern L, Bard H, Friis-Hansen B (eds) Intensive care of the newborn, vol 4. Masson, New York, pp 247-258

Bottoms SF, Rosen MG, Sokol RJ (1980) The increase in the cesarean birth rate. N Engl J Med 302: 559-563

Brazelton TB (ed) (1984) Neonatal behavioral assessment scale, 2nd edn. SIMP, London (Clinics in developmental medecine, 2nd edn, no 88)

Chasnoff IJ, Bussey ME, Savich R, Stack CM (1986) Perinatal cerebral infarction and maternal cocaïne use. J Pediatr 108: 456-459

Cyr RM, Usher RH, McLean FH (1984) Changing patterns of birth asphyxia and trauma over 20 years. Am J Obstet Gynecol 148: 490-498

Erasmus C, Blackwood WA, Wilson J (1982) Infantile multicystic encephalomalacia after maternal bee sting anaphylaxis during pregnancy. Arch Dis Child 57: 785-787

Feldman GB, Freiman JA (1985) Prophylactic cesarean section at term? N Engl J Med 312: 1264-1267

Fitzhardinge PM, Flodmark O, Fitz CR, Ashby S (1981) The prognostic value of computed tomography as an adjunct to assessment of the term infant with postasphyxial encephalopathy. J Pediatr 99: 777-781

Gosseye S, Golaire MC, Larroche JC (1982) Cerebral, renal and splenic lesions due to fetal anoxia and their relationship to malformations. Dev Med Child Neurol 24: 510-518

Koffler H, Keenan WJ, Sutherland JM (1974) Hydranencephaly following elevated hematocrit values in a newly born infant. Pediatrics 54: 770-772

Lacomme M (ed) (1960) Pratique obstétricale. Masson, Paris

Lagercrantz H, Slotkin TA (1986) The "stress" of being born. Sci Am 254: 92-98

Larroche JC (ed) (1976) Developmental pathology of the neonate. Excerpta Medica, Amsterdam

Lebrun F, Cabrol D, Amiel-Tison C (1985) Sécurité de la naissance à terme et taux de césarienne. In: Blanc B, Thoulon JM (eds) 14 et 15èmes Journées Nationales de Médecine Périnatale. Arnette, Paris, pp 49-59

Mannino FL, Trauner DA (1983) Stroke in neonates. J Pediatr 102: 605-610

Ment LP, Duncan CC, Ehrenkranz RA (1984) Perinatal cerebral infarction. Ann Neurol 16: 559-568

Naidu S, Messmore H, Caserta V, Fine M (1983) CNS lesions in neonatal isoimmune thrombocytopenia. Arch Neurol 40: 552-554

Sarnat HB, Sarnat MS (1976) Neonatal encephalopathy following fetal distress. A clinical and electroencephalographic study. Arch Neurol 33: 696-705

Sureau C (1974) The stress of labor. In: Aladjem S, Brown AK (eds) Clinical perinatology. Mosby, St Louis, pp 291-335

Touwen B (ed) (1976) Neurological development in infancy. SIMP, London (Clinics in developmental medecine, no 58)

Valkeakari T (1973) Analysis of serial echoencephalograms in healthy newborn infants during the first week of life. Acta Paediatr Scand [Suppl] 242: 1-62

Voorhies TM, Ehrlich ME, Frayer W, Lee BCP, Vannucci RC (1984) Occlusive vascular disease in asphyxiated newborn infants. J Pediatr 105: 92-96

Yoshioka H, Kadomoto Y, Mino M, Morikawa Y, Kasabuchi Y, Kusunori T (1979) Multicystic encephalomalacia in liveborn twin with a stillborn macerated co-twin. J Pediatr 95: 798-800

Appendix

Neurological evaluation of the newborn infant (Amiel-Tison 1979)

Name: Sex:

Date of birth: Hour:

Gestational age:

Birthweight:

	Days	1	2	3	4	5	6	7
Head circumference (cm)								
Anterior fontanelle	Normal							
	Tense							
	Depressed							
Squamo-parietal suture	Normal							
	Separated							
	Overlapping							
Other sutures	Normal							
	Separated							
	Overlapping							
Caput succedaneum								
Cephalhematoma								
Molding								
Facial ecchymosis								
Alertness	Normal							
	Increased							
	Lethargic							
	Light coma							
	Deep coma							
Crying	Normal							
	Abnormal							
	+Stridor							
	+Color changes							
Jitteriness	Absent							
	Incessant tremor							
	Clonic movements							
	Others							
Motor activity	Normal							
	Diminished							
	Increased							
Seizures	Nil							
	Subtle							
	Focal clonic							
	Multifocal clonic							
	Tonic							
	Status epilepticus							
Hyertonia elevators of upper eyelids	No							
	Yes							

		Days 1	2	3	4	5	6	7
Ocular signs	Nil							
	Setting sun sign							
	Wandering movements							
	Conjugate deviation							
	Staring episodes							
	Sustained nystagmus							
	Marked strabismus							
Pupil	Normal							
	Constricted							
	Dilated							
	Irregular							
Pupillary light reflex	Present							
	Absent							
Pursuit of light	Yes							
	No							
"Deliberate" fixation of gaze	Yes							
	No							
Acoustic blink reflex	Yes							
	No							
Facial palsy	No							
	Yes							
Limb palsy	No							
	Yes							

Passive tone of limbs

		1	2	3	4	5	6	7
Lower limb								
Heal to ear angle	Right							
	Left							
Popliteal angle	Right							
	Left							
Dorsiflexion angle of the foot	Right							
	Left							
Ankle clonus	Right							
	Left							
Adductor angle. Indicate whether wider on right or left	(R,L)							
Symmetry of foot flapping	R > L							
	L > R							
Upper limb								
Full flexion at elbow	Right							
	Left							
Recoil of elbows following extension	Right							
	Left							
Scarf sign (1, 2, 3)	Right							
	Left							

	Days	1	2	3	4	5	6	7
Symmetry of wrist flexion	R>L							
	L>R							
Symmetry of hand flapping	R>L							
	L>R							

Enter conclusion for each day for this data, taking account of GA

	1	2	3	4	5	6	7
Normal							
Generalized hypertonia							
Generalized hypotonia							
Hypotonia predominating in upper part of the body							
Hemisyndrome							

Axial tone (passive and active)

		1	2	3	4	5	6	7
Spontaneous posture	Normal							
	Hyperextension of neck							
	Opisthotonos							
Free space behind neck	No							
	Yes							
Ventral flexion of the trunk	Normal							
	Exaggerated							
	Impossible							
Dorsal extension of the trunk	Normal (impossible)							
	Exaggerated							
Opisthotonos provoked by lifting shoulders	No							
	Yes							
Response to repeated ventral flexion of the head	No increase of stiffness							
	Increasing stiffness							
Active contraction of neck flexors on forwards movement of the trunk (from lying position)	Normal							
	Difficult							
	Absent (passive movement only)							
	Impossible (neck extensors active)							
Active contraction of neck extensors on backwards movement of the trunk (from leaning forward position)	Normal							
	Difficult							
	Absent (passive movement only)							
	"Too good"							
Straightening of lower limbs (in upright position)	Yes							
	No							
Straightening of trunk (in upright position)	Yes							
	No							

Primary reflexes

		1	2	3	4	5	6	7
Sucking swallowing	Normal							
	Poor							
	Absent							

	Days	1	2	3	4	5	6	7
Moro's reaction test	Normal							
	+Clonic movements							
	+Low threshold							
	No opening of hands							
	No crying							
	Absent							
Palmar grasp	Normal							
	Poor							
	Absent							
Response to traction (active tone)	Normal							
	Poor							
	Absent							
Plantar grasp	Normal							
	Poor							
	Absent							
Automatic walking	Normal							
	Poor							
	Absent							

Others

Laboratory findings

Spinal fluid	Normal							
	Yellowish							
	Hemorrhagic							
	Protein (mg/100 ml)							
	Glucose (mg/100 ml)							
	WBC per mm^3							
	RBC per mm^3							

Skull rays

Optic fundi

EEG

Subdural tap

Transfontanelar echography or CT scan

Others

Treatment

Phenobarbitone (mg/kg/24 h)							
Diazepam (mg/kg/24 h)							
Mannitol (g/kg/24 h)							
Others							

Days	1	2	3	4	5	6	7
General conclusions							
Head findings							
Probable intracranial hypertension							
Probable "catch-up growth" of head							
Insufficient growth of head							
Microcephaly							
Hydrocephaly							
Macrocephaly							
Seizures							
Status epilepticus							
Isolated seizures							
Hyperexcitability							
Lethargy							
Coma							
Passive tone abnormalities							
Generalized hypertonia							
Generalized hypotonia							
Hypotonia predominating in upper half of body							
Hemisyndrome							
Hyperextension of the neck (postural)							
Opisthotonos (postural or passive)							
Active tone abnormalities							
Hypertonia of neck extensors							
No active response of neck flexors							
No straightening of lower limbs							
No straightening of trunk							
Reflex activity							
Hyporeflexia							
Areflexia							
Intracranial hemorrhage							
Others							

Breech Delivery in the Term Fetus – Relation to Neuromotor Dysfunction and Mental Handicap

H. MANZKE

Causes of Cerebral Damage

The cerebral damage of infants born in breech presentation can be classified by cause into three major groups.

Cerebral Lesions Due to Birth Trauma, Specifically Caused by Hyperextension of the Fetal Head, Pressure on the Suboccipital Region, Traction of the Spinal Cord, and Damage of the Vertebral Arteries. About 5% of the breech presentations occur in conjunction with hyperextension of the fetal head. Follow-up studies (Caterini et al. 1975; Westgren et al. 1981) have revealed that more than 20% of these vaginally delivered infants had neurological sequelae referable to spinal, superspinal, and cerebellar injuries, but all infants born by cesarean section were normal. The diagnosis can be determined prior to delivery by X-ray or ultrasound but is frequently an unexpected finding. This has been in itself an indication for routine X-rays of every patient in labor with breech presentation (Kirchhoff and Neumeyer 1978), and, more recently, makes a careful ultrasonographic examination mandatory.

Wigglesworth and Husemeyer (1977) pointed to the occurrence of occipital osteodiastasis, tears of tentorium, and laceration of the cerebellum in term breech infants delivered vaginally. The injury is produced by increased pressure of the fetal subocciput against the symphysis pubis of the mother. Ataxic cerebral palsy would be the neurological disorder one might expect to find in survivors. Dyskinesia may occur in various forms such as unvoluntary choreoathetoid movements, nystagmus, and intention tremor.

As for lesions of the spine and spinal cord, strong traction exerted when the spine is hyperextended or when the direction of pull is lateral, may produce fracture and separations of the vertebrae. The injury occurs most commonly at the level of the seventh cervical or first thoracic vertebra. Infants who survive typically show hypotonia combined with hyperreflexia and dysesthesia of the arms (Haidvogl et al. 1978; Bucher et al. 1979).

In infants who died after breech delivery, Yates (1970) found various degrees of damage of the vertebral arteries, which carry the blood to the brain stem, the cerebellum, and the occipitotemporal regions of the brain. He assumed that, due to obstruction of these arteries in nonlethal cases, infarction might occur in parts of the brain not yet identifiably functioning at birth. At a later age this might lead to dysfunction of cranial nerves causing strabismus, sensory auditory disturbances, hyperkinesia, and cerebral palsy of the cerebellar ataxic type.

Although the etiology of the hypopituitary dwarfism is uncertain, a number of authors assume that perinatal lesions of the pituitary stalk may be a major factor. Nearly two-thirds of the patients with hypopituitarism were born in breech presentation (Van der Werff ten Bosch 1962; Bierich 1972).

Cerebral Lesions Caused by Hypoxia Following Either Intrapartal Asphyxia or Postnatal Respiratory Distress, Particularly in Premature Infants. Specific perils result from prolapse of the umbilical cord at the fetal membrane rupture, cord compression during the expulsion period, meconium aspiration, premature abruptio placentae (Koller 1983), and mechanical difficulties in the delivery of the shoulders and the arms as well as of the subsequently emerging head. Also, one often finds placenta anomalies, such as hypoplasia of the placenta or faulty insertion of the umbilical cord (Koller 1983).

According to Kubli et al. (1975, 1976) the risk of acidemia in vaginal breech delivery is three to ten times greater than in vertex delivery (pH of umbilical artery blood <7.10). The disastrous sequelae of severe birth asphyxia and postnatal respiratory distress are well known. They do not differ from hypoxic cerebral damage attributable to perinatal complications other than breech delivery.

Cerebral Lesions Often Associated with Breech Presentation, but not Caused by the Birth Process Itself. In such cases fetal abnormalities have favored breech presentation, for instance, in infants with spina bifida (48% of the cases) or with reduction malformations of the lower extremities (60% of the cases). Congenital malformations have been found almost three times as often in breech-delivered newborns as in cephalic ones (Brenner et al. 1974; Dunn 1976). Neuromuscular dysfunctions, in particular, may limit the ability of the fetus to assume vertex position because the rotation of the fetus requires active movements of the fetus itself. Therefore, great care must be taken to examine breech-born infants for malformations and functional disorders soon after delivery or, if possible, before delivery by ultrasonographic studies.

Nearly one-third of all infants born in breech presentation are premature. This is the principal cause why the perinatal mortality and early morbidity rates of the breech-delivered infants are markedly higher than those of the vertex-delivered infants. In order to eliminate the influence of prematurity on the child's development, only the findings of term breech-delivered infants will be considered in the following critical review of follow-up studies.

Follow-up Studies Without Specific Neurological Tests

There are many reasons why the breech infant is born asphyxiated more often than the cephalic one. The percentages of surviving infants with Apgar scores below 6 taken at 5 min after delivery are shown in Table 1 [from the prospective

Table 1. Apgar scores after 5 min in singleton infants born in breech ($n=239$) and in vertex presentation. Data from the prospective follow-up study *"Schwangerschaftsverlauf und Kindesentwicklung"* (DFG) 1966-1972

Apgar score after 5 min	Breech presentation				Vertex presentation	
	Vaginally born ($n=171$)		Cesarean section ($n=68$)		Vaginally born ($n=5096$)	
	(n)	(%)	*(n)*	(%)	*(n)*	(%)
<6	25	14.6	1	1.5	82	1.6
6- 8	20	11.7	5	7.4	107	2.1
9-10	126	73.7	62	91.2	4907	96.3

Table 2. Incidence of abnormal neurological findings in singleton infants up to 3 years of age born in breech and in vertex presentation. Data from the prospective follow-up study *"Schwangerschaftsverlauf und Kindesentwicklung"* (DFG) 1966-1972

Neurological findings Age		Breech presentation Vaginally born	Cesarean section	Vertex presentation Vaginally born	X^2 test p
At 6 weeks					
Abnormal neurological findings	(%)	9.6*	4.4	3.2	<0.01
	(n)	10/104	2/46	119/3763	
Cannot raise head from prone	(%)	5.0	2.2	2.8	NS
	(n)	5/100	1/46	105/3652	
At 9 months					
Abnormal neurological findings	(%)	5.2	2.2	3.9	NS
	(n)	5/96	1/45	144/3668	
At 18 months					
Abnormal neurological findings	(%)	2.1	2.2	1.3	NS
	(n)	2/95	1/46	47/3640	
At 3 years					
Abnormal neurological findings	(%)	2.0	2.0	1.3	NS
	(n)	2/98	1/49	48/3753	
Mental retardation	(%)	4.7	1.7	2.4	NS
	(n)	5/107	1/58	99/4157	

* Significant difference

follow-up study *"Schwangerschaftsverlauf und Kindesentwicklung"* (course of pregnancy and child development) *(Deutsche Forschungsgemeinschaft)*]. The overall incidence of cesarean sections within the group of breech infants was 28.5%.

Re-examinations of the same infants, carried out at regular intervals, revealed that there were significantly more frequent neurological abnormalities in the vaginally breech-born infants than in the cephalic ones only at the age of 6 weeks. The percentages are shown in Table 2. Neurological testing at the ages of 9 months, 18 months, and 3 years did not show any statistically significant differences between the breech and nonbreech groups. For instance, at the age of 3 years, 2%

of the breech-delivered infants had abnormal neurological signs against 1.3% of the vertex-delivered infants.

However, the neurological methods utilized to single out children with minor disabilities were rather crude. This is the reason why a great number of follow-up studies performed by other authors cannot hold up to critical evaluation (Manzke 1978; Faber-Nijholt et al. 1983). Furthermore, the younger the infants, the poorer the predictability of the test results obtained during the early years. The reason for this is that the growth of intelligence and of motor skills is a dynamic process. Even normal infants vary widely in their development rate. On the other hand, children with transient abnormal neurological signs in the first years of life may catch up when treated adequately.

A number of requirements have to be set down for perinatal follow-up studies: sufficiently large populations representing random selections of the whole population; appropriate control groups; collaboration between clinics; multidisciplinary and multi-institutional teamwork among different specialists; follow-up examinations at regular intervals over more than 3 years; collection of interval data by questionnaires between the examinations; standardized and age-specific tests on the physical, neurological, and psychological development of the children including their development of vision, hearing, and language. The registration of the drop-outs in the follow-up studies is an unsolved problem. According to our own experience, it is the late cases of neonatal morbidity and mortality that tend to be lost unless special means are devised. The background data should comprise the family history and the socioeconomic situation of the family. Furthermore, it is necessary to register in detail the course of pregnancy and labor and the management of delivery. If necessary, a macroscopic and histological examination of the placenta should be performed.

There are no follow-up studies which meet all these criteria, including the American prospective follow-up study "Collaborative Project on Cerebral Palsy, Mental Retardation and other Neurological and Sensory Disorders of Infancy and Childhood" (Berendes 1964) and the German prospective follow-up study *"Schwangerschaftsverlauf und Kindesentwicklung."*

Follow-up Studies Applying Sophisticated Methods

Taking these facts into account, nearly 2000 children of the prospective study *"Schwangerschaftsverlauf und Kindesentwicklung"* were re-examined thoroughtly at the age of 6 years by pediatricians, ophthalmologists, otolaryngologists, and psychologists. Among the children tested there were 58 singleton breech-born infants. In order to investigate the extent to which neurological or mental abnormalities in breech-born infants may be due to the mode of delivery itself, the subjects were subdivided into those born by vaginal delivery and those born by cesarean section. The first group comprised 43 children and the second group 15. For comparison, the first baby born in the same clinic by spontaneous cephalic delivery after each breech-born subject was taken as the control. Furthermore, the breech born infants were matched according to sex, birthweight, and socioeconomic background. No child had gross malformation. The intelligence test batteries consisted of the Columbia mental maturity scale, the Raven coloured matrices test and the Peabody picture vocabulary test. The motoric functional status was assessed via the Hamm-Marburger coordination test and a neurologic motoscopic score especially designed by us. The neurologic motoscopic score consists of 22 items such as standing on one foot for longer than 10 s or a finger-nose test. A low-score index of 22 points was the best, as against other tests where the higher the rates the better the achievements. As Table 3 shows, the mean values of the probands and their controls differ only slightly. For instance, in the Columbia mental maturity scale the mean value for the vaginally breech-born infants amounts to 59.1 points and for the controls it was 62.6 points. However, using the Wilcoxon matched pair test, the differences of the three intelligence tests as well as of the two fine motoric tests were significant between the vaginally breech-born infants and their controls. But, the differences between the cesarean section-delivered children and their controls did not show any significance.

The results of the psychometric tests of all children ($n = 1651$) at the age of 6 years are presented in Table 4 (Manzke 1984). It is noticeable, that all mean values (Tables 3 and 4) belong to the higher range of the age-specific standard values. This is undoubtedly due to the fact that children from the upper social classes were over-represented in our whole series.

Cerebral dysfunction, if the term is used diagnostically for different disorders such as learning or behavioral disabilities as well as neurological defects, could be diagnosed in six children. Three of these were vaginally breech-born infants, one was born by cesarean section, and two were controls. This rate of six children with cerebral dysfunction among a total number of 108 children is normal.

The electroencephalograms obtained from nearly all children showed no significant differences between the findings of the probands and their controls. None of the children had clinically manifested epilepsy. Also, the rate of visual and auditory disorders did not differ significantly between the study groups and the control groups (Manzke 1984).

Table 3. Results of psychological and neurological-motoscopic examination of 58 breech-born children and their controls at the age of 6 years. Data from the prospective study *"Schwangerschaftsverlauf und Kindesentwicklung"* (DFG) 1966-1972

Tests	Breech-born vaginally ($n = 43$)	Matched pairs ($n = 43$)	Breech-born by cesarean section ($n = 15$)	Matched pairs ($n = 15$)
Columbia mental maturity scale	59.1 ± 11.4*	62.6 ± 8.5	66.6 ± 12.7	67.1 ± 11.6
Raven (colored matrices) test	17.7 ± 4.3*	19.7 ± 4.8	22.2 ± 6.8	23.2 ± 6.9
Peabody picture vocabulary test	54.6 ± 5.8**	57.2 ± 5.7	60.1 ± 5.6	57.7 ± 5.4
Hamm-Marburger body coordination test	61.3 ± 22.9**	67.3 ± 23.8	60.5 ± 24.9	63.7 ± 26.1
Neurological-motoscopic score	25.4 ± 4.0*	24.0 ± 2.5	24.8 ± 3.3	26.2 ± 5.5

* Significance at 5% level
** Significance at 1% level (Wilcoxon matched pairs test)

Our results are consistent with two other prospective studies recently published. Both studies are based on thorough physical checkups of the children by experienced pediatricians, including standardized age-specific neurological tests aimed at also discovering minor to minimal neurological dysfunctions.

Table 5 demonstrates the results of the neurological examinations performed in 217 matched pairs at ages between 3 and 10 years. The data are from the Perinatal Project Groningen (Faber-Nijholt 1981). There is a significant difference in the frequency of neurological abnormalities between the group of the vertex- and the group of the breech-born infants to the disadvantage of the breech-born infants. The percentage of normal cases amounts to 64% and 52.5%, respectively. This difference is caused mainly by the cases with suspect abnormalities (19.4% and 28.6%, respectively) and to a lesser degree by the cases with mild abnormalities (16.1% and 18.4%, respectively), whereas only one severely handicapped child was found in both groups. The cesarean section rate of the breech-born infants was 20.0%.

A detailed study of the neurological abnormalities showed that the neurological syndrome dyskinesia appeared to be frequent both in the vertex group and in the breech group, that is 56% and 58%, respectively (Table 6). Sensorimotor distur-

Table 4. Results of psychometric and neurological-motoscopic examinations of all children (n=1651) tested at the age of 6 years. Data from the prospective study *"Schwangerschaftsverlauf und Kindesentwicklung"* (DFG)

Tests	$\bar{x}$ ±SD*	SE⁺	Range	Skewness	Kurtosis
Raven test (colored matrices)	18.82± 4.84	0.12	4- 35	0.413	0.178
Columbia mental maturity scale	63.85± 9.82	0.24	1- 97	−0.352	3.124
Peabody picture vocabulary test	56.62± 7.08	0.17	3- 94	−0.675	9.421
Hamm-Marburger body coordination test	65.82±25.41	0.64	4-147	0.330	−0.320

* standard deviation
\+ standard error

Table 5. Results of the neurological examinations in 217 matched pairs at ages between 3 and 10 years. Distribution of the neurological findings in both groups. Data from the perinatal project Groningen (Faber-Nijholt 1981)

Presentation	Normal		Suspect		Abnormal				Total	
					Mild		Severe			
	(n)	(%)	*(n)*	(%)	*(n)*	(%)	*(n)*	(%)	*(n)*	(%)
Vertex	139	64.0	42	19.4	35	16.1	1	0.5	217	100.0
Breech	114	52.5	62	28.6	40	18.4	1	0.5	217	100.0
Total	253	58.3	104	23.9	75	17.3	2	0.5	434	100.0

X^2=6.62; df=2; p<0.05 (combination of the classes mild and severe)

Table 6. Neurological syndromes in the group of abnormal children and number of syndromes per child in this group. Comparison between vertex- and breech-born infants. Data from the Perinatal Project Groningen (Faber-Nijholt 1981)

Neurological syndromes	Vertex presentation (n=36)		Breech presentation (n=41)	
	(n)	(%)	(n)	(%)
Nature				
Dyskinesias	20	56	24	58
Coordination difficulties	12	33	21	51
Sensorimotor disturbances	18	50	19	46
Sensory disturbances	4	11	11	27
Hemisyndrome	7	19	6	15
Number				
One syndrome	16	44	15	37
Two syndromes	15	42	14	34
Three syndromes	5 (1[a])	14	10	24
Four syndromes	–		2 (1[a])	5
Total	36	100	41	100

[a] Handicapped child

bances and coordination difficulties also occurred rather frequently in both groups. The syndrome "sensorimotor disturbances" consists of double-sided dysfunctions in muscle tone, muscle consistency, muscle power, and reflex anomalies. A hemisyndrome occurred in seven vertex-born and six breech-born children, and sensory disturbances, i.e., auditory and visual disturbances, were found in four vertex- and 11 breech-born children. In summary, the frequency of dyskinesia, sensorimotor disturbances, and hemisyndromes did not differ in the two groups. Coordination difficulties and sensory disturbances, however, were encountered two to three times more often among the breech-born than among the vertex-born children.

The second prospective study was conducted in Lund. In this 4-year follow-up study the Swedish authors (Svenningsen et al. 1985) evaluated the long-term outcomes of 709 singleton term breech-born infants. The outcome was related to different management protocols during two consecutive study periods. In the first period from 1971 to 1974 the rate of cesarean section was 16.1% and in the second period from 1974 to 1977, 37.1%. In the first period an elective cesarean section was performed routinely if the anteroposterior diameter of the pelvic inlet was less than 11 cm and in the second period if the diameter of the inlet was less than 12 cm or less than 2 cm above the biparietal diameter measured with ultrasound. Finally, at the end of the second period, hyperextension of the fetal head became an additional indication for cesarean section. The follow-up examinations were carried out according to neurodevelopmental scales for Swedish children.

Table 7 shows the neurodevelopmental sequelae at 4 years of age in 480 breech-born infants. The total incidence of pathological findings (cerebral palsy, psychomotor retardation, minimal brain damage syndrome, epilepsy) decreased from 5.3% in the first period to 2.4% in the second period. The percent-

Table 7. Neurodevelopmental sequelae at 4 years of age in 480 breech-born infants. Data from the Prospective Follow-up Study Lund (Svenningsen et al. 1985)

	Period A (n=233)		Period B (n=247)		Vertex (n=1202)
	VD	CS	VD	CS	VD
Number of infants	185	48	155	92	1202
Cerebral palsy	5		2	1	3
Psychomotor retardation	2	1	1		4
MBD syndrome	3	1	1	1	10
Epilepsy	1				1
Total *(n)*	11	2	4	2	18
(%)	6.0	4.2	2.9	2.2	1.5
Combined total in each period (%)	(5.3)		(2.4)		(1.5)

p values: A vs. BNS; A vs. vertex <0.05; B vs. vertex NS
Period A, 1971-1974; Period B, 1974-1977
VD, vaginal delivery; CS, cesarean section; MBD, minimal brain damage

age of pathological findings within a control group of 1202 children born in vertex presentation was 1.5%.

Comparing these three groups, there was only a significant difference of the incidence of neurodevelopmental sequelae between the breech-born infants of the first period and the vertex-born infants. The rates of visual and auditory disorders as well as of behavioral problems did not differ between the study groups and the control groups. In most cases the neurodevelopmental sequelae of the first period could be related to labor problems such as footling, hyperextension of the fetal head and/or inadequate antero-posterior diameter at the brim. The results of the Swedish authors are in accordance with the findings of Hochuli et al. (1977), who also used routine X-ray pelvimetry and ultrasound fetal cephalometry (and thoracometry) in breech deliveries. With a cesarean section rate of 34.3%, they found no difference in the mortality and morbidity rates in breech-born infants delivered vaginally or by cesarean section.

Conclusions

An analysis of the literature reveals that the fetal mortality and morbidity rates of the infants born in breech presentation have decreased about two to three times over the last 30 years (Manzke 1978). At the same time, an increased cesarean section rate is evident. But it is not this technique itself, but more sophisticated indication that has produced better results. Characteristic cerebral damages caused by the pathomechanism of the vaginal breech delivery have become rare.

From the results of the two prospective follow-up studies in Groningen and Lund as well as from our results of the prospective study *"Schwangerschaftsverlauf und Kindesentwicklung"* we can conclude that, today, there are only slight differences in the late morbidity rate between the infants born in breech and those born in vertex position, which can be discovered only by applying sophisticated neurological and psychological tests.

It is uncertain if these differences are referable to the mechanism of the breech delivery itself. Some infants are born in breech delivery because of a certain congenital abnormality or because they have got orthopedic and neurological problems from their long-term pathological position in utero. Thus, it seems doubtful that a further increase of the cesarean section rate could improve the prognosis for the development of the infants born in breech position.

References

Berendes HW (1964) Obstetrical complications and mental deficiency. International Copenhagen Congress on the Scientifique Study of Mental Retardation, vol 1, pp 308-316

Bierich JR (1972) On the aetiology of hypopituitary dwarfism. Growth and growth hormone. Excerpta Med Int Congr Ser 244: 408-414

Brenner WE, Bruce R, Hendricks CH (1974) The characteristics and perils of breech presentation. Am J Obstet Gynecol 118: 700-712

Bucher HU, Bolshauser E, Friderich J, Isler W (1979) Birth injury to the spinal cord. Helv Paediatr Acta 34: 517-527

Caterini H, Langer A, Sama JC, Devanesan M, Pelosi MA (1975) Fetal risk in hyperextension of the fetal head in breech presentation. Am J Obstet Gynecol 123: 632-636

Dunn PM (1976) Maternal and fetal aetiological factors. In: Rooth G, Bratteby L-E (eds) Perinatal medicine. Almquvist and Wiksell, Stockholm, pp 76-81

Faber-Nijholt R (ed) (1981) Breech-presentation and neurological morbidity. A comparative study. Dissertation, University of Groningen

Faber-Nijholt R, Huisjes HJ, Touwen BCL, Fidler VJ (1983) Neurological follow-up of 281 children born in breech presentation: a controlled study. Br Med J 286: 9-12

Haidvogl M, Borkenstein M, Stix H, Fritsch G (1978) Geburtstraumatische Rückenmarksläsionen. Wien Med Wochenschr 128: 63-67

Hochuli E, Dubler O, Bornhauser E, Schoop E (1977) Die kindliche Entwicklung nach vaginaler und abdominaler Entbindung bei Beckenendlagen. Geburtshilfe Frauenheilkd 37: 4-11

Kirchhoff H, Neumeyer H (1978) Über den gravierenden Aussagewert der seitlichen Röntgenaufnahme für die Leitung der Geburt aus Beckenendlage. Geburtshilfe Frauenheilkd 38: 895-903

Koller S (1983) Risikofaktoren der Schwangerschaft. Springer, Berlin Heidelberg New York, pp 264-268

Kubli F, Rüttgers H, Meyer-Menk M (1975) Die fetale Azidosegefährdung bei vaginaler Geburt aus Beckenendlage. Z Geburtshilfe Perinatol 179: 1-16

Kubli F, Boos W, Rüttgers H (1976) Caesarean section in the management of singleton breech presentation. In: Rooth G, Bratteby LE (eds) Perinatal medicine. Almquvist and Wiksell, Stockholm, pp 69-75

Lilienfeld AM, Pasamanick B (1955) The association of mental and fetal factors with the development of cerebral palsy and epilepsy. Am J Obstet Gynecol 70: 93-103

Manzke H (1978) Morbidity among infants born in breech presentation. J Perinatol Med 6: 127-140

Manzke H (1984) Entwicklungsprognose von Kindern mit perinatalen Risikofaktoren. Fischer, Stuttgart

Neligan GA (1976) The quality of the survivors of breech delivery in a geographically defined population. In: Rooth G, Bratteby LE (eds) Perinatal medicine. Almquvist and Wiksell, Stockholm, pp 61-64

Svenningsen NW, Westgren M, Ingemarsson I (1985) Modern strategy for the term breech delivery - a study with a 4-year follow-up of the infants. J Perinatol Med 13: 117-126
Van der Werff ten Bosch JJ (1962) Hypofysaire dwerggroci. Ned T Geneeskd 106: 1282-1286
Westgren M, Grundsell H, Ingemarsson I, Mühlow A, Svenningsen NW (1981) Hyperextension of the fetal head in breech presentation: a study with long-term follow-up. J Obstet Gynaecol 88: 101-104
Wigglesworth JS, Husemeyer RP (1977) Intracranial birth trauma in vaginal breech delivery: the continued importance of injury to the occipital bone. Br J Obstet Gynaecol 84: 684-691
Yates PO (1970) In: Angle CR, Bering EA (eds) Physical trauma as an etiologic agent in mental retardation. Government Printing Office, Washington, p 167

Intracranial Hemorrhage and Ischemia

Pathological Anatomy of Intraventricular Haemorrhage in the Preterm Baby

J. S. WIGGLESWORTH

Introduction

To discuss the pathological anatomy of a haemorrhage is a somewhat uninteresting task as the main feature is blood which differs little from one bleed to another! I shall therefore be discussing the lesion complex of the preterm infant within which bleeding into the ventricles is a characteristic feature. I shall outline the main accepted structural components and evolution of this lesion complex and the theories on pathogenic mechanisms which can be derived mainly from consideration of the structure. I shall not stray too far into cerebral circulatory physiology however as this falls within the area to be discussed by Dr. Lou.

Historical Aspects

During the early part of this century when, as I discussed in my earlier paper, cranial trauma and asphyxia were the most important forms of perinatal pathology, bleeding into the ventricles was regarded as an uncommon occurrence. The condition was recognised by Yllpo (1919) as a problem of the preterm infant, to be separated from traumatic forms of intracranial bleeding, and a series of 20 cases was collected by Hemsath (1934). Hemsath described and illustrated clearly the bleeding into the subependymal matrix near the foramen of Monro, rupture into the lateral ventricle and spread throughout the ventricular system. As the frequency of death in term infants declined, so the relative importance of lesions in preterm infants increased. Grontoft (1953) claimed that the bleeds were derived from the thalamostriate vein and postulated that rupture of this vein occurred as a result of raised venous pressure. Harcke et al. (1972) showed an association of the haemorrhage with respiratory distress syndrome and Towbin (1968) claimed, on the basis of examining whole brain sections, that the lesion was a form of venous infarction. Larroche (1977) recognised both rupture of vein branches and venous thrombosis in association with the bleeds. Coen et al. (1970) suggested that the bleeding might be of arterial origin, but could not determine the nature of the small vessels which ruptured. Leech and Kohnen (1974) pointed out that the bleeds, although originating most often in the area of the foramen of Monro, might occur from any site of subependymal matrix including the temporal horn and roof of the fourth ventricle. By the mid-1970s, with considerable expenditure on neonatal intensive care, the frequency of death with massive intraventricular haemorrhage (IVH) in mechanically ventilated preterm infants prompted further urgent investigation into its pathogenesis. The vascular injection studies of Hambleton and Wigglesworth (1976) indicated that the haemorrhage represented a disruption of the microcirculation within the subependymal matrix, although the bleeds often developed near the capillary-vein junctions seen in this tissue and mimicked primary vein rupture. Since that time pathological studies have been overshadowed by imaging studies carried out in life and physiological studies on cerebral circulation.

Current Patterns of Presentation of Subependymal/Intraventricular Haemorrhage to the Pathologist

The earlier stages of the lesion complex are seen in very low birth weight infants who die in the first few hours after birth. In fetuses aborted in the 20–24-weeks age group the bleeding may commence during birth as we find early subependymal and intraventricular bleeds in a high proportion of such cases. The initial subependymal haemorrhage is most often situated over the head of the caudate nucleus opposite to the foramen of Monro, but may appear more posteriorly over the body of the caudate in infants below 28 weeks' gestation (Hambleton and Wigglesworth 1976). Careful study of the brain may show additional subependymal bleeds elsewhere and there is often an associated bleed into the choroid plexus (Leech and Kohnen 1974; Larroche 1977). The relatively large size of the subependymal bleed in the classic site often causes coincidental bleeds elsewhere to be overlooked. In infants of 34 weeks', or more, gestation, primary choroid plexus bleeds are the most frequent site of origin of IVH (Pape and Wigglesworth 1979). There are a number of possible modes of spread of the initial subependymal bleed. Small bleeds often remain localised and gradually become transformed into a subependymal pseudocyst which eventually disappears. Larger bleeds may rupture into the lateral ventricle at an early stage. Following rupture, there is a variable spread of blood through the ventricular system. A clot usually forms around and attached to the choroid plexus as well as to the site of origin and may spread through the foramen of Monro to the opposite ventricle or third ventricle. In some cases the foramen of Monro appears to be occluded by the clot and there may be a mass of clot filling and dilating one ventricle with little spread beyond it. In cases with bilateral haemorrhages filling the whole ventricular system the blood extends variably into the subarachnoid space forming a clot over the inferior surface of the cerebellum or extending over the base of the brain and into the sylvian fissures.

In addition to these well-known patterns of spread through the ventricular system, sequential studies have shown the frequent occurrence of apparent extensions of the primary subependymal bleed out into the parenchyma (Levene and De Vries 1984). These extensions are regarded as of particular clinical importance as they involve destruction of brain parenchyma and might therefore be expected to lead to greater handicap in survivors than uncomplicated ventricular bleeds. The possible nature of these extensions will be discussed below.

At a later stage, the initial clot becomes discoloured and slowly breaks down although dilatation of the ventricular system may persist, and obstruction of the aqueduct by necrotic debris or development of an arachnoiditis around the cerebellum may lead to a progressive posthaemorrhagic hydrocephalus (Larroche 1972).

The microscopic anatomy of subependymal haemorrhage is banal, comprising lakes of blood within the cellular subependymal matrix. In some areas the blood may be seen to cuff the congested thin-walled veins. Small masses of fibrin are sometimes present within the primary bleed. Hambleton and Wigglesworth (1976) related such fibrin masses to areas where there had been rupture at a capillary-vein junction. One of the features of the subependymal matrix noted by these authors was the presence of small capillaries entering directly into the large thalamostriate vein branches. These appeared to represent a possible point of weakness, as an artificial injection mass infused through the arteries at postmortem examination also tended to leak from this site.

Deductions on Pathogenesis Derived from Pathological Anatomy

Recognition of the primary subependymal bleed as being due to breakdown of the microcirculation rather than rupture of a particular larger vessel caused attention to be shifted away from the pressures which might be inflicted on major vein walls and towards the problems of cerebral blood flow and circulatory control in the preterm infant. From the anatomy of the cerebral vessels, as shown in the injection studies of Hambleton and Wigglesworth (1976), it was apparent that any increase in cerebral blood flow in the preterm infant would tend to be directed towards the central portions of the cerebrum and might well cause a dramatic increase in flow through the subependymal matrix. It was also recognised that most of the infants seen with IVH, and virtually all those of more than 30 weeks' gestation, had respiratory distress syndrome associated with hypercapnia and hypoxia which would be expected to abolish autoregulatory mechanisms if present and increase cerebral blood flow. The recognition of the frequent association of ischaemic lesions with the haemorrhages, and the physiological studies carried out by Lou et al. (1977), indicated that high and low flow conditions must alternate in various ways to lead to the mixture of pathological lesions seen (Wigglesworth and Pape 1978).

Pathology of Parenchymal Extension from Subependymal Haemorrhage

The extensions of subependymal bleeding into the adjacent white matter were regarded by Pape and Wigglesworth (1979) as venous infarcts on the basis of study of specimens which had been cleared into methylsalicylate in order to show the vessel pattern. Large dilated vein branches could be seen extending beyond the haemorrhagic zone. As the size and extent of the parenchymal haemorrhage seemed directly related to the size of the initial subependymal bleed, it was considered that the thalamostriate vein branches had been obstructed by the primary haemorrhage with consequent venous infarction. This sequence would explain the finding of venous infarction reported by Towbin (1968). It had previously been pointed out by Armstrong and Norman (1974) that massive bleeding into the periventricular white matter of newborn infants might represent bleeding into an area of periventricular leucomalacia. A recent paper (Rushton et al. 1985) suggests that parenchymal extensions of subependymal bleeds occur by a similar process of bleeding into areas of periventricular leucomalacia.

The importance of the distinction between the two possibilities is that the presence of underlying cerebral ischaemia would imply more extensive cerebral damage, and probably more severe permanent neurological deficit, than localised venous infarction. Studies currently in progress at University College Hospital support the concept of venous infarction as the underlying mechanism, as do the positron emission tomography studies of Volpe et al. (1983).

In our own recent material we have found that in cases where periventricular flares have been recognised on ultrasound before the development of subependymal and parenchymal bleeds there is indeed evidence of bleeding into a pre-existing area of periventricular leucomalacia, whereas in the more usual case, where the subependymal bleed is the first form of pathology to become apparent, the subsequent extension has the characteristics of a venous infarct. On microscopy an area of underlying periventricular leucomalacia is recognised as an area of coagulative necrosis with associated proliferation of astroglia and infiltration of macrophages. Haemorrhage into such an area appears in the form of coalescent petechiae unrelated to any larger vessels. In contrast, venous infarction is seen as areas of haemorrhage surrounding dilated thalamostriate vein branches with acute necrosis only of surrounding cerebral tissue without significant cellular reaction. Haemorrhages into areas of periventricular infarction are bilaterally symmetrical while those due to venous infarction may be unilateral.

Changing Birthweight-Gestation Patterns

One reason for the changing emphasis in the pathological findings relating to IVH may be the changing gestational age range over which the condition is seen. At Hammersmith Hospital, a steady decline in the gestational age and birthweight of infants who came to postmortem with IVH over successive periods between 1966 and 1976 was observed (Pape and Wigglesworth 1979). For the years 1974-1976 the mean gestation had fallen to 28.9 ± 0.4 weeks and the mean birthweight had fallen to 1206 ± 52 g. An examination of the figures for Hammersmith Hospital for the period 1981-1985 shows a mean gestation of 27 ± 0.28 weeks and a mean birthweight of 889 ± 40 g. Although many older and heavier infants still develop the condition, they mostly survive so that the pathology seen at autopsy is mainly that of a selected subgroup of very immature infants. It would not be surprising for the pathology to differ in some respects from that described in the larger and more mature infants who came to postmortem examination a few years ago.

The tendency to observe ischaemic lesions in the form of periventricular leucomalacia in a significant proportion of those infants with IVH who die (Nwaesei et al. 1984; Rushton et al. 1985) may be a manifestation of this change. It is also possible that pathological appearances may be influenced by the level of intensive care which is considered justifiable by the neonatologist. Thus an increase in the proportion of associated ischaemic lesions may indicate that clinicians are resuscitating and attempting to maintain alive a group of infants who would formerly have been classed as spontaneous late abortions.

References

Armstrong D, Norman MG (1974) Periventricular leucomalacia in neonates. Arch Dis Child 49: 367-375

Coen et al. (1970) Anatomic and epidemiologic features of the stroke lesion of newborn infants. Trans Neurol Assoc 95: 36-40

Gröntoft O (1953) Intracerebral and meningeal haemorrhages in perinatally deceased infants. I. Intracerebral haemorrhages: a pathologico-anatomical and obstetric study. Acta Obstet Gynaecol Scand 32: 308-334

Hambleton G, Wigglesworth JS (1976) Origin of intraventricular haemorrhage in the preterm infant. Arch Dis Child 51: 651-659

Harcke et al. (1972) Perinatal cerebral intraventricular hemorrhage. J Pediatr 80: 37-42

Hemsath FA (1934) Ventricular cerebral hemorrhage in the newborn infant. Am J Obstet Gynecol 28: 343-354

Larroche JC (1972) Post-hemorrhagic hydrocephalus in infancy: anatomical study. Biol Neonate 20: 287-299

Larroche JC (1977) Developmental pathology of the neonate. Excerpta Medica, Amsterdam

Leech RW, Kohnen P (1974) Subependymal and intraventricular hemorrhages in the newborn. Am J Pathol 77: 465-475

Levene MI, de Vries L (1984) Extension of neonatal intraventricular haemorrhage. Arch Dis Child 59: 631-636

Lou et al. (1977) Low cerebral blood flow in hypotensive perinatal distress. Acta Neurol Scand 55: 343-352

Nwaesei CG et al. (1984) Periventricular infarction diagnosed by ultrasound. A post mortem correlation. J Pediatr 105: 106-110

Pape KE, Wigglesworth JS (1979) Haemorrhage, ischaemia and the perinatal brain. Clinics in Developmental Medicine Nos 69/70, Heinemann, London, pp 128-129

Rushton et al. (1985) Structure and evolution of echo dense lesions in the neonatal brain. Arch Dis Child 60: 798-808

Towbin A (1968) Cerebral intraventricular haemorrhage and subependymal matrix infarction in the fetus and premature newborn. Am J Pathol 52: 121-134

Volpe et al. (1983) Positron emission tomography in the newborn. Extensive impairment of regional cerebral blood flow with intraventricular haemorrhage and haemorrhagic intracerebral involvement. Pediatrics 72: 589-601

Wigglesworth JS, Pape KE (1978) An integrated model for haemorrhagic and ischaemic lesions in the newborn brain. Early Hum Dev 2/2, 179-199

Ylppö A (1919) Pathologisch-anatomische Studien bei Frühgeborenen. Zschr Kinderh 20: 212-431

Hypoxia, Loss of Autoregulation and Intracranial Hemorrhage

H. C. Lou, G. Greisen, and A. Tweed

In recent years there has been a growing awareness of the significance of hemodynamic factors in the pathogenesis of perinatal neurologic disorders. In particular, the "lost autoregulation hypothesis" has received attention as a key to the understanding of the development of hypoxic-ischemic encephalopathy and periventricular hemorrhage: in normal conditions the adult as well as the unstressed newborn is capable of regulating vascular resistance to obtain a constant cerebral perfusion during quite wide changes of perfusion pressure. This autoregulation of cerebral blood flow (CBF) is lost in the stressed newborn, exposing the brain to ischemia in even moderate hypotension and to an increased pressure gradient across the capillary wall in even moderate hypertension, with increased risk of intracranial hemorrhage as a result (Lou et al. 1979a, b, c; Lou 1980). This has stimulated interest in the definition of factors which regulate cerebral perfusion in utero and the stresses surrounding the birth process.

Using an animal model, a chronically prepared near-term fetal lamb, we examined the autoregulation of CBF in utero in normoxic and hypoxic conditions (Tweed et al. 1983). CBF was measured using isotope-labeled 15 μm microspheres 24–48 h after surgical preparations. Seventeen animals were studied, eight considered to be normoxic (ascending aortic O_2 saturation – SaO_2 – 57% or higher) and nine spontaneously hypoxic (SaO_2 less than 50%) – the fetal hemoglobin averaged 11.5 g/100 ml. CBF autoregulation was assessed in four regions: telencephalon, right and left (grey + white matter), diencephalon, cerebellum, and brain stem. Autoregulation was found to be functionally active in all regions of the normoxic fetuses but abolished in the mildly hypoxic fetuses.

The demonstrated threshold of SaO_2 for impairment of autoregulation of 50%–60% corresponds to an arterial O_2 concentration of about 3 mmol per liter, which is very similar to the threshold for impairment of autoregulation in newborn lamb (Tweed et al. 1986) (Fig. 1) and adult dog (Häggendal and Johansson 1965). This threshold is a little higher than the level required for fetal hypoxic hyperemia (Johnson et al. 1979) in which a hyperbolic relationship between CBF and arterial O_2 concentration has been reported (Jones et al. 1984).

It may be concluded from these observations that the regulation of fetal CBF is fragile, apparently due to the relatively hypoxic conditions in utero: a minor additional hypoxic insult is sufficient to abolish this protective mechanism. The normal birth process may constitute such an insult, and this may explain why a number of investigators find that vaginally born premature infants are more prone to developing periventricular hemorrhages than premature infants born by cesarean section (Dolfin et al. 1982; Lou et al. 1982).

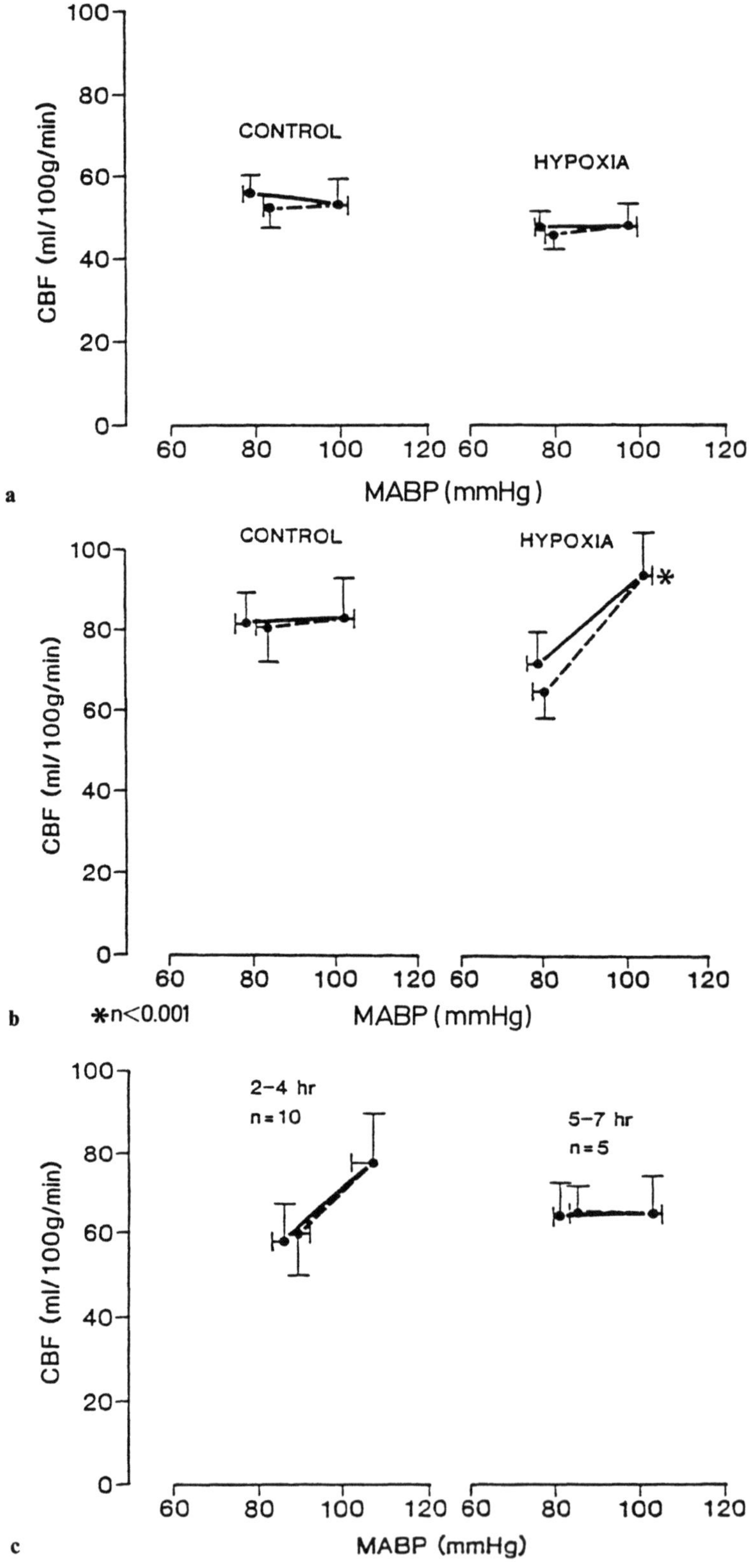
CBF (ml/100g/min)
CONTROL
HYPOXIA
MABP (mmHg)
a
CBF (ml/100g/min)
CONTROL
HYPOXIA
*
MABP (mmHg)
b
*n<0.001
CBF (ml/100g/min)
2–4 hr
n=10
5–7 hr
n=5
MABP (mmHg)
c

Mild periventricular hemorrhage probably carries a good prognosis. However, if the hemorrhage penetrates into the ventricular system there is a substantial risk of hydrocephalus developing due to impaired cerebrospinal fluid (CSF) outflow (Papile et al. 1979). But the most serious turn of events develops if the hemorrhage spreads into the brain parenchyma. The clinical condition of the infant is likely to deteriorate abruptly, in many cases resulting in death.

There is some evidence that ischemic lesions of the brain parenchyma precede this development. In our original series of 19 patients in whom CBF had been measured a few hours after birth, four died with clinical signs of hemorrhage verified at autopsy at the ages of 2-37 days. In all four, very low values of CBF had been measured immediately after birth. In a subsequent study we found a low-flow state prior to detectable intracranial hemorrhage, accompanied by electrophysiologic signs of ischemic brain dysfunction (Greisen et al. 1986): 15 infants, 32 weeks of gestation or less, were studied with continuous recording of amplitude-integrated electroencephalogram (aEEG) and repeated Doppler ultrasound determination of mean blood flow velocity in the internal carotid artery (cMFV). The recording was started after initiation of mechanical ventilation for respiratory distress if no signs of germinal layer hemorrhage (GLH) was found by ultrasound scanning. Seven of the 15 infants had cMFV increases of 100% or more associated with blood pressure increases following volume expansion (group I) indicating absence of autoregulation. Initial minimum blood pressure and minimum cMFV were lower in these infants compared with the remaining eight infants in whom the cMFV was stable (group II). Six of the infants in group I, all with low Apgar scores at birth, later developed GLH, whereas only two infants in group II bled ($p=0.039$). In all infants the aEEG showed suppression burst activity whereas no period of sustained electric silence was seen in any infant. In group II the burst rate increased over the first 6 h to 150 bursts per hour. In group I the burst rate increased less and seemed unaffected by the increased blood flow, indicating an abnormal function of neural tissue which was not readily reversed with improved energy supply (Fig. 2). Timing of eventual GLH by repeated ultrasound scanning showed this abnormality to be present before any hemorrhage in most of the infants, indicating that hemorrhage occurs in brains which have already been damaged by ischemia.

The hemorrhage itself may, in its turn, aggravate ischemia. Volpe et al. (1983) have shown with positron emission tomography (PET) scanning that intraparenchymal hemorrhage is surrounded by a zone of severe ischemia. In order to obtain a better understanding of the mechanisms of this regional ischemia, we examined the effect of blood admixture to mock spinal fluid on its ion composition in vitro (Edvinsson et al. 1986). It was found that during the first 2-3 days the K^+ concentration increased dramatically up to about ten-fold, depending upon the concen-

Fig. 1a–c. Impairment and recovery of autoregulation in newborn sheep after hypoxic insult (SaO_2 50%). **a** Preserved autoregulation after 10 min of hypoxia ($n=7$). **b** Impaired autoregulation after 20 min of hypoxia ($n=11$). **c** Recovery of impaired autoregulation over 2-7 h after hypoxia

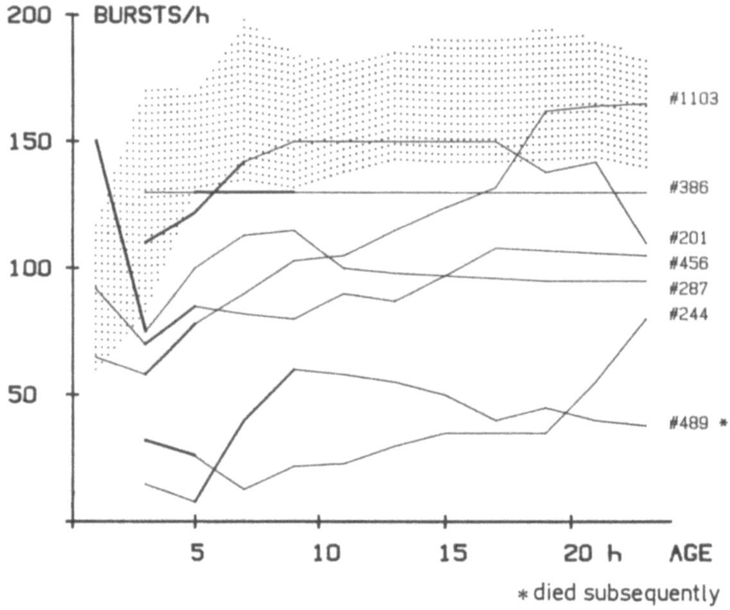

Fig. 2. EEG bursts per hour in premature infant (gestational age <32 weeks) prior to eventual intracranial hemorrhage. *Shaded area* represents eight infants with stable mean flow in carotid artery. Seven infants with unstable carotid flow (see text) are depicted individually. *Bold parts of the lines* indicate the periods of flow increase (>100%). Flow increase is not regularly accompanied by increase in burst rate

tration of blood in the mixture with mock spinal fluid. This level was maintained for at least 2 weeks. Such a K^+ concentration of about 20-50 mEq has a marked vasoconstrictor effect, which could very well be responsible for the perihemorrhagic ischemia. Likewise, it should be mentioned that a similar K^+ concentration is capable of inducing neuronal depolarization and spreading depression. Spreading depression is known to be accompanied by a considerable *increase* in glucose utilization (Shinohara et al. 1979). Hence, not only does the hemorrhage induce, or aggravate, ischemia in surrounding tissue, it may also greatly increase its energy demand.

In summary, the following sequence of events may be hypothesized:

1. Hypoxemia impairs autoregulation
2. Lack of autoregulation and initial hypotension induce hypnotic-ischemic infarction
3. Subsequent blood pressure increase leads to periventricular hemorrhage
4. Which may then spread into infarcted tissue
5. And induce the perihemorrhagic ischemia
6. Which is then aggravated by increased energy demand due to spreading depression

References

Dolfin T, Skidmore MB, Fong KW, Hoskins EM, Milligan JE, Moore DC, Shennan AT (1982) Perinatal factors that influence the incidence of subependymal and intraventricular hemorrhage in low birthweight infants. Syllabus-Second Special Ross Laboratories conference on perinatal intracranial hemorrhage, Washington DC, December 2-4

Edvinsson L, Lou HC, Tvede K (1986) On the pathogenesis of regional cerebral ischemia in intracranial hemorrhage. A causal role of K^+? Pediatr Res 20: 478-480

Greisen G, Lou HC, Rosen I (1986) Cerebral blood flow velocity increases and EEG during the first 24 hours of life in mechanically ventilated preterm infants. (to be published)

Häggendal E, Johansson B (1965) Effects of arterial carbon dioxide tension and oxygen saturation on CBF autoregulation in dogs. Acta Physiol Scand [Suppl] 258: 27-53

Johnsson GN, Palahniuk RJ, Tweed WA, Jones MV, Wade J (1979) Regional cerebral blood flow changes during severe fetal asphyxia produced by slow partial umbilical cord compression. Am J Obstet Gynecol 135: 48-52

Jones PM, Sheldon RE, Peeters LL, Makowski EL, Meschia G (1981) Regulation of cerebral blood flow in the ovine foetus. Am J Physiol 235: H162-H166

Lou HC (1980) Perinatal hypoxic-ischemic brain damage and intraventricular hemorrhage. A pathogenetic model. Arch Neurol 41: 825-829

Lou HC, Lassen NA, Friis-Hansen B (1979 a) Impaired autoregulation of cerebral blood flow in the distressed newborn infant. J Pediatr 94: 118-121

Lou HC, Skov H, Pedersen H (1979 b) Low cerebral blood flow: a risk factor in the neonate. J Pediatr 95: 606-609

Lou HC, Lassen NA, Friis-Hansen B (1979 c) Is arterial hypertension crucial for the development of intraventricular haemorrhage in the neonate? Lancet I: 1215-1217

Lou HC, Lassen NA, Tweed WA, Johnson GB, Jones MW, Palahniuk RJ (1979 d) Pressure passive cerebral blood flow and breakdown of the blood-brain barrier in experimental fetal asphyxia. Acta Paediatr Scand 68: 57-63

Lou HC, Phibbs RH, Wilson SL, Gregory GA (1982) Hyperventilation at birth may prevent early periventricular hemorrhage. Lancet I: 1407

Papile LA, Munsick G, Weaver N, Pecha S (1979) Cerebral intraventricular hemorrhage in infants < 1500 g. Developmental follow-up at one year. Pediatr Res 13: 528

Shinohara M, Pollinger B, Brown G, Rapoport S, Soholoff L (1979) Cerebral glucose utilization: Local changes during and after recovery from spreading cortical depression. Science 203: 188-190

Tweed WA, Coté J, Pash M, Lou HC (1983) Arterial oxygenation determines autoregulation of cerebral blood flow in fetal lamb. Pediatr Res 17: 246-249

Tweed WA, Coté J, Lou HC, Gregory GA, Wade J (1986) Impairment and recovery of autoregulation of cerebral blood flow in the newborn lamb. Pediatr Res (to be published)

Volpe II, Herscovitch P, Perlman JM, Raichle ME (1983) Position emission tomography in the newborn: Extensive impairment of regional cerebral blood flow with intraventricular hemorrhage and hemorrhagic intracerebral involvement. Pediatrics 72: 589-601

Obstetrical Factors and Intracranial Hemorrhage

M. BRAND and E. SALING

Introduction

Owing to the increasing survival rate even of very low birthweight infants, intracranial hemorrhage (ICH) is a more frequent problem today than in former years. According to the investigations of Larroche (1982), the incidence of ICH rose from 28% to 50% in premature babies of the 26th-33rd week of pregnancy and from 4.4% to 16.55% in those of the 34th-35th week of pregnancy between 1967 and 1981. In the newborn infants older than 36 weeks of gestation the incidence remained unchanged.

Despite successful clarification of numerous risk factors of ICH in recent years, the contribution and significance of obstetric factors in the etiopathogenesis are still unclear. A review of the literature and our own investigation results on the role of obstetric factors in the etiology of ICH are intended to contribute to the clarification of this important question.

Risk Factor Analysis (Review of the Literature)

In numerous publications from the first decade of this century, the action of force on the baby's cranium was regarded as the most important cause of perinatal brain damage: mechanical factors of labor lead to molding and compression of the head, tearing of the falcine dura and tentorium cerebelli, tearing and compression of the venous sinus, and to injury of extracerebral structures (Schwartz 1926; Müller 1973).

Hypoxia as the cause of ICH has been emphasized by many authors since 1920. Negative pressure during labor does not only result in a displacement of the cranial bones but also in an impeded cerebral outflow from the deep intracranial veins (Schwartz 1926) inducing stasis and hypoxia. In hypoxia, fetal metabolic acidosis arises due to anaerobic glycolysis (Saling 1963).

In 1979 Lou described for the first time the impaired cerebral autoregulation in asphyxiated newborn infants with ICH. This pathogenetic principle was confirmed by other investigators: Goddard-Finegold et al. (1982) and Ment et al. (1984) observed in animal models that acute hypoxia leads to loss of cerebral autoregulation. The initial fall in blood pressure is propagated into the now pressure-passive capillary network of the germinal layer where the following luxury-perfusion initiates the hemorrhage.

The significance of these mechanic, hypoxic, and hemodynamic risk factors for ICH during delivery is the question of many recent studies, diagnosing ICH by cranial computerized tomography (CT) or sonography.

Table 1. Obstetric and neonatal factors in very low birthweight infants with ICH

Authors	Risk factor analysis (preterm <1500 g)		Obstetric factors		Neonatal factors Association
	n	ICH (%)	No association	Association	
Strauss (1985)	119	24	+	Fetal heart rate patterns	Condition at birth
Szymonowicz et al. (1985)	100	36	+	Severe bruising of the head	Admission state
Rumack et al. (1985)	49	45		Longer labor, vaginal delivery from breech presentation, intrapartum hemorrhage	Apgar <5
v. Loewenich et al. (1985)	105	23		Difficult delivery	
Ment et al. (1984)	30	61	+		Resuscitation, ventilation therapy, CBF↓
Bada (1984)	150	79	+		Condition at birth, GA, BW
Rayburn et al. (1983)	103	44	+		
Horbar et al. (1983)	77	55		Duration of labor, vaginal delivery; presentation	
Dolfin (1983)	95	34		Presentation (vertex/breech), mode of delivery, 29 weeks GA	
Clark et al. (1981)	60	56	+		Outborn
Cooke (1981)	39	51	−		RDS, ventilation therapy, hypercapnia
Kosmetatos et al. (1980)	64	58	+		Low Apgar score, RDS, acidosis, ventilation therapy
n=12	991		7		

GA, gestational age; BW, birthweight; RDS, respiratory distress syndrome; CBF, cerebral blood flow

Obstetric Factors and ICH in Preterm Infants Weighing Less than 1500 g

Table 1 gives an overview of the most important investigations of obstetric factors in very low birthweight infants under 1500 g. The role of the following parameters was examined: presentation of the fetus, mode of delivery, duration of labor, course of labor, umbilical artery pH, Apgar score and intrapartum hemorrhage. In a total of 12 studies comprising in all 991 very low birthweight infants, seven authors (Strauss et al. 1985; Szymonowicz et al. 1985; Bada et al. 1984; Ment et al. 1984; Rayburn et al. 1983; Clark et al. 1981; Kosmetatos et al. 1980) did not find any association with antepartum and intrapartum complications and mode of delivery. In the investigation of Strauss et al. (1985), premature rupture of membranes, breech presentation, mode of delivery and transport before birth were not significantly different in newborn infants with and without ICH. But ominous fetal heart rate patterns occurred in 50% of monitored infants less than 1500 g with severe ICH, compared to 7% of matched controls.

Rayburn et al. (1983) checked many obstetric factors without finding any association with cerebral bleeding.

Szymonowicz et al. (1985) compared in two consecutive studies the incidence of ICH in preterm infants with a birthweight of less than 1250 g. Of the many obstetric factors they looked for, only severe bruising of the head (external hematomas) was significantly different in preterm infants with and without ICH. As described in Table 2, the state on admission was significantly associated with ICH ($p<0.001$): a low PO_2, low hematocrit, hypoxemia, hypercapnia, hypothermia, and hyaline membrane disease. They demonstrated that a reduction of ICH from 60% to 36% could be attained in these tiny preterm infants by strict guidelines on neonatal care with elective intubation, avoidance of hypothermia, careful monitoring of the blood gases and compensation of metabolic acidosis. In a similar way Bada et al. (1984) showed that it is not the obstetric factors but the neonatal condition, the birthweight, and the gestational age which correlate with ICH.

On the other hand, von Loewenich et al. (1985) consider mechanically difficult delivery as the most important obstetric factor in the etiology of ICH in very low birthweight infants.

Table 2. Differences between two studies in Melbourne (Szymonowicz et al. 1985)

	Previous study $n=50$	Present study $n=100$
Preventricular hemorrhage *(n)*	30	36
(%)	60	36*
Temperature (°C)	35.2 ± 1.2	35.8 ± 0.9*
Mean BP (mmHg)	35 ± 10	43 ± 13*
Severe bruising at birth *(n)*	7	2
(%)	19	3

* $p<0.001$

With regard to the mode of delivery, Rumack et al. (1985) and McDonald et al. (1984) found that vaginal delivery in vertex as well as in breech presentations and the duration of labor was correlated with ICH in preterm infants with a birthweight of less than 1500 g.

Dolfin et al. (1983) observed that newborn infants who were delivered from vertex presentation by cesarean section after the 29th week of gestation displayed significantly less ICH than babies delivered vaginally. Before the 29th week of gestation there was no difference between vertex and breech presentation. Both groups had a 50% incidence of ICH. Up to now, studies on the mode of delivery of very low birthweight infants in breech presentations do not permit an unequivocal recommendation (Leviton et al. 1977; Duenhoelter et al. 1979; Westgren et al. 1982; Bodmer et al. 1986).

Obstetric Factors in Preterm Infants Weighing More Than 1500 g

Table 3 shows an overview of the most important studies and results of obstetric factors and ICH in preterm infants over 1500 g. In a total of seven studies comprising, in all, 750 premature infants with a birthweight more than 1500 g, five authors (Beverley et al. 1984; Tejani et al. 1984; Thorburn et al. 1982; Levene et al.

Table 3. Obstetric factors and ICH in premature newborn infants weighing more than 1500 g

Authors	Gestational age (weeks)	*n*	ICH (%)	Obstetric factors		Neonatal factors
				No association	Association	
Meidell et al. (1985)	35	40	42		Pattern of labor	
Beverley et al. (1984)	34	150	26	+	Low Apgar score	RDS, metabolic acidosis, ventilation therapy
Tejani et al. (1984)	32	126	21	+ Fetal heart rate monitoring		
McDonald et al. (1984)	33	50	30		Vaginal delivery, longer labor, intrapartum hemorrhage	RR fluctuation >100%, rapid colloid infusions
Thorburn (1982)	33	95	34	+		RDS, pneumothorax
Levene et al. (1982)	34	146	36	+	Outborn	Severe acidosis; $pCO_2\uparrow$, hypothermia, RDS, buffer
Dykes et al. (1980)	35	151	64	+		Alveolar rupture, hypercapnia, buffer, hypotension, ventilation therapy
n=7		758		5		

1982; Dykes et al. 1980) were unable to demonstrate any significant correlation of presentation, mode of delivery, duration and pattern of labor, umbilical artery pH, and intrapartum bleedings to ICH. Meidell et al. (1985) found that the course of labor, namely long-lasting intrauterine contractions, was typical in babies with ICH of early onset.

Beverley et al. (1984) checked 16 obstetric factors and found only that a lowered Apgar score was associated with cerebral hemorrhage.

Tejani et al. (1984) observed that neither the presentation nor the mode of delivery and the umbilical artery pH showed any correlation with ICH. He did not find a typical fetal heart rate pattern to be associated with cerebral hemorrhage. In contrast, McDonald et al. (1984) reported that the mothers of babies with ICH experienced intrapartum hemorrhages more frequently and that their labor lasted longer. In addition, she found a correlation with vaginal delivery.

Levene et al. (1982) checked 30 different obstetric factors and found only the variable "outborn" to be significantly associated with ICH.

Obstetric Factors in Mature Infants and ICH

Investigations into the significance of obstetric factors in mature infants with ICH were reported by Fouche et al. (1982), Brockerhoff et al. (1981) and Fenichel et al. (1984). They found no dependence of ICH on presentation, mode of delivery, Apgar score, and umbilical artery pH. Brockerhoff et al. (1981) noticed that a short duration of the second stage of labor, lasting less than 15 min, to be associated with ICH.

Obstetric Factors and ICH in Selected Mature and Immature Newborn Infants

A recent study reported by Low et al. (1986) investigated 220 selected newborn infants; of these, 70 had a birthweight of less than 1500 g, 79 of more than 1500 g and 71 infants were mature. They found ICH in 21% of newborn infants who had not experienced any complications and in 56% of infants with complications. No association with maternal, fetal complications, fetal hypoxia, duration of labor, and mode of delivery were demonstrated. The statistical analysis revealed a correlation of ICH only with immaturity, severe respiratory complications, and major infections.

Risk Factor Analysis (Our Own Results: Berlin-Neukölln Prospective Study)

Obstetric Factors and ICH in Unselected Immature and Mature Newborn Infants

The significance of obstetric and neonatal risk factors for perinatal ICH was examined for the first time in a large number of unselected cases at the Berlin-Neukölln Women's and Children's Hospital in 1982-1983. In a total of 1251 newborn infants - 1090 mature and 161 immature - we performed prospectively serial cranial sonography and neurological examinations according to the scheme of Prechtl (1977). In selected cases cranial CT was applied additionally.

Mode of Delivery and ICH

Table 4 demonstrate the total incidence of ICH in our patients: it reached 3.9% in mature newborn infants and 24.2% in immature children. No significant dependence on the mode of delivery in the newborn infants with and without ICH could be demonstrated overall. Only in the premature infants with vaginal delivery from breech presentation was the frequency of hemorrhage higher (61%) than in the remaining modes of delivery.

By differentiation of vaginal operative deliveries according to the stage of the presenting part, shown in Table 5, the incidence of ICH was 10.5% in term infants delivered from the pelvic inlet and/or mid-pelvic plane, as compared to 4.5% in newborn infants delivered from the pelvic floor or pelvic outlet. The difference was not statistically significant ($p < 0.2$).

A short comment is necessary concerning vaginal operative delivery from the pelvic inlet. Such deliveries - after direct measurements of applied forces during vacuum extraction as published by Saling and Hartung (1973) - are, as we later

Table 4. Incidence of ICH and mode of delivery, total = 1251, ICH = 81 = 6.5%. (According to Brand and Saling 1985)

Mode of delivery	≥37 weeks of gestation (mature)			<37 weeks of gestation (premature)		
	Total (*n*)	Intracranial hemorrhage		Total (*n*)	Intracranial hemorrhage	
		(*n*)	(%)		(*n*)	(%)
	1090	42	3.9	161	39	24.2
Spontaneous	801	21	2.6	87	19	21.8
Vaginally operative from vertex presentation	194	15	7.7	24	3	12.5
Cesarean section	88	5	5.7	37	9	24.3
Breech presentation, vaginal	7	1	14	13	8	61.5

Table 5. Vaginal operative deliveries and ICH, $n=218$, ICH $=18=8.3\%$. (According to Brand and Saling 1985)

	Mature infants (≥37/0)			Premature infants (<37/0)		
	Total	ICH		Total	ICH	
	(n)	*(n)*	(%)	*(n)*	*(n)*	(%)
Pelvic inlet	30	2	6.7	1	0	0
Mid-pelvic plane	75	9	12.0	5	1	20.0
Early second stage	105	11	10.5	6	1	16.7
Mid-pelvic plane - pelvic floor	37	2	5.4	7	1	14.3
Pelvic floor + pelvic outlet	52	2	3.8	11	1	9.1
Late second stage	89	4	4.5	18	2	11.1
*Σ	194	15	7.7	24	3	12.5

found, often less difficult than extractions from the mid-pelvic plane. The number of cases with ICH from the pelvic inlet (two out of 30) is lower than in the cases with extraction from the mid-pelvic plane (nine out of 75). The reason is that in selected cases, vacuum extraction from the pelvic inlet, particularly in multiparae, can be an easy procedure.

Looking more closely at the 2.6% incidence of ICH in spontaneous deliveries compared to 10.5% in vaginal operative deliveries from the pelvic inlet or mid-pelvic plane, the difference reaches statistical significance ($p<0.02$).

According to these results, a mechanically difficult delivery raises the risk of cerebral hemorrhage for mature and immature newborn infants. The kind of hemorrhage which predominated in this group was subarachnoidal bleeding, representing the traumatic cause in 11 out of 18 patients.

We found a dependence of ICH on the mode of delivery in the group of very low birthweight infants. Of 44 preterm infants under 1500 g, 17 out of 31 had had more than grade II hemorrhage after vaginal delivery. On the other hand, only two out of 13 premature babies delivered by cesarean section experienced more than grade II hemorrhage ($p<0.02$).

Presentation, Mode of Delivery and Time of Onset of ICH

How important it is to know the time of onset of ICH in evaluating the influence of a single-risk factor like the presentation can be appraised with reference to 52 newborn infants after delivery from breech presentation. Of 22 babies born between the 23rd and 31st week of gestation, 68% had an ICH of early onset, before the 3rd day of life, as compared to an incidence of 82% after the 3rd day of life. The situation is similar when considering premature infants with vaginal and with cesarean section delivery from breech presentation. Immediately after birth, ICH could be detected in 48% of preterm infants delivered vaginally. In babies delivered by cesarean section this was diagnosed only in 7% ($p<0.001$). Between the 1st and 2nd days of life, 52% of the babies delivered from breech presentation had an ICH, as did 21% of the premature infants who had been delivered by cesarean section. After the 3rd day of life, the difference between the modes of delivery was no longer found to be so significant ($p < 0.2$).

The influence of the mode of delivery can only be estimated in the early diagnosed hemorrhages.

Acidosis and ICH

The connection between acidosis and ICH is shown in Table 6. Acidosis during labor, with an umbilical artery pH of less than 7.20, led to an 8.5% incidence of hemorrhage in mature babies as compared to 3.7% in normacidic infants ($p < 0.05$). In premature babies the incidence of ICH with an umbilical artery pH of less than 7.20 was 42% as compared to 21% with a balanced acid base status ($p < 0.05$).

Apgar Score and ICH

The Apgar score in premature babies differs from that in mature infants. Premature babies with an Apgar score under 7 had a ventricular hemorrhage in 62% of cases (Table 7). When the Apgar score was normal the frequency was only 20% ($p < 0.001$). This correlation cannot be confirmed in mature infants.

Table 6. Acidity in umbilical artery and ICH

pH \ Gestational age	≥37 weeks Total (*n*)	≥37 weeks ICH (*n*)	≥37 weeks ICH (%)	<37 weeks Total (*n*)	<37 weeks ICH (*n*)	<37 weeks ICH (%)
≥7.30	599	24	4.0	80	15	19
7.20–7.29	374	12	3.2	49	12	25
<7.20	71	6	8.5	19	8	4.2
		$p < 0.05$		$p < 0.05$		

Table 7. Apgar score and ICH

Score \ Gestational age	≥37 weeks Total (*n*)	≥37 weeks ICH (*n*)	≥37 weeks ICH (%)	<37 weeks Total (*n*)	<37 weeks ICH (*n*)	<37 weeks ICH (%)
9–10	989	33	3.3	107	19	18
7– 8	79	7	9.0	40	11	28
≤6	22	2	9.0	13	13	62
		$p < 0.3$			$p < 0.001$	

Fetal Heart Rate Patterns and ICH

The evaluation of fetal heart rate patterns in infants with and without ICH revealed cerebral bleeding in 9% of mature newborn infants with a tachycardia over 160 per minute without acidosis. On the other hand, term infants without tachycardia displayed a hemorrhage in only 1.8% of cases ($p<0.05$). This could not be demonstrated for preterm babies. Other ominous fetal heart rate patterns, such as bradycardia without acidosis, were not more frequently associated with ICH.

Peripartum Risk Factors and ICH

All the peripartum risk factors tested and significantly different in the χ^2 test in newborn infants with and without ICH are shown in Table 8. Above all, the gestational age and tocolysis were the most important variables. During labor, the mature infants with and without ICH differed in fetal heart rate patterns, namely tachycardia. The frequency of hemorrhage was higher in premature infants weighing less than 1500 g after vaginal delivery and in premature babies delivered vaginally from breech presentation.

The significantly different parameters postpartum with and without ICH were the 5-min Apgar score, the umbilical artery pH less than 7.20, the need for intubation and artificial ventilation, medication, and buffering in the next few days of life. In the newborn infants who were transported to a neonatal unit, hypercarbia, hypothermia, fluctuations in blood pressure, infection, and complications in the course of diseases such as pneumothorax, patent ductus arteriosus and bronchopulmonary dysplasia were significantly different in newborn infants with ICH.

Table 8. Peripartum risk factors and ICH

Risk factors	<37 weeks gestational age	≤37 weeks gestational age
Tocolysis	s	ns
Tachycardia	ns	s
Vaginal breech delivery	s	ns
Umbilical artery pH <7.20	s	s
5-min Apgar score	s	–
Intubation	s	ns
Buffer PP	ns	ns
Buffer during intensive care	s	ns
Temperature on admission	s	ns
pH on admission	s	ns
Mechanical ventilation	s	ns
$PcO_2\uparrow$	s	ns
Medication	s	ns
Complications	s	ns

s, significant; ns, not significant

Summary of Our Results

Compared with the studies reported in the literature, in our patients obstetric factors - like the mode of delivery, presentation, acidosis, and tachycardia in fetal heart rate patterns - could be found to be more frequently associated with ICH. The significance could be proven in subgroups like very low birthweight infants, preterm infants delivered from breech presentation, premature infants only, or mature infants only, or mature infants vaginally delivered from the mid-pelvic plane. Determining the exact time of onset of ICH (Brand and Saling 1985) is a further important point for differentiating the influence of the single-risk factors.

Conclusions

On the basis of the results reported in the literature and our own investigations as to the role of obstetric factors in the etiopathogenesis of ICH, the following can be concluded: despite mechanical birth injury and the frequent findings of extracerebral hemorrhages in a total of 23 investigations in the literature, comprising in all more than 1500 newborn infants, and our own study of 1251 unselected newborn infants, obstetric factors were not associated with ICH to the extent expected. Only in subgroups, such as very low birthweight infants, preterm infants in breech presentation or mature newborn infants who had been vaginally operatively delivered from the mid-pelvic plane, could an association with the mode of delivery be demonstrated. An important point in the prevention of ICH in the studies in the literature and in our own investigations seems to be the condition of the preterm infant at birth and its stabilization by strict monitoring of all vital parameters: blood gases, blood pressure, and body temperature. Further detailed examinations with regard to the single obstetric factors in correlation to the exact time of the onset of ICH are still to be done.

References

Bada HS, Krones SB, Anderson GD, Magill HL, Wong SP (1984) Obstetric factors and relative risk of neonatal germinal layer/intraventricular hemorrhage. Am J Obstet Gynecol 148: 798-803

Beverley DW, Chance GW, Coates CR (1984) Intraventricular haemorrhage - timing, occurrence and relationship to perinatal events. Br J Obstet Gynaecol 91: 1007-1013

Bodmer B, Benjamin A, McLean FH, Usher RH (1986) Has use of cesarean section reduced risks of delivery in the preterm breech presentation? Am J Obstet Gynecol 154: 244-250

Brand M, Saling E (1985) The timing of perinatal intracranial hemorrhage. Ross, Syllabus, pp 51-62

Brockerhoff P, Brand M, Ludwig B (1981) Untersuchungen zur Häufigkeit perinataler Hirnblutungen und deren Abhängigkeit vom Geburtsverlauf mit Hilfe der cranialen Computertomographie. Geburtshilfe Frauenheilkd 41: 597-600

Clark CE, Cylmlan RI, Roth RS, Sniderman SH, Lane B, Ballard RA (1981) Risk factor analysis of intraventricular hemorrhage in low birthweight infants. J Pediatr 99: 625-628
Cooke RWI (1981) Factors associated with periventricular haemorrhage in very low birthweight infants. Arch Dis Child 56: 425-431
Dolfin T, Skidmore MB, Fong KW, Hoskins EM, Shennan AT (1983) Incidence, severity and timing of subependymal and intraventricular hemorrhages in preterm infants born in a perinatal unit as detected by serial real-time ultrasound. Pediatrics 71: 541-546
Duenholter JH, Wells CE, Reisch JS, Santos-Ramos R, Jimenez JM (1979) A paired controlled study of vaginal and abdominal delivery of the low birthweight breech fetus. Obstet Gynecol 54: 310
Dykes FD, Lazzara A, Ahmann P, Umenstein B, Schwartz J, Brann AW (1980) Intraventricular haemorrhage: a prospective evaluation of etiopathogenesis. Pediatrics 66: 42-49
Fenichel GM, Webster DL, Wong WK (1984) Intracranial hemorrhage in term newborn. Arch Neurol 41 (1): 30-34
Fouche S, Sevely A, Rolland M, Mantelfe C, Regnier C (1982) Hemorraghies intra-cerebrales non traumatiques du nouveau ne a terme. Pediatrie 37 (3): 185-193
Goddard-Finegold J, Armstrong D, Zeller RS (1982) Intraventricular hemorrhage following volume expansion after hypovolemic hypotension in newborn. J Pediatr 100: 796-799
Horbar J, Pasnick M, McAuliffe TL (1983) Obstetric events and risk of periventricular hemorrhage in premature infants. Am J Dis Child 137: 678-681
Kosmetatos N, Dinter C, Williams ML, Lourie H, Berne AS (1980) Intracranial hemorrhage in the premature. Its predictive features and outcome. Am J Dis Child 134 (9): 855-859
Larroche JC (1982) Intraventrikuläre Blutung - Neue morphologische und epidemiologische Aspekte der Intensivpflege. In: Huch A, Huch R (eds) Klinisches Management des "kleinen Frühgeborenen" <1500 g. Thieme, Stuttgart, pp 165-169
Levene MI, Fawer CL, Lamont RF (1982) Risk factors in the development of intracranial haemorrhage in the preterm neonate. Arch Dis Child 57: 410-417
Leviton A, Gilles F, Strassfeld R (1977) The influence of route of delivery and hyaline membranes on the risk of neonatal intracranial hemorrhages. Ann Neurol 2 (6): 451-454
Lou HC, Lassen NA, Friis-Hansen B (1979) Impaired autoregulation of cerebral blood flow in the distressed newborn infant. Pediatrics 94: 118-121
Low JP, Galbraight RS, Sauerbrei E, Muir DW, Killen HL, Pater EA, Karchmar EJ (1986) Maternal, fetal and newborn complications associated with newborn intracranial hemorrhage. Am J Obstet Gynecol 154 (2): 345-351
McDonald MM, Koops BL, Johnsson ML, Guggenheim MA, Rumack CM, Mitchell SA, Hathaway WE (1984) Timing and antecedents of intracranial hemorrhage in the newborn. Pediatrics 74: 32-36
Meidell R, Marinelli P, Pettett G (1985) Perinatal factors associated with early onset intracranial hemorrhage in premature infants. Am J Dis Child 139: 160-163
Ment LR, Duncan CC, Ehrenkranz RA, Lange RC, Taylor KJ, Kleinman CS, Scott DT, Sivo J, Gettner P (1984) Intraventricular hemorrhage in the preterm neonate - timing and cerebral blood flow changes. J Pediatr 104: 419-435
Müller D (1973) Die subakute Massenverschiebung des Gehirns unter der Geburt. Thieme, Leipzig
Prechtl H (1977) Neurological examination of the fullterm newborn infant. Spastics international medical publication. Heinemann, London
Rayburn WF, Donn SM, Kolin MG, Schork MA (1983) Obstetric care and intraventricular hemorrhage in the low birthweight infant. Obstet Gynecol 62: 408-413
Rumack CM, Mancojohnson MI, Koops BL, Hathaway WE, Appareti K (1985) Timing and course of neonatal intracranial hemorrhage using real-time ultrasound. Radiology 154: 101-105
Saling E (1963) Die Blutgasverhältnisse und der Säure-Basen-Haushalt des Feten bei gestörtem Geburtsablauf. Z Geburtshilfe Gynäkologie 162: 262-292
Saling E, Hartung M (1973) Analyses of tractive forces during the application of vacuum extraction. J Perinat Med 1: 245
Schwartz P (1926) Geburtstraumatische Schädigungen des Kopfes Neugeborener und ihre Bedeutung für die Pathologie. Monatsschr Kinderheilkd 34: 511-537

Schwartz P (1956) Birth injuries of the newborn. Morphology, pathogenesis, clinical pathology and prevention of birth injuries of the newborn. Arch Pediatr 73: 429-451

Strauss A, Kirz D, Modanlu HD, Freeman R (1985) Perinatal events and intraventricular/subependymal hemorrhage in the very low birthweight infant. Am J Obstet Gynecol 151: 1022-1027

Szymonowicz W, Wilson F, Yu VYH, Walker A (1985) Reduction in periventricular haemorrhage in preterm infants associated with change in neonatal care. Ross, Syllabus, pp 99-113

Tejani N, Rebold B, Tuck S, Ditroia D, Sutro W, Verma U (1984) Obstetric factors in the causation of early periventricular-intraventricular hemorrhage. Obstet Gynecol 64: 510-515

Thorburn RJ, Lipscomb AP, Stewart AL, Reynolds EO, Hope PL (1982) Timing and antecedents of periventricular hemorrhage and of cerebral atrophy in very preterm infants. Ear Hum Dev 7: 221-238

v Loewenich V, Halberstadt E, Brand M, Saling E (1985) Die intracraniellen Blutungen des Neugeborenen. Gynäkol Geburtshilfe 2: 31-34

Westgren M, Ingemaarsson I, Ahlström H, Lindroth M, Svenningsen NW (1982) Delivery and long-term outcome of very low birthweight infants. Acta Obstet Gynecol Scand 61: 25-30

Prevention of Intraventricular Hemorrhage: Role of Atraumatic Birth and Sedation

V. VON LOEWENICH and E. HALBERSTADT

Intraventricular hemorrhage (IVH) is a rather common autopsy finding in premature infants. Therefore, IVH has been studied since the early beginnings of scientific neonatology (Ylppö 1919). Since noninvasive imaging techniques, such as computerized tomography (CT) or ultrasound scanning, have become available, it has also been possible to visualize and follow up IVH in survivors. IVH can be found in small premature infants at a frequency of 30%-50% or even higher, depending on the weight or gestational age cut-off points of the study group, and on other risk factors which will be discussed later (Clark et al. 1981; Dolfin et al. 1983; Garcia-Prats 1982; Hill and Volpe 1986; Hutchinson et al. 1982; McDonald et al. 1984; Perlman and Volpe 1986; Van de Bor 1986). Because IVH may be the cause of lifelong handicap, the prevention of this cerebral pathology is one of the most urgent tasks in perinatal medicine.

Definition of IVH. The origin of IVH is in the germinal layer, a highly vascularized tissue situated in the groove between the caudate nucleus and the thalamus. As Hambleton and Wigglesworth (1976) could clearly show, this hemorrhage is due to arterial leakage and not to rupture of the terminal vein, as had been previously believed. The hemorrhage may be limited to the germinal layer (germinal layer hemorrhage, or subependymall hemorrhage, or first degree IVH), but bleeding can also penetrate into the ventricular cavity (true IVH or second to fourth degree IVH). Second degree IVH means blood in the ventricles, third degree: additional dilatation of the ventricles, and fourth degree: penetration of hemorrhage into periventricular tissue [staging according to the nomenclature of Papile et al. (1978)].

Role of Birth Trauma

The origin of our study was a very simple clinical observation: small premature infants looking bruised and covered with hematomas had an obviously bad prognosis, i.e., a high incidence of IVH and a high mortality rate. In contrast, "nice looking" premature infants suffered less often from IVH and had a higher survival rate. Our hypothesis was that very immature infants with their thin skin and their jelly-like subcutis were not up to the mechanics of a natural birth and were, therefore, born polytraumatized. This was the reason for developing our concept of "mechanically soft delivery" (a mechanical variant of the so-called delivery without violence). Vaginal delivery is allowed only if a singleton is found in cephalic presentation, the membranes are intact, and there is enough time to perform epidural anesthesia. Then the baby is delivered within the membranes via a broad retractor after doing an extensive episiotomy. Without these conditions a cesarean section (CS) is performed. Because before 30-32 weeks of gestational age (postmenstrual - p.m.) a lower uterine segment has not yet been established, extracting the infant through a transverse lower uterotomy may become difficult. Therefore we decided during the course of our study to inject a betamimetic intravenously immediately before the uterotomy. In fact the extraction of the infant then becomes easier and less traumatic, and a longitudinal incision can be avoided.

Patients. We examined 132 premature infants with a gestational age (p.m.) of under 211 days. We chose this limit because we had not seen one IVH in babies born after 30 weeks of gestation. Mean birthweight was 1069 g, mean gestational age p.m. 28 weeks + 1 day. The patients were born in our hospital, i.e., they did not have to be transported after birth, between December 1981 and June 1982 and between February 1983 and January 1986. Of these, 31 (23%) had second to fourth degree IVH. IVH was diagnosed by CT at the end of the first postnatal week during the first study period (1981-1982), and by ultrasound (Technicare Sector scan 5 or 7.5 MHz) during the second study period. At least one scan was performed at the end of the 1st week of life.

Classification of Birth Mechanics. The obstetrician classified the mode of delivery as mechanically easy of difficult without knowing the infant's outcome. This classification was done for vaginal delivery and CS as well.

Statistics. Frequencies were compared by means of the χ^2 test or, if not adequate, by Fisher's exact test; means by Student's *t* test.

Results

Table 1 shows the impact of birth mechanics on the frequency of IVH irrespective of the route of delivery. Nearly the same impact of mechanical load can also be seen in CS infants (Table 2). There is no significant difference between frequency

Table 1. IVH $\geqslant$ II° vs. mode of delivery

	(*n*)	(%)
Difficult	19/28	68
Easy	12/104	12

$p < 10^{-6}$

Table 2. IVH $\geqslant$ II° vs. mode of cesarean section

	(*n*)	(%)
Difficult	11/20	55
Easy	11/80	14

$\chi^2 = 15.7$
$p < 0.000{,}1$ (2-tailed)

of IVH in CS infants with cephalic or noncephalic presentation (Table 3). Although the numbers are rather small, mechanically difficult vaginal delivery might be the worst way of delivery for very immature infants (see Table 4).

Comparing natural ("traditional") vaginal delivery, easy or difficult, with mechanically soft vaginal delivery, it turns out that the retractor technique offers some clear benefit in avoiding IVH (Table 5). CS reduces the frequency of IVH in noncephalic presentations compared to vaginal delivery (see Table 6). Although CS also seems to be better than traditional vaginal delivery in cases of cephalic presentation, this difference is not statistically significant (Table 7). However, when we compared both modes of delivery in infants of less than 1500 g birthweight, pooling our data with the data of Von Loewenich et al. (1985), we could show a significant advantage of CS in case of cephalic presentation.

On the other hand, vaginal delivery via retractor, our so-called mechanically soft delivery, seems to be better than CS. However, this difference cannot be confirmed mathematically (Table 8). It is no surprise that delivery via retractor offers better results than traditional vaginal delivery from cephalic presentation (Table 9).

There was no significant difference in birthweight between infants born vaginally or by CS (Table 10). However, mean gestational age of infants born by CS

Table 3. IVH $\geq$ II° vs. presentation, delivery by cesarean section

	(n)	(%)
Cephalic	12/62	19
Others	10/38	26

Ns

Table 4. IVH $\geq$ II° vs. mode of vaginal delivery

	(n)	(%)
Difficult	8/8	100
Easy	1/24	4

$p < 10^{-6}$

Table 5. IVH $\geq$ II° vs. method of vaginal delivery

	(n)	(%)
Traditional	8/14	57
Retractor	1[a]/18	6

[a] Breech presentation.
$p = 0.002$

Table 6. IVH $\geq$ II° in noncephalic presentations - cesarean section vs. vaginal delivery

	(n)	(%)
CS	10/36	28
Vaginal	5/6	83

$p = 0.016$

Table 7. IVH $\geq$ II° in cephalic presentation - cesarean section vs. traditional vaginal delivery (TV)

	(n)	(%)
CS	12/64	19
TV	4/9	44

$p < 0.09$ NS

Table 8. IVH $\geq$ II° in cephalic presentation - cesarean section vs. retractor delivery (R)

	(n)	(%)
CS	12/64	19
R	0/17	0

$p < 0.06$ NS

was significantly higher than in infants born vaginally (Table 11). On the other hand, no differences in gestational age could be found between infants with or without IVH, or with difficult vs. easy delivery (Tables 12 and 13).

Other Risk-Associated Factors.

Only two symptoms of intrapartum asphyxia could be identified as risk-associated factors of IVH in our study group: an umbilical artery pH below 7.20 and a 5-min Apgar score below 6 (Tables 14 and 15).

Impact of Postnatal Transport

In a small sample of infants with birthweights below 1500 g examined by CT during a 9-month period in 1981-1982, we found IVH in four out of eight outborn infants and in one out of 31 inborn infants (Bielicki et al. 1984). This study could not be continued because all pregnant women in our region in danger of premature delivery are now referred to centers where postnatal transport is not necessary. Therefore we pooled our few data with the data published by two other

Table 9. IVH ≥ II° in cephalic presentation - traditional vaginal delivery (TV) vs. retractor delivery (R)

	(n)	(%)
TV	4/9	44
R	0/17	0

$p = 0.008$

Table 10. Mean birthweight vs. method of delivery

	(g)
CS	1090
Vaginal	1002

NS (t test)

Table 11. Mean gestational age vs. method of delivery

	(weeks + days)
CS	28 + 3
Vaginal	27 + 1

$p < 0.01$ (t test)

Table 12. Mean gestational age (GA) vs. IVH ≥ II°

	(weeks + days)
IVH	28 + 0
Ø*	28 + 1

NS (t test)
* no hemorrhage

Table 13. Mean gestational age vs. mode of delivery

	(weeks + days)
Difficult	27 + 6
Easy	28 + 2

NS (t test)

Table 14. IVH ≥ II° vs. umbilical pH

	(n)	(%)
< 7.20	9/22	41
> 7.20	17/89	19

$p < 0.04$

Table 15. IVH $\geq$ II° vs. 5-min Apgar score

	(n)	(%)
≤ 5	12/23	52
>5	19/105	18

$p<0.001$

Table 16. IVH in very low birthweight infants. (Data from Bielicki et al. 1984; Clark et al. 1981; Garcia-Prats 1982)

	%)	
Outborn	50 ± 6	(90% CL)
Inborn	18 ± 6	

$p<10^{-6}$ ($n=319$)

Table 17. Reduction of IVH in very low birthweight infants by regionalization. (Data from Bielicki et al. 1984; Clark et al. 1981; Garcia-Prats 1982)

2.8-fold ($p=0.025$)
or
1.8–4.7-fold (95% CL)

$n=319$

authors (Clark et al. 1981; Garcia-Prats 1982). The results can be seen in Tables 16 and 17.

Sedation

Phenobarbitone is widely used in neuro-intensive care for lowering intracranial pressure as well as brain metabolism. Good results are seen in the treatment of posthypoxic and post-traumatic brain edema. Whether phenobarbitone also reduces the incidence of IVH is still debatable: some authors found a lower frequency of IVH after prophylactic treatment of the immature newborn infant (Bedard et al. 1984; Donn et al. 1981; Ruth et al. 1986) or the fetus just before birth (Shankaran et al. 1986). Other studies could not find any effect (Anwar et al. 1986; Kuban et al. 1986; Whitelaw et al. 1983). Therefore routine prophylaxis with phenobarbitone cannot be recommended at the present time.

Another interesting approach is paralyzing. Perlman et al. (1985) observed infants with fluctuations of brain perfusion following analog fluctuations of arterial blood pressure. These infants showed a very high incidence of IVH. Paralyzing these infants eradicated the fluctuations of CBF and lowered the frequency of IVH markedly.

Discussion

CBF is regulated by pH, pCO_2, and, less than by the other parameters, also by pO_2. Within wide limits CBF is independent of mean arterial pressure. This autoregulation of CBF prevents fluctuations of CBF with fluctuations of mean arterial pressure. On the other hand, autoregulation of CBF may be disturbed or even stopped in human or animal newborns by asphyxia (Lou et al. 1979) or by shock (Goddard-Finegold and Michael 1984). Breakdown of CBF autoregulation means that CBF, or cerebral perfusion pressure becomes linearly dependent on mean arterial pressure. Then high arterial pressure may cause IVH by rhexis of arterioles, and low arterial pressure could be the first step to periventricular leukomalacia. The observation of Perlman et al. (1985) may be interpreted in this way.

Interestingly, asphyxia is identified as a risk-associated factor of IVH in nearly all publications about the causes of IVH (Brand and Saling, this volume; Dolfin et al. 1983; Garcia-Prats 1982; Hill and Volpe 1986; Von Loewenich et al. 1985; McDonald et al. 1984; Szymonowicz et al. 1985; Van de Bor et al. 1986); its impact on autoregulation of CBF was clearly shown by Lou et al. (1979). Peri- or postnatal shock, which causes IVH in beagle puppies also disturbs autoregulation of CBF (Goddard-Finegold and Michael 1984). Although shock parameters have not been well documented in recent papers, it seems justified to assume that immature infants, bruised by a mechanically difficult delivery and showing extended hematomas, are suffering from shock. Indeed, a strong correlation between mechanical load during birth and frequency of IVH was not only found in our own material, but also in the data from Berlin-Neukoelln (Brand and Saling, this volume; Von Loewenich et al. 1985) and in the extensive material from Melbourne (Szymonowicz et al. 1985). Our hypothesis that intrapartum events are correlated with the occurrence of IVH may be supported by the common experience that IVH appears almost always during the first 3 days of postnatal life (Brand and Saling, this volume; Hill and Volpe 1986; Von Loewenich and Birkle 1981; McDonald et al. 1984; Perlman and Volpe 1986; Van de Bor 1986), with a peak between the 1st and 2nd days.

More difficult to explain is the impact of postnatal transport of the just-born immature baby to a neonatal intensive care unit (Bielicki et al. 1984; Clark et al. 1981; Garcia-Prats et al. 1982). During car transport the infant's head is exposed to incredibly high vertical accelerations (Boenisch et al. 1985). But further investigation is needed as to whether avoiding these accelerations reduces the frequency of IVH, or whether, in animal studies, accelerating the head provokes IVH. One has to bear in mind that prenatal transport of the fetus in utero not only lowers the postnatal mortality rate but also the frequency of IVH, although it is not known which component of the "baby transport" might be detrimental.

References

Anwar M, Kadam S, Hiatt IM, Hegyi T (1986) Phenobarbitone prophylaxis of intraventricular haemorrhage. Arch Dis Child 61: 196-197

Bedard MP, Shankaran S, Slovis TL, Pantoja A, Dayal B, Poland RL (1984) Effect of prophylactic phenobarbital on intraventricular hemorrhage in high risk infants. Pediatrics 73: 435-439

Bielicki M, v Loewenich V, Halberstadt E, Grau H (1984) Intraventrikuläre Blutungen bei sehr kleinen Frühgeborenen. In: Kowalewski S (ed) Pädiatrische Intensivmedizin VI, Vol.47 INA. Thieme, Stuttgart, pp 150-152

Boenisch H, Gaden W, Mau D, Gurbandt U, Teuteberg H-O, Braun H, Beermann HJ (1985)

Mechanische Belastung Neugeborener bei Inkubatortransporten. Monatsschr Kinderheilkd 133: 471-475

Clark CE, Clymann RI, Roth RS, Sniderman SH, Lane B, Ballard RA (1981) Risk factor analysis of intraventricular hemorrhage in low birthweight infants. J Pediatr 99: 625-628

Dolfin T, Skidmore MB, Fong KW, Hoskins EM, Shennan AT (1983) Incidence, severity, and timing of subependymal and intraventricular hemorrhages in preterm infants born in a perinatal unit as detected by serial real-time ultrasound. Pediatrics 71: 541-546

Donn SM, Roloff DW, Goldstein GW (1981) Prevention of intraventricular hemorrhage in preterm infants by phenobarbitone: a controlled trial. Lancet II: 215-217

Garcia-Prats JA, Procianoy RS, Adams JM, Rudolp AJ (1982) The hyaline membrane disease - intraventricular hemorrhage relationship in the very low birth weight infant. Perinatal aspects. Acta Paediatr Scand 71: 79-84

Goddard-Finegold J, Michael LH (1984) Cerebral blood flow and experimental intraventricular hemorrhage. Pediatr Res 18: 7-11

Hambleton G, Wigglesworth JS (1976) Origin of intraventricular haemorrhage in the preterm infant. Arch Dis Child 51: 651-659

Hill A, Volpe JJ (1986) Intracranial haemorrhage. In: Roberton NRC (ed) Textbook of neonatology. Churchill Livingstone, Edinburgh, pp 559-570

Hutchison AA, Barrett JM, Fleischer AC (1982) Intraventricular hemorrhage in the preterm infant. N Engl J Med 307: 1272-1273

Kuban KCK, Leviton A, Krishnamoorthy KS, Brown ER, Littlewood-Teele R, Baglivo JA, Sullivan KF, Huff KR, White S, Cleveland RH, Allred EN, Spritzer KL, Skouteli HN, Cayea P, Epstein MF (1986) Neonatal intracranial hemorrhage and phenobarbital. Pediatrics 77: 443-450

Lou HC, Lassen NA, Friis-Hansen B (1979) Impaired autoregulation of cerebral blood flow in the distressed newborn infant. J Pediatr 94: 118-121

McDonald MM, Koops BL, Johnson ML, Guggenheim MA, Rumack CM, Mitchell SA, Hathaway WE (1984) Timing and antecedents of intracranial hemorrhage in the newborn. Pediatrics 74: 32-36

Morgan MEI, Benson JWT, Cooke RWI (1981) Ethamsylate reduces the incidence of periventricular haemorrhage in very low birth weights babies. Lancet II: 830-831

Papile LA, Burstein J, Burstein R, Koffler H (1978) Incidence and evolution of subependymal and intraventricular haemorrhage: a study of infants with birth weight less than 1500 gm. J Pediatr 92: 529-534

Perlman JM, Volpe JJ (1986) Intraventricular hemorrhage in extremely small premature infants. Am J Dis Child 140: 1122-1124

Perlman JM, Goodman S, Kreusser KL, Volpe JJ (1985) Reduction in intraventricular hemorrhage by elimination of fluctuating cerebral blood-flow velocity in preterm infants with respiratory distress syndrome. N Engl J Med 312: 1353-1357

Ruth V, Virkola K, Paetau R, Raivio KO (1986) Prevention of hypoxic-ischemic cerebral damage in preterm infants by phenobarbital. Pediatr Res 20: 1054, abstract 124

Shankaran S, Cepeda EE, Ilagan N, Mariona F, Hassan M, Bhatia R, Ostrea E, Bedard MP, Poland RL (1986) Antenatal phenobarbital for the prevention of neonatal intracerebral hemorrhage. Am J Obstet Gynecol 154: 53-57

Szymonowicz W, Wilson F, Yu VYH, Walker A (1985) Reduction in periventricular haemorrhage in preterm infants associated with changes in neonatal care. In: Proceedings of Ross Labs Special Conference, Washington DC, Dec 15-17 1985, Syllabus 99-113

Van de Bor M, Van Bel F, Lineman R, Ruys JH (1986) Perinatal factors and periventricular-intraventricular hemorrhage in preterm infants. Am J Dis Child 140: 1125-1130

Von Loewenich V, Birkle C (1981) Survivors of intracranial hemorrhage. J Perinat Med 9: Suppl 1: 154-157

Von Loewenich V, Brand M, Halberstadt E, Saling EZ (1985) Die intracraniellen Blutungen des Neugeborenen. Arch Gynecol 238: 263-270

Whitelaw A, Placzek M, Dubowitz L, Lary S, Levene M (1983) Phenobarbitone for prevention of periventricular haemorrhage in very low birthweight infants. Lancet II: 1168-1170

Ylppö A (1919) Pathologisch-anatomische Studien bei Frühgeborenen. Z. Kinderheilkd 20: 212-431

Prediction of Outcome: Periventricular Hemorrhage Versus Ischemia

A. STEWART and P. HOPE

Introduction

Prior to the formation of FIGO in 1954, obstetrical care was judged according to maternal, foetal and infant mortality only. The importance of the quality of survival was not fully appreciated until later; and even when it was recognised, definition of "quality" proved to be very difficult. Lesions, particularly haemorrhagic ones, were noted at autopsy in the brains of infants who had died in the perinatal period. Indices of brain damage were therefore chosen as outcome measures of quality. The choice was reasonable, but there were two problems. First, the majority of relevant CNS impairments could only be diagnosed when the infants were many months - even years - old. Secondly, it was difficult, if not impossible, to distinguish so long after birth between congenital or antenataly acquired CNS conditions and those which resulted from perinatal insults or environmental circumstances in early childhood. The introduction of brain imaging techniques for use in the neonatal period (Papile et al. 1978; Pape et al. 1979) appeared to offer a solution to both problems and to provide an objective measure of the state of the brain in the immediate neonatal period with which outcome could be predicted. We should like to review what has been learnt in the 7 years since these techniques were introduced, paying particular attention to prediction of outcome and the relative roles of haemorrhage and ischaemic lesions.

Methods

Infants Studied. Investigators tended to concentrate on infants believed to be at high risk of brain damage, including that due to cerebral or intraventricular haemorrhage. The infants were usually undergoing intensive neonatal care because they were very sick or very immature, defined according to short gestation (<33 weeks - or occasionally $\leqslant 34$ weeks) or very low birthweight (<1500 g).

Ultrasound. Because this technique was believed to be safe and the equipment was portable, it was the most widely used procedure and has provided the majority of information. Since the technique was introduced in 1978, the equipment has undergone major technological changes resulting in great improvements in the quality of imaging and of resolution. These changes, however, caused problems of interpretation which will be referred to later. From the beginning, germinal layer/intraventricular haemorrhages (IVH) were diagnosed and ventricular characteristics and dimensions were described. Markedly increased echo densities in the periventricular region (see Rushton et al. 1985 for definition) were also noted, and these usually developed into cystic areas due to local loss of cerebral tissue (one form of atrophy). Accuracy of imaging was investigated using computerised tomography (CT) scanning or autopsy findings as standards for comparison (e.g. Silverboard et al. 1980; Thorburn et al. 1982a; Levene et al. 1985). More recently, using mechanical sector scanners, less marked increased echo densities have also been reported in the periventricular region, typically seen posteriorly to the body of the lateral ventricle. These moderately dense echoes were thought not to be due to haemorrhage; they were transient and were believed possibly to represent the early changes of periventricular leucomalacia (PVL) (Preston et al. 1983) and in some cases, frank cystic PVL was later observed to develop at the same site (Fawer et al. 1985). These findings were also investigated with autopsy and CT comparisons (Fawer et al. 1985; Rushton et al. 1985; Laub and Ingirich 1986), and more recently with measures of cerebral energy metabolism using magnetic resonance spectroscopy (Hamilton et al. 1986) which Professor Reynolds will discuss later in this volume. Unfortunately, every group of investigators prepared its own definitions, and most have felt the need to revise the definitions as increased knowledge has led to a better understanding of the observations. Interpretation of the various reports has been further complicated by differences in timing and frequency of scanning, with recent studies including more scans for longer periods - and this will also be referred to later.

Data Analysis. In order to understand the implications of the imaging findings and to derive information which could be used for predictive purposes, perinatal data including obstetric factors and mortality statistics were collated and infants were followed up. Outcome among survivors was defined according to neurodevelopmental status based on neurological examination and developmental testing at ages ranging from 1-2 years (after correction for preterm birth). Abnormality was defined as "major" when serious impairments or disorders which interfered with function and caused disability were identified. The majority of these disorders were cerebral palsies and delayed development, thought to represent impaired cognitive functioning. The problems sometimes occurred together. Other diagnoses included sensory neural hearing loss and cortical blindness. Some investigators included a second category of minor impairments or disorders (Stewart et al. 1986). These were usually abnormalities of tone and reflexes present at the end of the 1st year of life but which, nevertheless, were not causing frank disability. They were included because such findings were believed to be associated with poor performance on tests of cognitive function and of fine motor skills at school age and therefore likely to indicate children at risk of learning difficulties and school failure (Amiel-Tison et al. 1984).

Statistical Analysis. Procedures included χ^2 testing, one-way analysis of variance, multiple stepwise regression and logistical regression analyses. Predictions were based on probability estimates *(p)*, defined as the proportion of infants with an abnormal neurodevelopmental outcome, and 95% confidence intervals or the lowest to the highest probability compatible with the data and within which the result would fall if the study were repeated.

Results

Periventricular Haemorrhage

The earliest studies concentrated almost entirely on these haemorrhages. They were easily recognised - and were what the investigators expected to find in very preterm infants!

Mortality. All studies reported a significant association between PVH and perinatal or neonatal death, particlarly death within 7 days of birth (e.g. Ahman et al. 1980; Shankaran et al. 1982; Thorburn et al. 1982b). Mortality tended to be higher in infants with larger haemorrhages. In our own study (Table 1), only large haemorrhages and those associated with marked periventricular echo densities carried an increased risk of death.

Neurodevelopmental Outcome. In all studies, PVH was significantly associated with neurodevelopmental disorders (e.g. Thorburn et al. 1981; Shankaran et al. 1982; Stewart et al. 1983; Stewart 1985) at follow up in infants aged 1-2 years, but the proportion of affected infants appeared to depend upon several factors, including the development of ventricular dilatation as well as the extent of the haemorrhage (Palmer et al. 1982) (Table 2). Infants who developed posthaemorrhagic hydrocephalus had a particularly bad prognosis. This complication occurred most often following a large IVH - and in fact probably accounted for the bad outcome in these infants (Stewart et al. 1986). Infants who had markedly

Table 1. Mortality according to US diagnosis of PVH in 579 very preterm (<33 weeks) infants, born 1979 and 1981-1984

US	*n*	Mortality		
		≤7 days (%)	8-28 days (%)	>28 days (%)
No PVH	310	11	3	6
Small PVH	192	15	4	7
Large PVH	45	29	4	11
PVH + marked parenchymal echo densities	32	31	16	13

Table 2. Neurodevelopmental abnormalities at 12 months according to PVH alone and with other US lesions in 342 very preterm (<33 weeks) infants born 1979-83

US	*n*	Neurodevelopmental abnormality	
		Major (%)	Total (%)
No PVH	184	4	10
Small PVH only	98	4	19
Large PVH only	3	0	0
PVH + ventricular dilatation	40	35	45
PVH + hydrocephalus	8	50	75
PVH + marked parenchymal echo densities	9	89	100

increased periventricular echo densities (as described by Rushton et al. 1985) also had a very bad prognosis (Stewart et al. 1983; McMenamin et al. 1984; Stewart et al. 1986), with disorders (usually predominantly neuromotor) in most, if not all, affected infants.

Hypoxic-Ischaemic Lesions

Because ultrasound (US) diagnosis of these lesions has only recently become possible and the interpretation of some findings remains controversial, there are limited data available to review. Conclusions, therefore, can only be regarded as tentative. The two lesions believed with certainty to represent hypoxic-ischaemic damage, cystic PVL or generalised cerebral atrophy, could only be diagnosed at a late stage with US, so mortality studies proved impossible. Almost all reported cases of cystic PVL were neurodevelopmentally abnormal at 9-24 months (Bozynski et al. 1985; Calâme et al. 1985; de Vries et al. 1985; Weindling et al. 1985). The prognosis for infants with generalised atrophy was almost as bad (Stewart et al. 1983), and de Vries et al. (1985) have pointed out that infants with frank loss of brain tissue presumed to be due to PVL were usually the most seriously disabled with global developmental delay in addition to neuromotor disorders. Ventricular dilatation almost invariably accompanies PVL (Dubowitz et al. 1985). Very few reports give the follow-up results for these infants separately, those that did indicated a relatively poor prognosis with more than 25% neurodevelopmentally abnormal (Stewart et al. 1983, 1986) (Table 3).

The outcome for infants with moderately increased periventricular echo densities remains controversial. From the little information available, when the US findings were transient and no cysts, ventricular dilatation or generalised cerebral atrophy developed, the prognosis was good and equivalent to that of small, uncomplicated PVH (Stewart et al. 1985). Support for this opinion based on the

Table 3. Neurodevelopmental abnormalities at 12 months according to US scan findings in 342 very preterm (<33 weeks) infants born 1979–83

US	n	Neurodevelopmental abnormality	
		Major (%)	Total (%)
Normal scan	174	3	7
Uncomplicated PVH	101	4	19
Ventricular dilatation	41	27	34
Hydrocephalus	8	50	75
Cerebral atrophy –			
Cystic[a]	10	80	100
General	8	38	88
	18	61	94

[a] Following marked parenchymal echo densities or cystic PVL

findings among very few infants, comes from Laub and Ingirich (1986) who reported that similar US findings which did not proceed to cyst formation or general atrophy, occurred commonly in normal, potentially healthy term infants.

Haemorrhage Versus Ischaemia as Determinants of Outcome

Several investigators have inferred from their findings that ischaemic lesions are the most important cause of neurodevelopmental disorders in very preterm infants (e.g. Calâme et al. 1985; de Vries et al. 1985). In an attempt to quantify the relative importance of haemorrhage and ischaemic lesions, Stewart et al. (1983) speculated from their data that PVH accounted for only 19% of the neurodevelopmental disorders diagnosed by 18 months among very preterm infants (<33 weeks) whereas ischaemic lesions were either noted, or thought likely to have been present on the basis of the neurodevelopmental status, in up to 66% of affected infants (Table 4). Exclusion of small degrees of hypoxic-ischaemic injury on the basis of US findings was not possible with the quality and resolution of imaging available in the early studies and insufficient follow-up data have been reported, since lesions thought to represent the early changes of PVL began to be recognised, to allow satisfactory statistical analysis. These deductions were based on oversimplified interpretations of US scan findings but they indicated the need for a non-invasive measure of hypoxic-ischaemic injury at or shortly after the insult in order to investigate the aetiology and pathogenesis of ischaemic lesions of the brain in the perinatal period, as Professor Reynolds will discuss later in this volume.

Table 4. Details of very preterm (<33 weeks) infants admitted to the neonatal unit of University College Hospital London in 1979-83

Admitted within 1 week of birth	485
Neonatal death (<28 days)	104
"Late" death (1-9 months)	30
Total survivors	*351*
Disabling congenital defect	6
Unclassified US lesion	1
Lost to follow up	2
Total for analysis	*342*

Predictions

Ultrasound Brain Scans

Prediction of outcome was perceived as an important function of US brain scanning from the time it was introduced. From the data reviewed so far it is clear that US has limitations but it is widely available and it will be a long time before sufficient data accumulate from other, potentially more accurate measures, to be used for the purposes of prediction in individual infants. We have used the results from a study of 485 very preterm (<33 weeks) infants who had prospective US brain scans to calculate probability estimates *(p)* and 95% confidence intervals for neurodevelopmental outcome at 12-18 months which may be applied to other similar, individual infants (Stewart et al. 1986). Of the 485 infants, 342 survived without serious congenital malformations known to affect neurodevelopmental outcome and have been followed up to more than 12 months of age (Table 5). Results from these 342 infants provided the data base for the calculations which were made according to scan findings at the end of the 1st week of life and at discharge from the neonatal unit (Table 5).

First Week of Life. Although prediction of outcome would be of most use in the first days of life, US diagnoses were confined at that age to PVH and markedly

Table 5. Perinatal details of 342 very preterm (<33 weeks) infants who survived, without serious congenital defects, following admission to the neonatal unit of University College London (UCH) in 1979-83

Male/female	187/155	
Born in UCH/referred	197/145	
Vaginal delivery Caesarean section	189/153	
Median gestation (weeks)	30	(24-32)
Median birthweight (g)	1340	(535-2500)
Small for gestational age	21	
Hyaline membrane disease	164	
Mechanical ventilation	191	

increased periventricular echo densities (see Table 6 for definitions). On this basis, very preterm (<33 weeks) infants with no PVH or markedly dense echoes had small probabilities, within narrow confidence limits, of a major (4%; 2%-9%) or of any (10%; 6%-15%) neurodevelopmental disorder (Table 7). The probabilities increased according to the presence and extent of PVH. Infants who had markedly increased echo densities had the largest probabilities of neurodevelopmental disorders at 12-18 months with values of 89% (52%-99%) for major disorders and 100% (66%-100%) for either major or minor disorders; and these values were clearly separate from those for infants with no PVH or dense echoes (Table 8).

Table 6. Definitions of lesions in the brain diagnosed with US by the end of the 1st week of life in very preterm (<33 weeks) infants

Periventricular haemorrhage (PVH): germinal layer or intraventricular haemorrhage; *small:* causing little or no ventricular distension; *large:* markedly distending with blood one or both ventricles (e.g. casts)

Parenchymal echo density: extension of dense echoes from the germinal layer or ventricles into brain tissue, consistent with parenchymal extension of PVH or haemorrhagic infarction (e.g. haemorrhagic periventricular leucomalacia)

Table 7. Probability estimates and 95% confidence intervals from major, or major and minor neurodevelopmental disorders at 12 months according to US findings in the 1st week of life among 342 very preterm (<33 weeks) infants

US	*n*	Probability of neurodevelopmental disorders[a]	
		Major	Major/minor
No PVH/parenchymal echo densities	184	4 (2- 9)	10 (6- 15)
Small PVH	133	11 (6-18)	26 (19- 35)
Large PVH	16	31 (11-59)	44 (20- 70)
Parenchymal echo densities	9	89 (52-99)	100 (66-100)

[a] 95% confidence interval.

Table 8. Definitions of lesions in the brain diagnosed with ultrasound at discharge from the neonatal unit in very preterm (<33 weeks) infants

Uncomplicated periventricular haemorrhage (PVH): germinal layer or intraventricular haemorrhage not associated with parenchymal echo densities, or followed by ventricular dilatation or hydrocephalus

Ventricular dilatation: 1979-82, dilatation of one or both lateral ventricles with cerebrospinal fluid (CSF), insufficient to meet criteria of hydrocephalus; 1983, dilatation with CSF such that the depth of the frontal horn immediately anterior to the thalamo-caudate notch exceeded 3 mm

Hydrocephalus: marked dilatation of a lateral ventricle such that the width increased to more than 2 standard deviation plus 5 mm above the mean for comparable normal infants

Cerebral atrophy: local or general loss of brain tissue from any cause

Table 9. Probability estimates and 95% confidence intervals for major, or major and minor neurodevelopmental disorders at 12 months according to US findings at discharge among 342 very preterm (<33 weeks) infants)

US	*n*	Probability of neurodevelopmental disorders[a]	
		Major	Major/minor
Normal/uncomplicated PVH	275	4 (2- 7)	11 (8-17)
Ventricular dilatation	41	27 (14-43)	34 (20-51)
Hydrocephalus/cerebral atrophy[b]	26	58 (37-77)	88 (70-97)

[a] 95% confidence intervals
[b] Includes cysts following parenchymal echo densities, PVH and general loss of brain tissue

At Discharge from Intensive Care Unit. By this age, more lesions were diagnosed with US, including those believed to be due to hypoxic-ischaemic injury (see Table 8 for definitions). On the basis of these findings, logistical multiple regression analysis indicated that very preterm (<33 weeks) infants could be divided into three main categories (Table 9) with small, intermediate or large probabilities of adverse outcomes at 12-18 months. For example, infants with normal scans and those with uncomplicated PVH had a 4% probability of a major disorder, with narrow confidence intervals of 2%-7%, and 11% (8%-17%) for both major and minor disorders. By contrast, infants with hydrocephalus or cerebral atrophy (cystic or generalised, from any cause) had a 58% (37%-77%) probability of major disorders and an 88% (70%-97%) probability of major or minor disorders. Infants with ventricular dilatation had intermediate probabilities of 27% (14%-43%) for major and 34% (20%-51%) for both major and minor disorders (Table 9). Thus, on the basis of US brain scan findings at discharge from the neonatal unit, it was possible to define a large group of infants, who comprised 80% of our study, and to whom we could confidently assign a good outcome at 12 months of age. None of these infants had definite US evidence of hypoxic-ischaemic injury. By contrast, the small group, 9% of infants assigned a bad outcome, including those with definite ischaemic lesions (cystic PVL or general cerebral atrophy); and the group (12%) assigned intermediate probabilities for adverse outcomes were defined on the basis of US diagnosis of ventricular dilatation which often indicates hypoxic-ischaemic injury (Gould et al. unpublished data).

Ultrasound and Neurological Examination

In an early study of US brain scanning and structured neurological examinations (as described by Amiel-Tison and Grenier 1985), we noted that neurological examination improved the recognition of very preterm (<33 weeks) infants who proved to be normal at 18 months (Stewart et al. 1984). We therefore carried out, in collaboration with Amiel-Tison, a prospective study designed to test the hypothesis that improved prediction of a normal outcome at 12 months could be achieved from a combination of US brain scans and neurological examinations at term. We found that infants with normal US scans or with uncomplicated PVH and a normal result on neurological examination at term had a 98% probability (with 95% confidence interval of 90%-99%) of normal neurodevelopment at 12 months of age. Thus for the first time, individual preterm (<33 weeks) infants who had an excellent prognosis were identified when they were discharged from the neonatal unit.

Conclusions

Neonatal US brain scanning provides predictive information which can be applied to similar individual infants. On the basis of scan findings at discharge from hospital, very preterm (<33 weeks) infants can be assigned small, intermediate or large probabilities of an adverse neurodevelopmental outcome at 12 months. US brain scanning in the neonatal period also provides some evidence that ischaemic lesions are the main determinants of neurodevelopmental abnormalities noted at follow up, at age 12-24 months, in very preterm infants.

Acknowledgements. Many people collaborated in the studies carried out at University College Hospital London which are referred to in this review. I should like particularly to acknowledge the contributions of Drs. J. Baudin, A. M. de L. Costello, P. A. Hamilton, Mr. D. Lowe, Prof. E. O. R. Reynolds, Miss J. Townsend, and the financial support of the Medical Research Council.

References

Ahman PA, Lazzara A, Dykes FD, Brann AW, Schwartz JF (1980) Intraventricular hemorrhage in the high-risk pre-term infant: Incidence and outcome. Ann Neurol 7: 118

Amiel-Tison C, Grenier A (1985) La Surveillance neurologique au cours de la premier année de la vie. Masson, New York

Amiel-Tison C, Dubé R, Garel M, Jequier JC (1984) Outcome at age 5 years of full term infants with transient neurologic abnormalities in the first year of life. In: Stern L (ed) Intensive care in the newborn, IV. Masson, New York, p 247

Bozynski MEA, Nelson MN, Matalon TAS, Genaze DR, Rosati-Skertich C, Naughton PM, Meier WA (1985) Cavitary periventricular leukomalacia: incidence and short-term outcome in infants weighing 1200 grams at birth. Dev Med Child Neurol 27: 572-577

Calâme A, Fawer C-L, Anderegg A, Perentes E (1985) Interaction between perinatal brain damage and processes of normal brain development. Dev Neurosci 7: 1-11

De Vries LS, Dubowitz LMS, Dubowitz V, Kaiser A, Lary S, Silverman M, Whitelaw A, Wigglesworth JS (1985) Predictive value of cranial ultrasound in the newborn baby: a reappraisal. Lancet II: 137-355

Dubowitz LMS, Bydder GM, Mushin J (1985) Developmental sequence of periventricular leukomalacia. Arch Dis Child 60: 349-355

Fawer C-L, Calâme A, Perentes E, Anderegg A (1985) Periventricular leukomalacia: a correlation study between real-time ultrasound and autopsy findings. Neuroradiology 27: 292-300

Hamilton PA, Hope PL, Cady EB, Delpy DT, Wyatt JS, Reynolds EOR (1986) Impaired energy metabolism in brains of newborn infants with increased cerebral echo-densities. Lancet I: 1242-1246

Laub MC, Ingrisch H (1986) Increased periventricular echogenicity (periventricular halos) in neonatal brain: a sonographic study. Neuropediatrics 17: 39-43

Levene MI, Williams JL, Fawer C-L (eds) (1985) Ultrasound of the infant brain. Spastics international medical publications. Blackwell, Oxford

McMenamin JB, Shackelford DG, Volpe JJ (1984) Outcome of neonatal intraventricular hemorrhage with periventricular echo-dense lesions. Ann Neurol 15: 285-290

Palmer P, Dubowitz LMS, Levene MI, Dubowitz V (1982) Development and neurological progress of pre-term infants with intraventricular haemorrhage and ventricular dilatation. Arch Dis Child 57: 748-753

Pape KE, Blackwell RJ, Cusick G, Sherwood A, Houang MTW, Thorburn RJ, Reynolds EOR (1979) Ultrasound detection of brain damage in pre-term infants. Lancet I: 1261-1264

Papile LA, Burstein J, Burstein R, Koffler H (1978) Incidence and evolution of subependymal and intraventricular hemorrhage: a study of infants with a birthweight of less than 1500 g. Pediatrics 92: 529-534

Preston PR, Rushton DI, Durbin GM (1983) Ultrasound periventricular echo-densities in neonatal brains. Lancet II: 847-848

Rushton DI, Preston PR, Durbin GM (1985) Structure and evolution of echo-dense lesions in the neonatal brain. Arch Dis Child 60: 798-808

Shankaran S, Slovis TL, Bedard MP, Poland RL (1982) Sonographic classification of intracerebral hemorrhage: prognostic indicator of mortality, morbidity, and short term neurologic outcome. J Pediat 100: 469-475

Silverboard G, Horder MH, Ahman PA, Lazzara A, Schwartz JF (1980) Reliability of ultrasound diagnosis of intracerebral hemorrhage and posthemorrhagic hydrocephalus: comparison with computed tomography. Pediatrics 66: 507-514

Stewart A (1985) Early prediction of neurological outcome when the very pre-term infant is discharged from the intensive care unit. Ann Pédiatr 32: 27-38

Stewart AL, Thorburn RJ, Hope PL, Goldsmith M, Lipscomb AP, Reynolds EOR (1983) Ultrasound appearance of the brain in very pre-term infants and neuro-developmental outcome at 18 months of age. Arch Dis Child 58: 598-604

Stewart AL, Thorburn RJ, Hope PL, Costello AM de L, Goldsmith M, Swain P, Reynolds EOR (1984) Prediction of neuro-developmental status at 18 months of age by ultrasound and neurological examination. Pediatr Res 18: 95 (abstract)

Stewart AL, Hope PL, Hamilton PA, Baudin J, Wyatt JS, Reynolds EOR (1985) Increased periventricular echo-densities in very pre-term infants and prediction of early neuro-developmental outcome. Pediatr Res 19: 1084 (abstract)

Stewart AL, Reynolds EOR, Hope PL, Hamilton PA, Baudin J, Costello AM de L, Bradord BC, Wyatt JS (1987) Probability of neuro-developmental disorders estimated from ultrasound appearance of brains in very pre-term infants. Dev Med Child Neurol 29: 3-11

Thorburn RJ, Lipscomb AP, Stewart AL, Reynolds EOR, Hope PL, Pape KE (1981) Prediction of death and major handicap in very pre-term infants by brain ultrasound. Lancet I: 1119-1121

Thorburn RJ, Lipscomb AP, Reynolds EOR, Blackwell RJ, Cusick G, Shaw DG, Smith JF (1982a) Accuracy of imaging of the brain of newborn infants by linear-array real-time ultrasound. Early Hum Dev 9: 31-46

Thorburn RJ, Lipscomb AP, Stewart AL, Reynolds EOR, Hope PL (1982b) Timing and antecedents of periventricular haemorrhage in very pre-term infants. Early Hum Dev 9: 221-238

Weindling AM, Rochefort MJ, Calvert SA, Fok T-F, Wilkinson A (1985) Development of cerebral palsy after ultrasonographic detection of periventricular cysts in the newborn. Dev Med Child Neurol 27: 800-806

Magnetic Resonance Spectroscopy of the Brain and Early Neurodevelopmental Outcome

E. O. R. Reynolds and P. A. Hamilton

Introduction

Newborn infants admitted to neonatal intensive care units are at risk for two major types of lesion in the brain, periventricular haemorrhage and hypoxic-ischaemic injury. If the incidence, timing, pathogenesis and prognostic significance of these lesions are to be explored, and methods of prevention and treatment rigorously tested, then objective techniques are required for the accurate diagnosis of the lesions as close as possible to the time when they arise.

In recent years, ultrasound scanning of the brain has provided a wealth of information about the evolution of periventricular haemorrhage which principally affects preterm infants. Ultrasound is, however, a poor technique for detecting the early changes of ischaemia - though the later consequences may become visible as cystic periventricular leucomalacia or other loss of brain tissue.

There is, therefore, an urgent need for the development of new techniques for the non-invasive investigation of the early changes of ischaemic injury. This need has recently been brought more sharply into focus by evidence that birth asphyxia is the commonest cause of perinatally acquired permanent neurodevelopmental disorders in newborn infants (Alberman 1982), and also that ischaemic injury is a more important cause than periventricular haemorrhage of neurodevelopmental disorders in preterm infants (Stewart et al. 1983) - who form the major workload of any neonatal intensive care unit. Magnetic resonance spectroscopy (MRS) is one technique which shows considerable promise for the investigation of ischaemic injury to the brain.

Magnetic Resonance Spectroscopy

Magnetic resonance spectroscopy (MRS) can be used to measure the intracellular concentrations of metabolites and intracellular pH (pH_i) inside the organs of the body (see Gadian 1982 for review). Because it is non-invasive and apparently safe, it is particularly suited to the investigation of newborn infants. MRS has been established for many years as a valuable analytical technique in laboratory chemistry, but it is only quite recently that the study of living animals and human subjects has become possible. This development depended on the production of the large and powerful superconducting magnets that are necessary for the provision of a sufficiently strong and uniform magnetic field. The principle of the technique is based on the tendency of certain atomic nuclei with magnetic moments to line up along the magnetic field. This alignment can be disturbed by applying a suitable radiofrequency pulse at right angles to the field. When the pulse ceases, the nuclei return to their previous alignment and in so doing emit radiofrequency signals which can be detected. The frequency and magnitude of the signals provide information about the chemical composition of the sample under investigation and the concentrations of the metabolites present. So far, the phosphorus (^{31}P) nucleus has been the one most studied in human subjects and it is of particular interest for the investigation of ischaemic injury, since the relative concentrations of the mobile phosphorus metabolites that are most important in energy metabolism can be measured, notably adenosine triphosphate (ATP), phosphocreatine (PCr) and inorganic orthophosphate (Pi). Furthermore, pH_i can be estimated from the frequency of the Pi resonance. In conditions where oxidative metabolism is inadequate, alterations in the concentrations of the phosphorus metabolites and in pH_i are to be expected. In particular, as energy failure develops, the concentration of PCr will fall in order to maintain ATP levels through the creatine kinase pathway, and the concentration of Pi will rise, causing a fall in the PCr/Pi ratio: later, when energy failure is severe, the concentration of ATP will also fall.

The Brain in Newborn Infants

Following pilot investigations on experimental animals (Delpy et al. 1982) and the development of a transport system which allowed infants to be studied safely in the bore of the magnet, ^{31}P spectra have been obtained from over 120 infants, often studied on several occasions. Details of the methods have been given elsewhere (Cady et al. 1983; Hope et al. 1984; Hope and Reynolds 1985; Hamilton et al. 1986). Briefly, an Oxford Research Systems TMR 32-200 spectrometer was used, operating at a field strength of 1.89 T. The infant's head lay on a 5 cm or 7.4 cm diameter radiofrequency coil, which both supplied the exciting radiofrequency pulse and detected the magnetic resonance signal returning from the sensitive volume of the magnet, which was centred on the adjacent temporo-parietal cortex. The pulse duration was 80 μs for the 5 cm and 100 μs for the 7.4 cm coil; the flip angle at the centre of the coil was between 90° and 100°, and the pulse interval was 2.256 s. The spectra were usually produced from the sum of the responses to 768 pulses. The relative concentrations of the phosphorus metabolites were calculated from the integrals of the spectral peaks after correction for the effects of saturation; and pH_i was estimated from the difference in chemical shift between the PCr and Pi resonances.

The major purpose of this presentation is to discuss the relation between the MRS results and early outcome; other findings can be summarised as follows:

1. In the brains of normal infants, spectral peaks were detectable from phosphomonoesters (probably largely phosphoethanolamine), Pi, phosphodiesters, PCr and ATP (Cady et al. 1983; Hope et al. 1984) (Fig. 1).
2. The relative concentrations of some of the metabolites changed with increasing gestational age (Hamilton et al. 1986) (Fig. 1). The main changes probably signify an increase in the phosphorylation potential or "energy state" of brain tissue.
3. A reduction in energy state implying impaired oxidative phosphorylation was found in the brains of infants with a wide range of conditions of suspected or proven ischaemic injury including birth asphyxia, periventricular leucomalacia and other forms of cerebral infarction (Cady et al. 1983; Hope et al. 1984; Hope and Reynolds 1985, Hamilton et al. 1986). Following birth asphyxia, there was often a latent period before energy failure developed, suggesting the possibility of effective early treatment (Hope et al. 1984). A deteriorating energy state was often accompanied by an intracellular alkalosis (Hope et al. 1984; Hamilton et al. 1986).
4. Certain inborn errors of metabolism caused very gross energy failure (Hope and Reynolds 1985).

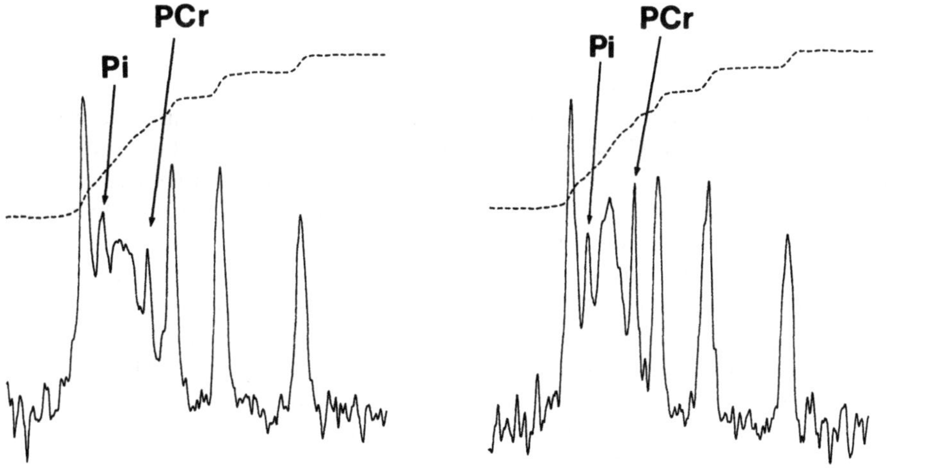

Fig. 1 a, b. Phosphorus spectra from two normal infants, **a** born at 28 weeks of gestation and studied 7 days after birth, **b** born at 40 weeks and studied aged 1 day. The *x-axis* is chemical shift (ppm) and the *y-axis* is signal intensity: the *interrupted lines* are the integrals of the spectra (concentration is proportional to the height of the steps in the integral curve). The peaks are attributable, from left to right, to phosphomonoesters, inorganic orthophosphate *(Pi)*, phosphodiesters, phosphocreatine *(PCr)* and the γ, α and β phosphorus nuclei of adenosine triphosphate. The PCr/Pi ratio in the preterm infant (a) was 0.74 and in the term one (b), 1.19. (Data from Hamilton et al. 1986)

Phosphorus Spectra and Early Outcome

Two studies have been carried out to investigate the relation between the results of MRS and early outcome: (a) a study of infants with cerebral ischaemic echodensities; (b) an investigation of the relation between the MRS findings and early neurodevelopmental outcome in the whole group of infants so far studied who had reached an age of at least 1 year.

Energy Metabolism in Infants with Cerebral Ischaemic Echodensities

Certain patterns of increased echodensity detected by ultrasound scanning in the brain are often attributed to ischaemic injury (Levene et al. 1985). Sometimes these echodensities evolve into cystic periventricular leucomalacia or other forms of cerebral atrophy - or they may disappear, apparently without adverse sequelae. The purpose of this investigation was to find out whether evidence of impaired energy metabolism could be found in the brains of infants with ischaemic echodensities, and if so, whether the MRS findings provided useful prognostic information, as judged by subsequent death or ultrasound evidence of cerebral atrophy. Full details of this study have been published elsewhere (Hamilton et al. 1986).

During a period of 33 months, increased cerebral parenchymal echodensities were detected by routine ultrasound scanning of the brains of 147 of the 979 infants admitted to the neonatal unit of University College Hospital. In 29 of the infants, the echodensities were very clearly delineated and confluent with intraventricular haemorrhage; they were therefore thought likely to be mainly or entirely due to haemorrhage rather than ischaemia. Increased echodensities in 62 of the other 118 infants were mild and transient but in the remaining 56 infants they were marked, persisted for at least 48 h in survivors and appeared consistent with ischaemic injury. MRS was performed in 27 of these latter infants, who had been born at 27-42 (median 40) weeks of gestation. The echodensities were diffuse and bilateral in 14 of the 27 and were usually associated with birth asphyxia: in ten they were largely confined to the periventricular region and were thought to be due to leucomalacia, and in three infants they were unilateral and consistent with cerebral arterial infarction. MRS was first carried out when the infants were 8 h-23 days (median 3 days) old, 0-8 days (median 1 day) after the echodensities were first noted and while these remained clearly visible: further MRS studies were performed on 19 of the infants at intervals of a few days. Ultrasound scanning was continued in the surviving infants to find out which ones developed cerebral atrophy, defined as any form of loss of brain tissue. MRS studies were also done on 18 control infants born at 28-42 (median 32) weeks of gestation when they were 1-61 (median 5) days old: these infants had no evidence of birth asphyxia or neurological abnormality and their ultrasound scans were normal.

Figure 2a shows an ultrasound scan and a ^{31}P spectrum from an infant with echodensities consistent with periventricular leucomalacia: the PCr/Pi ratio was abnormality low and cysts subsequently developed in brain tissue, as shown in Fig. 2b, although by then the spectrum had returned to normal. Figure 3 shows very similar echodensities in another infant: however, the spectrum obtained at the

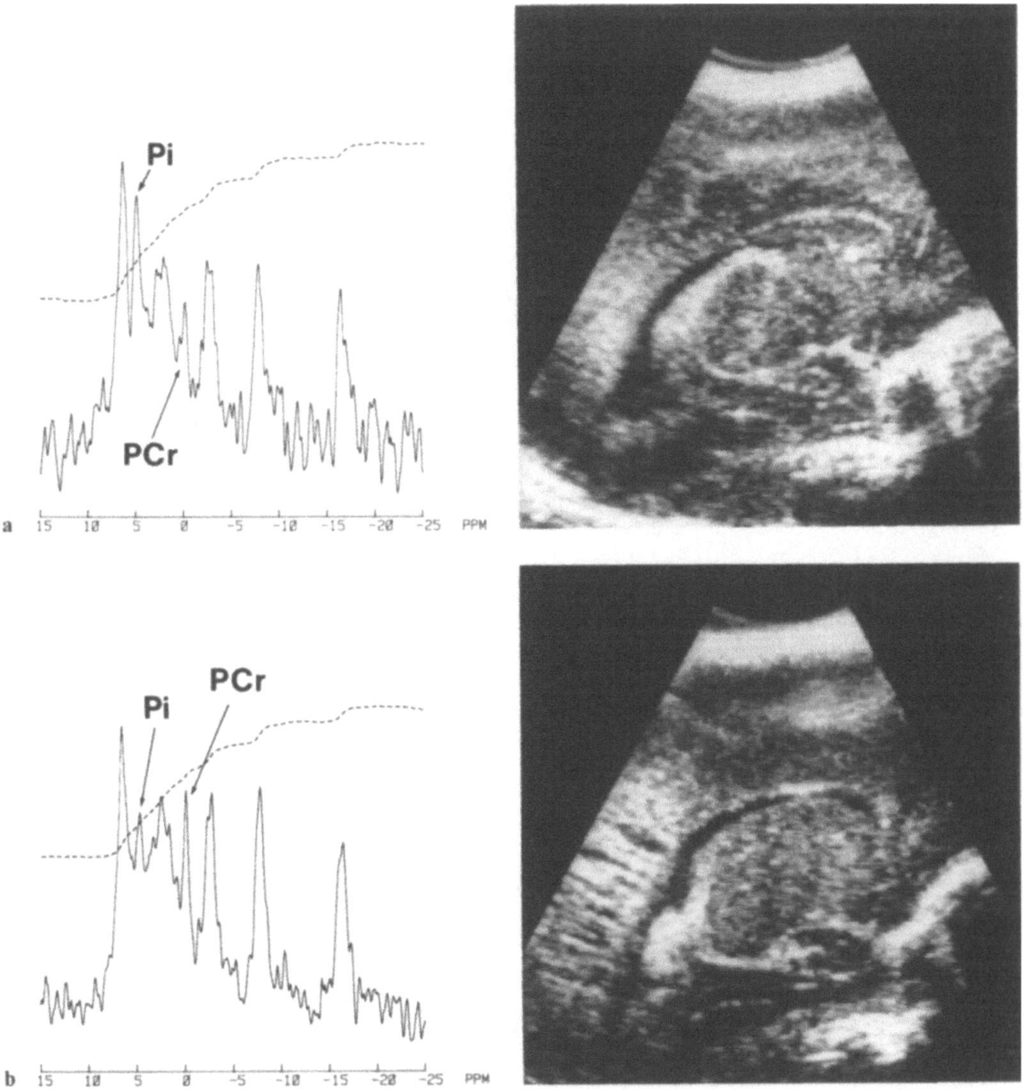

Fig. 2. a, b. Spectra and parasagittal ultrasound scans from an infant born at 33 weeks of gestation. **a** At 3 days of age: PCr/Pi was low, 0.60; the echo densities posterior to the lateral ventricle *(left)* are consistent with periventricular leucomalacia. **b** At 10 days (spectrum) and 27 days (scan): PCr/Pi was normal, 0.85; the scan shows periventricular cysts. (Data from Hamilton et al. 1986)

time was normal, and the echodensities resolved without any subsequent loss of brain tissue. Figure 4 shows spectra from two severely asphyxiated babies with diffuse echodensities, both of whom died later: the PCr/Pi ratio from the spectrum illustrated in Fig. 4a is grossly reduced and the ATP concentration (expressed as a fraction of total phosphorus) is also low. In the spectrum illustrated in Fig. 4b there are no clearly distinguishable signals from PCr or ATP.

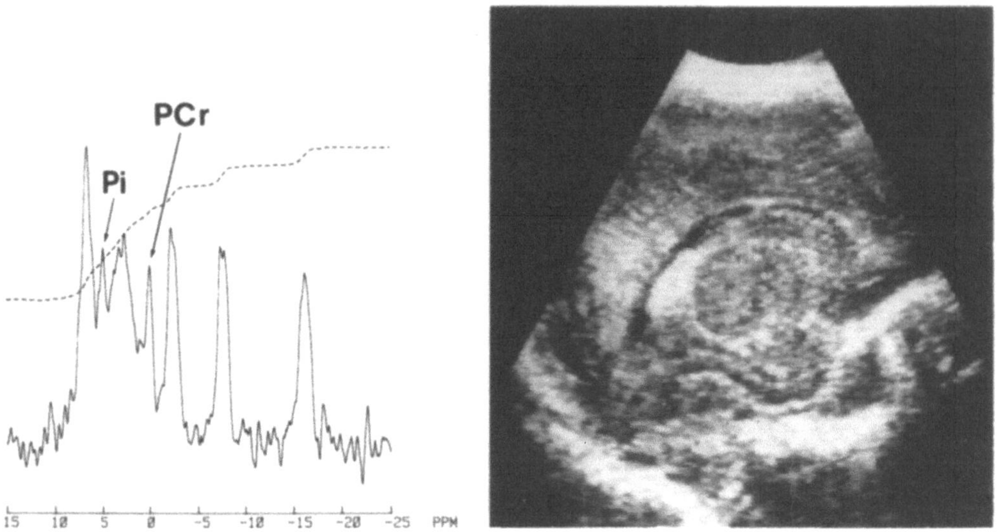

Fig. 3. Spectrum and parasagittal ultrasound scan from an infant born at 32 weeks of gestation and studied 8 days after birth. The scan shows echodensities very similar to those in Fig. 2, but PCr/Pi was normal, 0.84, and no cysts or other evidence or cerebral atrophy developed. (Data from Hamilton et al. 1986)

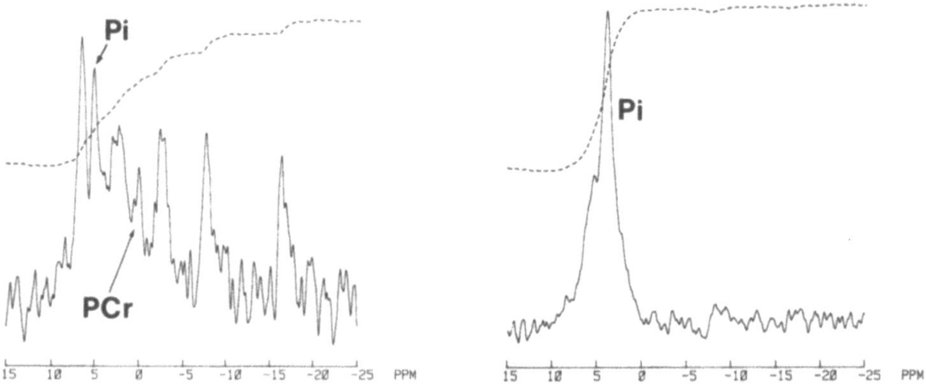

Fig. 4 a, b. Spectra from two infants, both of whom died, with diffusely increased echodensities and severe impairment of energy metabolism. **a** Born at 38 weeks of gestation and studied aged 2 days: she had been severely asphyxiated during delivery. PCr/Pi was 0.29 and ATP/total phosphorus was also low. **b** Born at 27 weeks of gestation and studied aged 8 days: he had suffered an extremely severe asphyxial episode aged 5 days; PCr and ATP were virtually absent. (Data from Hamilton et al. 1986)

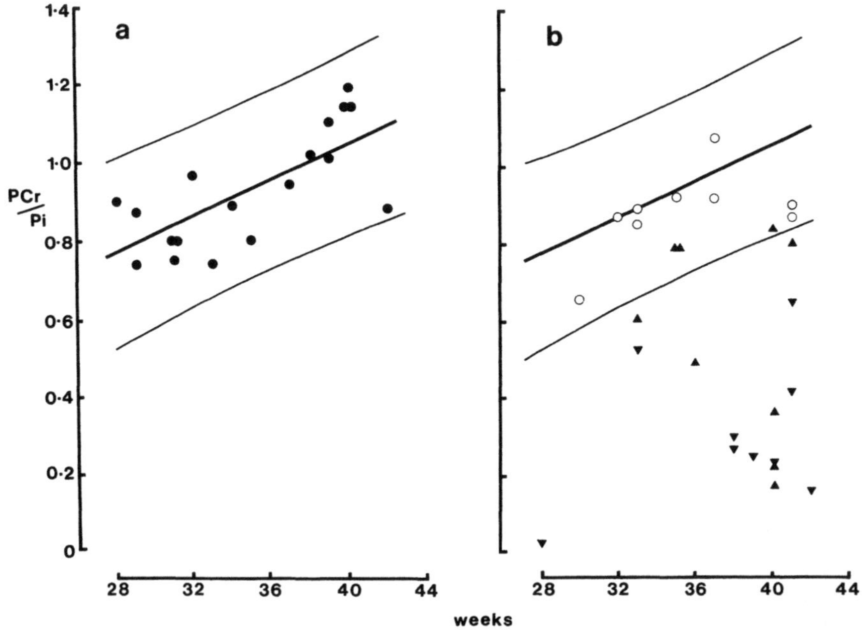

Fig. 5. **a** Relation between PCr/Pi ratio and gestational plus postnatal age in 18 normal infants. The regression line and 95% confidence limits are shown. **b** Data from 27 infants with increased cerebral echodensities. The regression line and 95% confidence limits from the normal infants are shown for comparison. ○, Survived without cerebral atrophy; ▲, survived with cerebral atrophy; ▼, died. (Data from Hamilton et al. 1986)

Figure 5a shows the relation between the PCr/Pi ratio and gestational plus postnatal age in the normal control infants, and Fig. 5b shows the values recorded from the infants with increased echodensities. It can be seen that low values were strongly associated with later death or cerebral atrophy. The difference in adverse outcome between infants whose PCr/Pi ratios were in the normal range and those with ratios below it was highly significant ($p < 0.001$, Fisher's exact test).

The results of this study showed that the prognosis for infants with increased echodensities whose PCr/Pi ratios were reduced was much worse than among infants whose ratios lay within the normal range.

MRS Results and Neurodevelopmental Outcome at 1 Year of Age

The progress of a heterogeneous group of 65 infants studied by MRS because of definite or possible cerebral abnormalities was assessed at 1 year of age. The infants were born at a median age of 37 weeks (range 24–42 weeks) and studied at a median postnatal age of 3 days (range 0–96 days). Many were studied on more than one occasion. The principal neonatal diagnoses and minimum PCr/Pi ratios

Table 1. Neonatal diagnoses and minimum PCr/Pi ratios in 65 infants studied by magnetic resonance spectroscopy

Diagnosis[a]	PCr/Pi	
	Normal	Low[c]
Birthweight < 10th centile	9	6
Birth asphyxia	9	14
Convulsions	10	20
Hyaline membrane disease	10	3
Polycythaemia (Hct > 65)	5	3
Ultrasound - evidence of		
Haemorrhage	4	4
Ischaemia	9	16
Inborn errors of metabolism[b]	0	2
Miscellaneous (e.g. meningitis, hydrocephalus, maternal heroin, collapse, blood loss)	18	1

[a] Most infants had more than one diagnosis.
[b] Propionic acidaemia, arginosuccinic acidaemia.
[c] Below 95% confidence limits as shown in Fig. 5 a.

Table 2. PCr/Pi ratio and early outcome in 65 infants studied by magnetic resonance spectroscopy

	Died	Cerebral palsy		Normal
		GQ[a] ≤ 85	GQ > 85	
PCr/Pi				
Normal, $n = 42$	5	6	8	23
Low, $n = 23$	16	5	1	1

[a] General quotient (Griffiths 1954).

are given in Table 1. All had repeated neurodevelopmental testing using methods that have been described elsewhere (Stewart et al. 1983). Outcome is related to PCr/Pi ratio in Table 2. It can be seen that infants whose ratios were low were much more likely to die or to suffer cerebral palsy with a low general quotient (GQ) than infants whose ratios were normal ($p < 0.001$, Fisher's exact test).

Conclusions

We conclude that phosphorus MRS is a valuable non-invasive technique for investigating hypoxic-ischaemic injury to the brain in newborn infants. As well as providing information about the pathogenesis of this type of injury, useful prognostic information can be obtained.

Current developments such as spectroscopy of other nuclei, especially protons (1H) for measurment of lactate and certain amino acids, and the combination of magnetic resonance imaging with spectroscopy seem certain to yield further important information about brain metabolism in newborn infants.

Acknowledgements. This work was done in collaboration with Dr. J. Baudin, Mr. E. B. Cady, Dr. A. M. de L. Costello, Dr. M. J. Dawson, Mr. D. T. Delpy, Dr. P. L. Hope, Dr. P. S. Tofts, Dr. A. L. Stewart, Prof. D. R. Wilkie and Dr. J. S. Wyatt. Support was provided by the Medical Research Council, the National Fund for Research into Crippling Disease, The Muscular Dystrophy Group, the Wellcome Trust and the Special Trustees of University College Hospital.

References

Alberman E (1982) The epidemiology of congenital defects: a pragmatic approach. In: Adinolfi M et al. (eds) Paediatric research: a genetic approach. SIMP, Heinemann, London, pp 1-28

Cady EB, Costello AM de L, Dawson MJ, Delpy DT, Hope PL, Reynolds EOR, Tofts PS, Wilkie DR (1983) Non-invasive investigation of cerebral metabolism in newborn infants by phosphorus nuclear magnetic resonance spectroscopy. Lancet I: 1059-1062

Delpy DT, Gordon RE, Hope PL, Parker D, Reynolds EOR, Shaw D, Whitehead MD (1982) Non-invasive detection of cerebral ischemia by phosphorus nuclear magnetic resonance. Pediatrics 70: 301-313

Gadian DG (1982) Nuclear magnetic resonance and its applications to living systems. Clarendon, Oxford

Griffiths R (1954) The abilities of babies. University of London Press, London

Hamilton PA, Hope PL, Cady EB, Delpy DT, Wyatt JS, Reynolds EOR (1986) Impaired energy metabolism in brains of newborn infants with increased cerebral echodensities. Lancet I: 1242-1246

Hope PL, Reynolds EOR (1985) Investigation of cerebral energy metabolism in newborn infants by phosphorus nuclear magnetic resonance spectroscopy. Clin Perinatol 12: 261-275

Hope PL, Costello AM de L, Cady EB, Delpy DT, Tofts PS, Chu A, Hamilton PA, Reynolds EOR, Wilkie DR (1984) Cerebral energy metabolism studied with phosphorus NMR spectroscopy in normal and birth-asphyxiated infants. Lancet II: 366-370

Levene MI, Williams JL, Fawer C-L (1985) Ultrasound of the infant brain. SIMP, Blackwell, Oxford

Stewart AL, Thorburn RJ, Hope PL, Goldsmith M, Lipscomb AP, Reynolds EOR (1983) Ultrasound appearance of the brain in very preterm infants and neurodevelopmental outcome at 18 months of age. Arch Dis Child 58: 598-604

Prognosis of the Very Low Birthweight and Very Preterm Infant

Outcome of Very Low Birthweight or Very Preterm Infants with Special Consideration of Perinatal Events

A. STEWART and P. HOPE

Introduction

Preterm birth with a birthweight below 1500 g (very low birthweight - VLBW) is still an important perinatal complication, although reports from France of reductions in prevalence are encouraging (e.g. Papiernik et al. 1985). On average in "developed" countries, fewer than 2% of live babies born weigh less than 1500 g, but these infants still account for a large proportion of deaths in the early weeks of life. For example, in the United Kingdom, although only 0.9% of live births weighed <1500 g in 1984, 48% of infants who died in the 1st week and 44% of those in the 1st month were of this low birthweight. This alone indicates that these pregnancies represent a major part of the perinatal workload, particularly for the staff of neonatal intensive care units. Estimates of the contribution from VLBW infants to childhood morbidity and disability are difficult to find. Alberman (1982) made some calculations, based on prevailing prevalence rates for various impairments and disabilities in the United Kingdom and estimated that VLBW infants accounted for about 1.9% of the major disabilities diagnosed in childhood in any 1 year in the United Kingdom, and she speculated that these infants probably contributed an even smaller proportion (0.8%) to the total of minor problems. More recently, there have been suggestions that VLBW infants, particularly those who weigh <1000 g (extremely low birthweight - ELBW), continue to be major users of health care services right through the 1st year of life. For example, hospital admissions for respiratory infections or repair of hernias have been reported to be much more frequent among these infants, although actual estimates of the effects of these needs on services are not generally available. We should like to review reports on the current outcome of VLBW infants and to discuss a little information concerning the relationship between outcome and perinatal events which has resulted from prospective ultrasound (US) brain scan studies in the past 5 years.

Outcome: Current Status

Since 1979 there have been several reviews of the published reports of the outcome for VLBW infants (e.g. Hack et al. 1979; Stewart et al. 1981; McDonald 1982; McCormick 1985). The majority of these reviews considered outcome in terms of both mortality and morbidity. Morbidity was usually judged solely on the basis of neurodevelopmental assessments, but McCormick (1985) also attemped to consider other aspects, including health in infancy and the impact of preterm birth on the family, particularly on the mother. In general, the conclusions drawn were similar and may be summarised as follows:

Mortality. Mortality rates continued to fall after the 1960s while the numbers of healthy survivors increased. The effect was noted among all birthweight groups, including those who weighed less than 1000 g.

Morbidity. The impairments and disorders diagnosed did not change from the earliest studies; nor did the relative frequency of the conditions. Cerebral palsy, mental retardation and sensory losses (hearing and vision) were the three most commonly found. After an initial reduction in the early 1960s - probably due to a fall in iatrogenic brain injury - the proportion of these neurodevelopmental disorders remainted unchanged at 5%-8% of total VLBW live births, or 10%-15% of the long-term survivors.

Year of Birth. Outcome at any point in time was consistent in all centres and appeared to reflect prevailing obstetric and paediatric expertise (Koops et al. 1982).

Limitations of Data. Almost all available reports were made at specialist centres and were not population based. Factors determining the selection of infants for treatment were thought to be liable to bias the results although they were usually unrecognised. The studies were mainly observational. The results and conclusions, therefore, could be challenged on the grounds that no properly designed, formal randomised studies had been done.

Deductions. Because of the sequence of events, obstetric, paediatric and other health care interventions were believed to be largely responsible for an overall improvement in outcome for VLBW infants. For proof, population-based studies were necessary.

Recent Developments

In the past 4 years, population studies have been reported which have largely confirmed the overall results of the earlier ones from specialist centres (e.g. Horwood et al. 1982; Koops et al. 1982; Saigal et al. 1982; Shapiro et al. 1983; Lloyd 1984; Rantakillio and Von Wendt 1985; Powell et al. 1986). Several studies have attempted to make comparisons of results before and after the introduction of modern methods of care (e.g. Horwood et al. 1982; Alberman et al. 1982). Although these studies seemed to indicate recent improvements following changes in care routines, interpretation was difficult. Follow-up information was limited, depending on parental report only in one study, and the age range of the children was too wide to allow meaningful comparisons. In contrast to these relatively unsatisfactory results, a study from New York City of mortality in LBW infants according to level of expertise of neonatal care (Paneth et al. 1982) clearly showed that standard of care determined outcome in VLBW infants, as judged by mortality.

Extremely Low Birthweight

The greatest changes have occurred among these tiniest infants. Since 1972, when the first report devoted entirely to this subgroup was made (Alden et al. 1972), mortality has fallen dramatically. Most specialist centres now report rates for deaths within 28 days of less than 50%. Neurodevelopmental morbidity, on the other hand, has changed little (Stewart et al. 1981) and the trend for overall outcome appears similar to that of the larger infants. In 1982, Orgill et al. pointed out that among ELBW infants, mortality depended upon birthweight and gestation but neurodevelopmental morbidity in survivors did not. Thus, the outcome for the very few tiniest survivors who weighed less than 750 g, for example, was the same as those who weighed 751-1000 g. This observation was confirmed by Saigal et al. (1984) in a regional study of ELBW infants and our own data from University College Hospital were similar. Dunn (1985) has shown how this type of experience led to increasing numbers of referrals of these infants once intensive care was selectively introduced on a regional basis in Avon County, United Kingdom. Concern, however, has been expressed at this trend (Amiel-Tison 1986) and cost effectiveness challenged. Whilst this is understandable on physiological grounds, data published so far do not support the reservations expressed.

The Future

In general, reports continue to give encouraging results for the outcome of the VLBW infants. Concern, however, has been expressed on several aspects of morbidity.

Cerebral Palsy. The most recent results of the Swedish cerebral palsy study (Hagberg et al. 1984) suggested that the incidence may be rising again among VLBW infants. These findings have not been confirmed by other studies.

Retinopathy of Prematurity. Blindness due to retinopathy of prematurity (ROP) may be increasing again. No satisfactory documentation of the validity of editorial comments has yet been published.

Health in Infancy. Several recent reports, notably from North America (see McCormick 1985), have indicated an excess of illness and hospital re-admissions among VLBW infants in the early months following discharge from neonatal intensive care units. ELBW infants were particularly affected. Reasons included minor surgery, for example repair of hernias, respiratory infections and other more serious, respiratory complications following mechanical ventilation. The last category included chronic lung disease with prolonged oxygen dependency (Bryan 1985). It seems likely that this condition is at least partly dependent on ventilator management. Since 1979, in our own unit at University College Hospital, about 20% of the infants born before 33 weeks were still oxygen-dependent at 28 days but only one child was sent home on oxygen at about 4 months of age. Such health problems may create additional demands upon health care resources but these demands are small compared to the cost, for example, of caring for life for a severely disabled individual and should not be regarded as an indication to withhold care for VLBW or even ELBW infants.

School Performance. There have been several reports (e.g. Calâme et al. 1983; Klein et al. 1985) of relatively large proportions of ex-LBW children with psychometric evidence of learning disorders. As a group, overall levels of functioning appear to be satisfactory but detailed testing has revealed deficits in specific areas of cognitive functioning, notably in language skills, which may be responsible for the difficulties experienced by the children.

In Summary. Mortality in VLBW infants continues to fall, particularly among ELBW infants; by contrast, morbidity, although low, has not changed for many years. Warnings of probable increases in some impairments indicate the need for continued monitoring of outcome as the children grow older.

Outcome: Aetiological Factors

It is both disappointing and surprising that the prevalence of neurodevelopmental morbidity among VLBW infants has not fallen in the same way as mortality. With the exception of blindness due to ROP, the conditions diagnosed at follow-up have not changed since the earliest reports, nor have their relative frequencies. Cerebral palsy is still the commonest impairment reported, and yet relatively little is known of the aetiology. Significant relationships have been noted between some neonatal factors and later morbitiy. For example, VLBW infants who have been acidaemic at birth or who had convulsions or reccurrent apnoeic spells were significantly more likely to have an adverse outcome than those who did not suffer these complications (e.g. Stewart et al. 1978; Jurgens-Van der Zee et al. 1979). The only antenatal or obstetrical factors associated with an adverse outcome were intrauterine growth retardation, gestation, birthweight, foetal presentation and type of delivery (see Zuspan and Christian 1983). Intrauterine growth retardation, however, is a symptom that a foetus is sick, but there are many causes, so associations can only be interpreted if a diagnosis is made. The apparent lack of antenatal or perinatal influences on the outcome of VLBW survivors was difficult to understand. Inappropriate methods of investigation seemed to be the most likely explanation! Some workers applied the "optimality concept" to the problem (Towen et al. 1980). Others considered that the introduction of objective non-invasive methods for the measurement of brain structure and function in the immediate neonatal period offered a more direct method of investigating the relationship between perinatal factors and brain injury.

Objective Measures of Brain Injury: Relationship with Outcome. In an earlier paper in this volume (Stewart and Hope), results of follow-up studies were discussed which showed associations between lesions diagnosed with US brain scans in the neonatal period in very preterm infants and adverse neurodevelopmental outcome at 1 year (Stewart et al. 1983). From these data, it was deduced that ischaemic lesions were the main determinants of an adverse outcome judged by neurodevelopmental assessments at 1-2 years in these infants. Reynolds (this volume) then described how magnetic resonance spectroscopy (MRS) investigations of cerebral energy metabolism identified infants in the early days of life who had sustained permanent hypoxic-ischaemic brain damage sufficient either to kill them or, if they survived, to affect their neurodevelopmental progress as they grew older (Hamilton et al. 1986).

Antecedents of Periventricular Haemorrhage. According to published reports of studies based on US diagnosis, these lesions generally occurred after birth, towards the end of the 1st day of life (see Cooke 1981; Thorburn et al. 1982), and they were significantly associated with early mortality. Prevalence depended upon gestation, birthweight and neonatal respiratory illness, particularly hyaline membrane disease (HMD), requiring treatment with mechanical ventilation and pneumothorax (Dykes et al. 1980; Lipscomb et al. 1981). Fluctuating cardiorespiratory variables associated with severe respiratory illness were believed to be responsible (Perlman et al. 1985). The only perinatal factor which appeared, in most reports, to affect the prevalence of periventricular haemorrhage (PVH) was place of birth. Presumably this was a measure of the standard of intrapartum care and of immediate access to intensive neonatal support. The effect on PVH of other perinatal and neonatal factors were controversial, particularly the influence of mode of delivery. In our own study, infants delivered by Caesarean section had the lowest risk of developing PVH and those delivered vaginally by the breech the highest; and the difference was highly significant ($p < 0.01$). Although infants delivered by section were significantly more mature and heavier than vaginally delivered infants, this did not fully account for the differences in prevalence of PVH. Vaginally delivered breech and vertex presentations were of equally low birthweight and short gestation, but the prevalence of PVH was much lower among the vertex deliveries. We therefore concluded from our experience that vaginal breech delivery carried an excess risk of PVH. Other investigators found no relationship between mode of delivery and PVH (e.g. Cooke 1981) but all agreed that PVH was mainly determined by neonatal events.

Antecedents of Ischaemic Lesions. As was discussed earlier, US is not a particularly efficient method of identifying ischaemic lesions. They tend to be diagnosed with US much later than PVH. Diagnosis depends upon changes which evolve over many days. The majority of neonatal deaths occur before this evidence appears, so mortality studies based on US diagnosis of ischaemic lesions are impossible. For the same reasons, studies of the antecedent factors of ischaemic lesions based on US diagnosis are difficult, and ischaemic lesions and PVH frequently occur together in the same infant which further complicates interpretation of results. In the absence of published data - and fully aware of these difficulties - we attempted to analyse data from our own study in two ways; to discover when hypoxic-ischaemic injury occurred and to investigate predisposing factors. Of 579 infants scanned in a 5-year period, US evidence of ischaemic damage was noted in just three infants at the first scan done within 12 h of birth and in eight between 12 and 119 h, giving a total of 11 (2%) infants in whom we speculated that the lesion was antenatally acquired. The remaining infants developed the evidence after the age of 5 days, implying that the result occurred at or after the onset of labour.

Only 21 of the 579 infants had definite evidence of ischaemic damage with lesions that could not be attributed to PVH on the basis of US scanning. Seven of these 21 infants were delivered vaginally by the breech compared with just 8% of the 298 infants with normal scans. The only other factors which differed significantly between these 21 infants and infants with normal US scans were initial low Apgar scores ($\leqslant 3$ at 1 min), the need for mechanical ventilation and indices of hypoxaemia. In contrast to PVH, HMD was not significantly associated with purely ischaemic lesions. It is obviously impossible to draw conclusions from such a study, but it is interesting that the findings are in accord with the earlier studies which indicated the importance of condition at birth as a predictor of neurodevelopmental outcome.

Conclusions and Implications

Paneth et al. (1982) showed that standard of neonatal intensive care was the main determinant of mortality in VLBW infants in a large study of all LBW births in New York City. The principal factors distinguishing the highest standards (level 3) of care included all aspects of the management of respiratory illness. Thus, it may be deduced that mortality in VLBW infants has been influenced to an important extent by neonatal management of the conditions which predispose particularly to PVH rather than to ischaemic lesions. In the future, improvements in morbidity will depend upon interventions designed particularly to prevent or to ameliorate hypoxic-ischaemic injury. Results of investigations using measures of cerebral energy metabolism or oxygenation as described by Reynolds should indicate what these might be. Meanwhile, perhaps we should be mindful of the results of the earlier studies and the hints from the more recent US data indicating the importance of the condition of the infant at birth as well as the prevention of hypoperfusion or hypoxaemia throughout the neonatal period.

These conclusions also have implications for the choice of methods for evaluating obstetric and neonatal management routines. PVH alone is not an appropriate outcome measure to use when testing the effects of interventions designed to affect morbidity in VLBW or preterm infants. Some early, objective measure of ischaemic damage must be used - or the results of follow up in survivors awaited.

References

Alberman E (1982) The epidemiology of congenital defects: a pragmatic approach. In: Adinolfi M, Benson P, Giannelli F, Seller M (eds) Paediatric research: a genetic approach. Spastics international medical publications. Heinemann, London, chapter 1, p 1

Alberman E, Benson J, McDonald A (1982) Cerebral palsy and severe educational subnormality in children with a birthweight of 4lbs or less: a comparison of births in 1951-1953 and 1970-1973. Lancet I: 606-608

Alden ER, Mandelkorn T, Woodrum DE, Wennberg RP, Parks CR, Hodson WA (1972) Morbidity and mortality of infants weighing less than 1000 g in an intensive care nursery. Pediatrics 50: 40-49

Amiel-Tison C (1986) Les nouveau-nés pesant 500 a 999 g. In: Encyclopedie Medicochirurgicale, 5114L 20, Les Editions Techniques, Paris

Bryan H (1985) Chronic lung disease in premature infants. In: Beard RW, Sharp F (eds) Pre-term labour and its consequences. Royal College of Obstetricians and Gynaecologists, London. Perinatology, Ithaca, pp 365-371

Calâme A, Ducret J, Jaunin L, Plancherel (1983) High risk appropriate for gestational age (AGA) and small for gestational age (SGA) pre-term infants. Helv Paediatr Acta 38: 39-50

Cooke RWI (1981) Factors associated with periventricular haemorrhage in very low birth-weight infants. Arch Dis Child 56: 425-431

Dunn PM (1985) Fetal viability: a perinatal viewpoint. In: Beard RW, Sharp F (eds) Pre-term labour and its consequences. Royal College of Obstetricians and Gynaecologists London. Perinatology, Ithaca, pp 295-301

Dykes FD, Lazzara A, Ahmann P, Blumenstein B, Schwartz J, Brann AW (1980) Intraventricular haemorrhage: a prospective evaluation of etiopathogenesis. Pediatrics 66: 42-49

Hack M, Fanaroff A, Merkatz IR (1979) The low birth weight infant - evolution of a changing outlook. N Engl J Med 301: 1162-1166

Hagberg B, Hagberg G, Olow I (1984) The changing panorama of cerebral palsy in Sweden 1954-70. IV. Epidemiological trends 1959-78. Acta Paediatr Scand 73: 433-440

Hamilton PA, Hope PL, Cady EB, Delpy DT, Wyatt JS, Reynolds EOR (1986) Impaired energy metabolism in brains of newborn infants with increased echo-densities. Lancet I: 1242-1246

Horwood SP, Boyle MH, Torrance GW, Sinclair JC (1982) Mortality and morbidity of 500-1499 gram birth weight infants live-born to residents of a defined geographic region before and after neonatal intensive care. Pediatrics 69: 613-620

Jurgens-Van Der Zee AD, Bierman-Van Eedenburg MEC, Fidler VJ, Olinga AA, Visch JH, Towen BCL, Huisjes HJ (1979) Pre-term birth, growth retardation and acidemia in relation to neurological abnormality of the newborn. Early Hum Dev 3: 141-154

Klein N, Hack M, Gallagher J, Fanaroff A (1985) Pre-school performance of children with normal intelligence who were very low birth weight infants. Pediatrics 75: 531-537

Koops BL, Morgan LJ, Battaglia FC (1982) Neonatal mortality risk in relation to birth weight and gestational age: update. J Pediatr 101: 969-977

Lipscomb AP, Thorburn RJ, Reynolds EOR, Stewart AL, Blackwell RJ, Cusick G, Whitehead MD (1981) Pneumothorax and cerebral haemorrhage in pre-term infants. Lancet I: 414-416

Lloyd BW (1984) Outcome of very-low-birthweight babies from Wolverhampton. Lancet II: 739-741

McCormick MC (1985) The contribution of low birth weight to infant mortality and childhood morbidity. N Engl J Med 312: 82-90

McDonald A (1982) Is the outcome of very low birth weight improving? In: Adinolfi M, Benson P, Giannelli F, Seller M (eds) Paediatric research: a genetic approach. Spastics international medical publications. Heinemann, London, chapter 2, p 13
Orgill AA, Astbury J, Bajuk B, Yu VYH (1982) Early development of infants 1000 g or less at birth. Arch Dis Child 57: 823-827
Paneth N, Kiely JL, Wallenstein S, Marcus M, Pakter J, Susser M (1982) Newborn intensive care and neonatal mortality in low-birth-weight infants. N Engl J Med 307: 149-155
Papiernik E, Bouyer J, Dreyfus J (1985) Risk factors for pre-term births and results of a prevention policy. The Haguenau perinatal study 1971-1982. In: Beard RW, Sharp F (eds) Pre-term labour and its consequences. Royal College of Obstetricians and Gynaecologists, London. Perinatology, Ithaca, pp 15-24
Perlman JM, Goodman S, Krevsser KL, Volpe JJ (1985) Reduction in intraventricular hemorrhage by elimination of fluctuating cerebral blood-flow velocity in pre-term infants with respiratory distress syndrome. N Engl J Med 312: 1353-1357
Powell TG, Pharoah POD, Cooke RWI (1986) Survival and morbidity in a geographically defined population of low birth weight infants. Lancet I: 539-543
Rantakallio P, Von Wendt L (1985) Prognosis for low birth weight infants up to the age of fourteen years, a population study. Dev Med Child Neurol 27: 655-663
Saigal S, Rosenbaum P, Stoskoff B, Milner R (1982) Follow-up of infants 501-1500 g birth weight delivered to residents of a geographically defined region with perinatal intensive care facilities. J Pediatr 100: 606-613
Saigal S, Rosenbaum P, Stoskoff B, Sinclair JC (1984) Outcome of infants 501-1000 gm birth weight delivered to residents of the McMaster Health Region. J Pediatr 105: 969-976
Shapiro S, McCormick MC, Starfield BH, Crawley B (1983) Changes in infant morbidity associated with decreases in neonatal mortality. Pediatrics 72: 408-415
Stewart A, Turcan D, Rawlings G, Hart S, Gregory S (1978) Outcome for infants at high risk of major handicap. In: Elliott K, O'Connor M (eds) Major mental handicap: methods and costs of prevention. Ciba foundation symposium no. 59 (new series). Elsevier, Amsterdam, pp 151-164
Stewart A, Reynolds EOR, Lipscomb AP (1981) Outcome for infants of very low birth weight: survey of world literature. Lancet I: 1038-1041
Thorburn RJ, Lipscomb AP, Stewart AL, Reynolds EOR, Hope PL (1982) Timing and antecedents of periventricular haemorrhage in very pre-term infants. Early Hum Dev 9: 221-238
Towen BCL, Huisjes HJ, Jurgens-Van Der Zee AD, Bierman-van Eendenburg MEC, Smrkovsky M, Olinga AA (1980) Obstetrical condition and neonatal neurological morbidity. An analysis with the help of the optimality concept. Early Hum Dev 4: 207-228
Zuspan FP, Christian CD (eds) (1983) Reid's controversy in obstetrics and gynaecology - III. Saunders, Philadelphia

Role of Transport for the Prognosis of the Very Low Birthweight Preterm Infant

H. T. VERSMOLD

Neonatal intensive care developed in pediatric hospitals usually separated from obstetrical institutions. The undoubted benefit of neonatal transport was to make appropriate care available to those who needed it (Swyer 1970; Usher 1977). This is still so for quite a number of newborn infants. It soon became obvious that the advantage of neonatal transport increased with the skill of transport teams, but also the slogan "The Uterus is the Best Transport Incubator" indicated the growing anticipation that infants born in hospitals with a connected neonatal intensive care unit (NICU) might be better off.

Extensive regionalization programs to concentrate mothers at risk in perinatal centers are now typical for those countries with a relatively low perinatal mortality (Piekkala et al. 1985; Riegel et al. 1985). But even today there is a controversy (Auld 1978; Editorial 1986) about whether antenatal maternal transport to a perinatal center really improves neonatal outcome.

The subject of this paper is an evaluation of recent literature with the following questions:

- What is the impact of neonatal transport, and of its components, resuscitation and transportation?
- What are the effects of neonatal transport to a NICU compared to maternal antenatal transport to a perinatal center?
- What is the proof that large-scale regionalization programs are effective?

The effect of transport will be discussed with respect to mortality and to morbidity. The focus will be on long-term outcome, but here only limited information is available. In the most recent literature, however, i.e., since the use of cranial ultrasound some data on intracranial hemorrhage (ICH) have been reported.

Neonatal Transport

Neonatal transport and its organization are now usually very well developed. Nevertheless, newborn infants are still frequently transported by untrained personnel. Qualified neonatal transport results in better outcome than nonqualified transport (Chance et al. 1978). Special aspects like equipment, personnel, and organization of transport services, or the potential hazard of noise and vibration

(Bönisch et al. 1985; Campbell et al. 1984, Shenai et al. 1981) are not the subject of this paper.

Neonatal transport has two major components, resuscitation and transportation itself, and it is difficult to analyze these separately.

Quality of Resuscitation

Volume overload during resuscitation (>10 ml/kg per resuscitation) has been identified as the cause of an increased incidence of ICH in outborn babies (Clark et al. 1981) in a study evaluating a variety of relevant risk factors. In another controlled study (Lazzara et al. 1985) a special training program in resuscitation decreased the incidence of ICH in transported newborn infants.

Quality of Transportation

In a controlled study of only the effects of transportion (Chance et al. 1978) significantly less hypothermia, hypotension, acidosis, mortality, death with hypothermia and duration of hospitalization occurred with expert than with nonexpert transport. These conditions represent risk factors for respiratory distress syndrome (RDS), ICH, and hypoxic ischemic encephalopathy.

Maternal Versus Neonatal Transport

To evaluate maternal antenatal transport, inborn and outborn infants of level 3 perinatal centers have been compared, and, more recently, also infants after maternal and neonatal transport. Three groups of studies will be discussed:

- Hospital-based comparisons - in hospital-based comparisons different standards of neonatal care are not a bias, but a selection of cases may occur
- Comparisons within a defined population - here a selection bias is less likely, and data are more relevant with respect to regionalization programs
- Comparisons of defined populations with and without a regionalization program

Hospital-Based Comparisons

Survival of very low birthweight (VLBW) infants was generally higher in the maternal transport group (Table 1). This is not always true for infants below a birthweight of 1000 g, probably because of more restrictive referral policies for the smallest and sickest outborn infants. The studies were controlled by comparing matched pairs (Modanlou et al. 1980) or mortality risk groups by gestational age and birthweight (Harris et al. 1978, 1981).

Table 1. Maternal vs. neonatal transport (hospital-based comparisons)

Author		Survival higher after maternal transport
Harris et al.	(1978)	< 1500 g
Modanlou et al.	(1980)	1001–1250 g
Harris et al.	(1981)	moderate risk
Huisman et al.	(1983)	500–1500 g

Table 2. Maternal vs. neonatal transport (population-based comparisons)

Author		Survival higher after maternal transport
Bakketeig et al.	(1978)	all birthweights
Cordero et al.	(1982)	< 1500 g
Paneth et al.	(1982)	501–2250 g
Miller et al.	(1983)	1000–1500 g
Sachs et al.	(1983)	> 1201 g
Kitchen et al.	(1984)	500– 999 g
Paneth et al.	(1984)	501–2250 g
Gortmaker et al.	(1985)	750–1500 g
Kollée et al.	(1985)	< 1500 g
Saule and Riegel	(1986)	< 2000 g
Verloove-Vanhorick and Verwey	(1987)	< 1500 g

Population-Based Comparisons

Again, survival of LBW infants was generally lower after neonatal transport to perinatal centers (Table 2), again not always for the smallest infants. Adjustment for perinatal risk factors showed a better outcome at similar, or despite increased risk (Miller et al. 1983; Paneth et al. 1982; P. Verloove, personal communication). The most extensive adjustments for risk factors were done in the New York (Paneth et al. 1982, 1984) and the Netherlands studies (Verloove-Vanhorick and Verwey 1987).

Consideration of a number of confounding perinatal risk factors and of the hospitals' standard by these authors validates their conclusion that antenatal transfer of VLBW infants to perinatal centers is superior to neonatal transport. The same appears true for morbidity, as discussed below.

A most careful and extensive analysis of 1300 newborn infants below 1500 g or 32 weeks of gestation, i.e., 94% of all such infants born in the Netherlands in 1983, was done by Verloove-Vanhorick and Verwey (1987) taking into account 22 perinatal confounding factors. Antenatal transport to a level 3 center significantly reduced the mortality risk. The adjusted mortality odds ratio was 0.6 times that without antenatal transport.

After these within-population comparisons, the next logical step would be a prospective, controlled comparison between populations with and without a defined regionalization program.

Regionalization of perinatal care

The effect of regionalization of perinatal care in geographically defined populations has recently been evaluated in three different studies.

McCormick et al. (1985) studied eight regions with a regionalization program and eight close by control regions. In infants below 1500 g he observed a sharp decline in neonatal mortality parallel to a shift of deliveries to level 3 centers with no difference between study and control areas. However, centralization of high-risk deliveries to level 3 centers had already been so widespread in both regions that a further program effect was not detectable.

Siegel et al. (1985) evaluated a rural regional perinatal care program and a control area of similar structure. Again a decline of yearly neonatal mortality trends (fetal, neonatal, birthweight-specific) was observed, particullarly for infants of 1500-2500 g, and again with no difference between the program and control areas. Unfortunately, the study does not consider at all infants delivered in level 3 perinatal centers because these data were not available.

Eksmyr (1986) compared two geographically defined regions in southern Sweden, one with a central hospital with neonatal intensive care services and the other a region without such facilities. Maternal risks were comparable. The unexpected result was a lower rate of early neonatal death in the control area. However, when adjusting for birthweight and excluding congenital malformations, these differences were no longer statistically significant, except for infants above 2500 g. In addition, a marked shift had occurred towards birth in the perinatal center, to which mothers in the control region also had access. So 74% of deaths of infants from mothers originating from the control region occurred in the perinatal center of the study region. The author concludes that "... specialized obstetric service but lacking neonatal wards may be justifiable ..., provided risk deliveries can be planned in hospitals with neonatal wards ..."

In conclusion, the limitations of these studies illustrate that definite experimental proof or disprood of the hypothesis that antental transport is superior to postnatal transport can hardly be expected in the future. We are left with the observational, quasi-experimental studies quoted above.

Transport and Morbidity

Inadequate resuscitation and neonatal transport lead to relevant early and late morbidity, as already mentioned above (Chance et al. 1978).

Early Morbidity

The factors hypothermia, hypoglycemia, hypercapnia, and hypotension have been documented in numerous descriptive studies. Each one of these factors is known to be associated with severe long-term morbidity.

Long-term Morbidity

Respiratory distress syndrome (RDS) is more frequent and more severe in hypothermic and hypotensive infants (Obladen et al. 1985). Hypercapnia is associated with ICH (Dykes et al. 1980). Hypotension and hypoxic ischemic encephalopathy are related (Volpe 1981), and the tolerance to hypoxia appears reduced with hypoglycemia. Perinatal asphyxia, via loss of autoregulation of cerebral blood flow, increases the risk of ICH (Lou et al. 1979).

In fact, it has been documented that RDS and ICH occur more frequently after neonatal transport compared to antenatal transport, or compared to inborns (Table 3). Also, death associated with patent ductus arteriosus, with bronchopulmonary dysplasia, and with necrotizing enterocolitis were more frequent in outborns than inborns (Huisman et al. 1983). Mean duration and cost of hospitalization of survivors, indirect indices of morbidity, were markedly lower after maternal transport (Anderson et al. 1981).

Combining 319 VLBW infants reported in San Francisco (Clark et al. 1981), Houston (Garcia-Prats et al. 1982), and Frankfurt (von Loewenich et al. 1984), the incidence of ICH in outborns was $50\% \pm 6\%$ (90% confidence level) compared to $18\% \pm 6\%$ ($p < 10^{-6}$) (von Loewenich et al. 1984).

Table 3. Maternal vs. neonatal transport - morbidity

Modanlou et al.	(1980)	less RDS
Clark et al.	(1981)[a]	less ICH
Harris et al.	(1981)	less RDS
Lazarra et al.	(1982)	less ICH
Garcia-Prats	(1982)[a]	less RDS, ICH
Huisman et al.	(1983)[a]	less mortality + PDA mortality + BPD mortality + NEC
Lamont et al.	(1983)[a]	less ICH
Verloove-Vanhorick and Verwey	(1987)	less RDS, ICH

[a] Inborn vs. outborn.
RDS, respiratory distress syndrome; ICH, intracranial hemorrhage; PDA, patent ductus arterious; BPD, bronchopulmonary dysplasia; NEC, necrotizing enterocolitis.

Table 4. How often is maternal transport impossible?

Auld	(1978)	40% not identifiable risks
Selbmann et al.	(1980)	17% unexpected risks
Kollée et al.	(1985)	18.5% maternal transport impossible (but 38.5% neonatal transports)
Riegel et al. (Yllpö-Study)	(1986)	S. Finland 94% inborns S. Bavaria 30% inborns
Verloove-Vanhorick and Verwey	(1987)	Level 3: 96% < 1500 g inborns

No published information is available on long-term neurodevelopemental outcome after maternal compared to neonatal transport.

Psychosocial Aspects

Maternal transport to a perhaps far-away perinatal center, away from her home surroundings and her family is also a psychosocial problem. On the other hand, neonatal transport represents separation of mother and child during the first postpartum days which have been shown to be the most important for maternal-infant bonding (Klaus et al. 1972).

The Impossible Maternal Transport

Maternal transport is not always possible because of nonidentifiable risks and acute emergency situations (Schoetzau et al. 1983). A rate of 40% not preidentifiable risks had been estimated by Auld (1978), which came down to 15%-20% in detailed single case analyses (Kollée et al. 1985; Selbmann et al. 1980).

In contrast to these numbers of "impossible" maternal transports, about 95% of the VLBW (Verloove-Vanhorick and Verwey 1987) or high-risk (Riegel et al. 1985) newborn infants of level 3 centers in the Netherlands and Finland are inborns.

Conclusion

Controlled hospital-based and population-based analyses indicate improved survival and quality of survival after maternal antenatal compared to neonatal transport. Three comparisons of populations in areas with and without regionalization programs appear to illustrate shortcomings of such studies rather than to provide arguments against this conclusion.

Qualified neonatal transport has been of unmeasurable benefit, and will always be necessary. Well-functioning neonatal transport systems should, however, not be an argument against the better solution: fetal transport in utero.

Acknowledgement. The help of Mrs. Heike Pohl and Mrs. Christine Pronold in the preparation of the manuscript is gratefully acknowledged.

References

Anderson C, Aladjem S, Ayuste O, Caldwell C, Ismail M (1981) An analysis of maternal transport within a suburban metropolitan region. Am J Obstet Gynecol 140: 499-504

Auld P (1978) Maternal transport is not the answer. Perinat Neonat 2: 8

Bakketeig LS, Hoffmann HS, Steinthal PM (1978) Obstetric service and perinatal mortality in Norway. Acta Obstet Gynecol Scand 57 [suppl 77]: 3-19

Bönisch H, Gaden W, Mau D, Gurbrandt U, Teuteberg HO, Braun H, Beermann HJ (1985) Mechanische Belastung Neugeborener bei Inkubatortransporten. Monatsschr Kinderheilkd 133: 471-475

Campbell AN, Lightstone AD, Smith JM, Kirpalani H, Perlman M (1984) Mechanical vibration and sound levels experienced in neonatal transport. Am J Dis Child 138: 967-970

Chance GW, Mathew JD, Williams G, Cunningham K (1978) Neonatal transport: a controlled study of skilled assistance. J Pediatr 93: 662-666

Clark CE, Clymann RI, Roth RS, Sniderman SH, Lane B, Ballard RA (1981) Risk factor analysis of intraventricular haemorrhage in low birthweight infants. J Pediatr 99: 625-628

Cordero L, Backes C, Zuspan F (1982) Very low birth weight infant: I. Influence of place of birth on survival. Am J Obstet Gynecol 143: 533-537

Dykes FA, Lazzarra A, Ahmann P, Blumenstein R, Schwarz J, Brann AW (1980) Intra ventricular hemorrhage. Pediatrics 66: 42-49

Editorial (1986) Perinatal care: organization and outcome. Lancet I: 777-778

Eksmyr R (1986) Two geographically defined populations with different organization of medical care. Cause-specific analysis of early neonatal deaths. Acta Paediatr Scand 75: 10-16

Garcia-Prats JA, Procianoy RS, Adams JM, Rudolp AJ (1982) The hyaline membrane disease - intraventricular hemorrhage: Relationship in the very low birth weight infant. Perinatal aspects. Acta Paediatr Scand 71: 79-84

Gortmaker S, Sobol A, Clark C, Walker DK, Geronimus A (1985) The survival of very low-birth weight infants by level of hospital of birth: a population study of perinatal systems in four states. Am J Obstet Gynecol 152: 517-524

Harris TR, Isaman J, Giles HR (1978) Improved neonatal survival through maternal transport. Obstet Gynecol 52: 294-300

Harris BA, Wirtschafter DD, Huddleston JF, Perlis HW (1981) In utero versus neonatal transportation of high risk perinates: a comparison. Obstet Gynec 57: 496-499

Huisman A, Visser GHA, Okken A, van der Wagen A, Huisjes HJ (1983) Intrauteriene verwijzingen; een overzicht van vier jaar ervaring, 1978-1981. Ned Tijdschr Geneeskd 127: 1525-1530

Kitchen W, Ford G, Orgill A, Rickards A, Astbury J, Lissenden J, Bajuk B, Yu V, Drew J, Campbell N (1984) Outcome in infants with birth weight 500 to 999 gm: a regional study of 1979 and 1980 births. J Pediatr 104: 921-927

Klaus MH, Jerauld R, Kreber NC, McAlpine W, Steffa M, Kennell JH (1972) Maternal attachement: importance of the first post-partum days. N Engl J Med 286: 460-463

Kollée LAA, Eskes TKAB, Peer PGM, Koppes JFP (1985) Intra- or extrauterine transport? Comparison of neonatal outcomes using a logistic model. Eur J Obstet Gynecol Reprod Biol 20: 393-399

Lamont RF, Dunlop PDM, Crowley P, Levene M, Elder MG (1983) Comparative mortality and morbidity of infants transfered in utero or postnatally. J Perinat Med 11: 200-202

Lazzara A, Kanto WP, Dykes FD, Ahmann PA, West K (1985) Continued education in the community hospital and reduction in the incidence of intracerebral hemorrhage in the transported preterm infant. J Pediatr 101: 757-761

Lou HC, Lassen NA, Friis-Hansen B (1979) Impaired autoregulation of cerebral blood flow in the distressed newborn infants. J Pediatr 94: 118-121

McCormick M, Shapiro S, Starfield B (1985) The regionalization of perinatal services. Summary of the evaluation of a national demonstration program JAMA 253: 799-804

Miller TC, Densbager M, Koragman J (1983) Maternal transport and the perinatal denominator. Am J Obstet Gynecol 147: 19-24

Modanlou HD, Dorchester W, Freeman RK, Rommal C (1980) Perinatal transport to a regional perinatal center in a metropolitan area: maternal versus neonatal transport. Am J Obstet Gynecol 138: 1157-1164
Obladen M, Heemann V, Hennecke KH, Hanssler L (1985) Ursachen neonataler Letalität 1981-1983: Eine regionale Analyse. Z Geburtshilfe Perinatol 189: 181-187
Paneth N, Kiely JL, Wallenstein S, Marcus M, Pakter J, Susser M (1982) Newborn intensive care and neonatal mortality in low-birthweight-infants. N Engl J Med 307: 149-155
Paneth N, Kiely JL, Susser M (1984) Age at death used to assess the effect of interhospital transfer of newborns. Pediatrics 73: 854-861
Piekkala P, Erkkola R, Kero P, Tenovuo A, Sillanpaa M (1985) Declining perinatal mortality in a region of Finland, 1968-82. Am J Public Health 75: 156-160
Riegel K, Selbmann HK, Österlund K (1985) Perinatalrisiken und kindliche Mortalität und Morbidität. Arvo-Ylppö-Studie. BPT-Bericht 5/85. Gesellschaft für Strahlen und Umweltforschung, München
Sachs BP, Marks JS, McCarthy BJ, Burton A, Rochat RW, Terry J (1983) Neonatal transport in Georgia. Implications for maternal transport in high-risk pregnancies. South Med J 76: 1397-1400
Saule H, Riegel K (1986) Effectiveness of neonatal transport systems. J Perinat Med (in press)
Schoetzau A, Schöber JG, Selbman HK (1983) Läßt sich die Indikation für den Abruf des Neugeborenen-Notarzt-Dienstes vor der Geburt stellen? Z Geburtshilfe Perinatol 187: 138-141
Selbman HK, Brach H, Elser K, Holzmann J, Johannigmann K, Riegel K (1980) Münchner Perinatalstudie 1975-1977. Dtsch Ärzteverlag, Köln
Shenai JP, Johanson GE, Varney RV (1981) Mechanical vibration in neonatal transport. Pediatrics 68: 55-57
Siegel E, Gillings D, Campbell S, Guild P (1985) A controlled evaluation or rural regional perinatal care: Impact on mortality and morbidity. Am J Public Health 75: 246-253
Swyer PR (1970) The regional organisation of special care for the neonate. Pediatr Clin North Am 17: 761-776
Usher R (1977) Changing mortality rates with perinatal intensive care and regionalization. Semin Perinatol 1: 309-319
Verloove-Vanhorick SP, Verwey RA (1987) Project on preterm and small for gestational age infants in the Netherlands 1983. Thesis, Rijksuniversiteit Leiden (ISBN 90-9001620-1)
Volpe JJ (1981) Neurology of the newborn. Saunders, Philadelphia
Von Loewenich V, Bielicki M, Halberstadt E, Grau H (1984) Wie weit ist die intraventriculäre Blutung sehr unreifer Frühgeborener vermeidbar? In: Dudenhausen JW, Saling E (eds) Perinatale Medizin X. Thieme, Stuttgart, pp 308-309

Improved Outcome of Very Low Birthweight Infants 1977–1986. Critical Analysis of Results and Possible Mechanisms

H. MENTZEL

Outcome of very low birthweight (VLBW) infants depends to a high degree on optimal cooperation between obstetricians and neonatologists. Until recently this necessity had not been recognized in many countries. Years ago there was very little chance of finding a position as a neonatologist because neonatology was almost unknown. This is still true in the Federal Republic of Germany. It was D.V.I. Fairweather (1981) who first in Europe emphasized the urgent need for close cooperation between the obstetrician and the neonatologist and stated that he enjoyed this successful "symbiosis."

In Tübingen there is a similar close cooperation between the obstetricians of the Universitäts-Frauenklinik and the neonatologists of the Universitäts-Kinderklinik. The following results regarding the outcome of VLBW infants represent the product of the continuous combined efforts.

Outcome is usually defined in terms of mortality and morbidity. These should not be evaluated isolated. The mortality rates in VLBW infants in Tübingen during the last 14½ years are listed in Table 1, separated into specific weight groups. The years were divided into three consecutive time periods. Death before discharge was included; infants with lethal malformations were excluded. In all weight groups a continuous decrease in mortality could be shown. Only in the very tiny infants below 750 g mortality increased again during the last period. This was due to a growing number of extremely hypotrophic infants who still have a bad prognosis.

For the obstetrician and for the parents, prognosis correlated with weeks of gestation is of even more importance. We therefore classified in a next step the VLBW infants according to gestational age at birth. Instead of mortality we calcu-

Table 1. Mortality of VLBW infants 1972–May 1986, to discharge, lethal malformations excluded, Department of Neonatology, Tübingen

Birthweight (g)	1972–1976			1977–1981			1982–May 1986		
		Deaths			Deaths			Deaths	
	(n)	*(n)*	(%)	*(n)*	*(n)*	(%)	*(n)*	*(n)*	(%)
500– 750	10	9	90	30	17	57	27	18	66
751–1000	35	22	63	61	29	48	59	14	24
1001–1500	122	33	27	130	11	8	124	9	7
1501–2000	241	26	11	231	5	2	221	3	1.3

Table 2. Survival of VLBW infants according to week of gestation, 1981-May 1986, to discharge, lethal malformations excluded

Gestational age (weeks)	Live borns Total (*n*)	Survivals (*n*)	Survivals (%)
24.-25.	12	5	42
26.-27.	37	19	51
28.	38	28	74
29.	36	32	89
30.	44	38	86
31.	56	51	91
32.	105	103	98

lated the gestational age-specific survival rates for the years 1981-May 1986 (Table 2). This allowed a comparison with results recently published in the literature. Goldenberg et al. (1984) published favorable data from eleven Perinatal Centers. The mean survival rate for the 28th week of gestation reached 75%, and for the 29th week of gestation 81%. The results in Tübingen correspond closely with the published data.

In the following studies we tried to find specific factors which contributed mainly to the dramatic reduction in mortality of VLBW infants in Tübingen in recent years. We searched for changes in the causes of death, comparing two time periods: 1977-1981 versus 1982-1986. In defining causes of death we abandoned the old classification that immaturity was the most preferred cause of death in VLBW infants and even more so in very preterm infants. In our experience, immaturity as the main or single cause of death in infants of 24-30 weeks of gestation should no longer be used. In reality most of those tiny infants suffer from substantial diseases or die as a result of severe complications during ventilation or intensive care treatment. In many places in Germany, most of these highly compromized infants still die because of insufficient or refused medical care.

For our studies of possible changes in the causes of death, we assigned all infants with a birthweight of 1000 g or less who died during the last 9 years to one of five possible causes contributing mainly to deterioration. Infants with lethal malformations were excluded. Fetal bacterial infections hours or days prior to delivery with early manifestation of sepsis or pneumonia after birth presented as a full-blown disease with poor outcome. Initial postnatal asphyxia with severe acidosis puts a great load on VLBW infants which they can hardly cope with. Acute complications during arteficial ventilation, e.g., air leak, worsen the outcome to a great extent. The same is true for infants with long-time ventilation and development of bronchopulmonary dysplasia. Extremely hypotrophic infants represent a special group of prematurity with severe malnutrition superimposed on immaturity. Even with the application of modern neonatal intensive care, the prognosis is still poor.

The results for infants with a birthweight of 500-750 g are displayed in Table 3. Total mortality has increased in this group between 1977 and 1986 because the number of extremely hypotrophic infants doubled during this time. There has

Table 3. Causes of death in infants with a birthweight of 500–750 g, disease- or treatment-related in two consecutive time periods

Birthweight 500–750 g	1977–1981		1982–May 1986	
	(n)	(%)	*(n)*	(%)
Total number	30	100	27	100
Deaths	17	57	18	66
Cause of death				
Early infection	3	10	5	18
Severe asphyxia	9	30	5	18
Ventilation complications				
Acute	2	6	1	4
Chronic	1	3	2	7
Extreme hypotrophy	2	6	5	18

Table 4. Causes of death in infants with a birthweight of 751–1000 g, disease- or treatment-related in two consecutive time periods

Birthweight 751–1000 g	1977–1981		1982–May 1986	
	(n)	(%)	*(n)*	(%)
Total number	61	100	59	100
Deaths	29	47	14	24
Cause of death				
Early infection	7	11	4	7
Severe asphyxia	10	16	0	-
Ventilation complications				
Acute	6	10	7	12
Chronic	5	8	1	2
Extreme hypotrophy	1	2	2	3

been a remarkable reduction in the incidence of severe asphyxia at birth. In the next weight group, 751–1000 g, total mortality decreased from 47% to 24% (Table 4). Severe initial asphyxia was no longer observed in the last time period. Chronic lung disease following long-time ventilation contributed to death of only one infant.

The decrease in total mortality is predominantly a consequence of the reduction in treatment-related causes of death. These could be reduced by half (36% to 19%), whereas the disease-related causes of death increased slightly (14% to 19%). These results give strong evidence for the marked positive influence of optimal neonatal intensive care on the survival chances of very tiny infants. The dramatic changes in mortality during the last 10 years have been summarized in Fig. 1. VLBW infants with a birthweight of 500–750 g have now reached the same mortality rates as infants weighing 751–1000 g in the 1970s. In Tübingen today the latter group has the same survival chances as the group of 1001–1250 g 10 years ago.

After presenting the favorable data on outcome according to mortality, we now come to morbidity. The most important morbidity in VLBW infants is character-

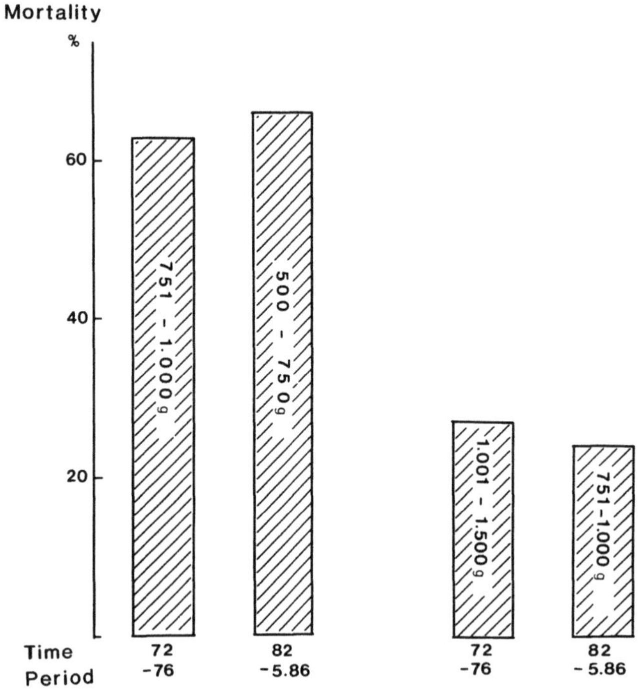

Fig. 1. Change of birthweight groups with approximately 60% or 20% mortality over 10 years

Table 5. Incidence of cerebro-ventricular hemorrhage (CVH) in very preterm infants, born 1981-May 1986

Gestational age (weeks)		CVH		IVH/IPH		PHH	
	(n)	*(n)*	(%)	*(n)*	(%)	*(n)*	(%)
24.-25.	12	5	42	1	8	–	–
26.-27.	42	17	40	12	28	2	5
28.	37	8	21	5	13	2	5
29.	39	10	25	6	15	–	–
30.	46	7	15	5	11	–	–
24.-30.	176	47	27	29	16	4	2

ized by irreversible cerebral damage. The development of cerebral hemorrhage in the first hours and days of life plays a predominant role in cerebral handicap (Stewart 1982; Leidig 1985; Leidig et al. 1984). The incidence of total cerebroventricular hemorrhage (CVH) observed during 1981-May 1986 was 27% in infants from 24 to 30 weeks of gestation (Table 5). Intraventricular hemorrhage (IVH) plus intraparenchymous hemorrhage (IPH) occurred in 16%. The later development of posthemorrhagic hydrocephalus (PHH) was observed in 2%.

Table 6. Incidence of CVH in survivors according to gestational age, 1981–May 1986

Gestational age (weeks)	Survivors Total	CVH		IVH/IPH		PHH	
	(*n*)	(*n*)	(%)	(*n*)	(%)	(*n*)	(%)
24.-25.	5	1	20	1	20	-	-
26.-27.	19	10	52	8	42	2	10
28.	28	6	21	5	18	2	7
29.	32	7	22	4	12	-	-
30.	38	6	16	5	13	-	-
24.-30.	122	30	24	23	19	4	3

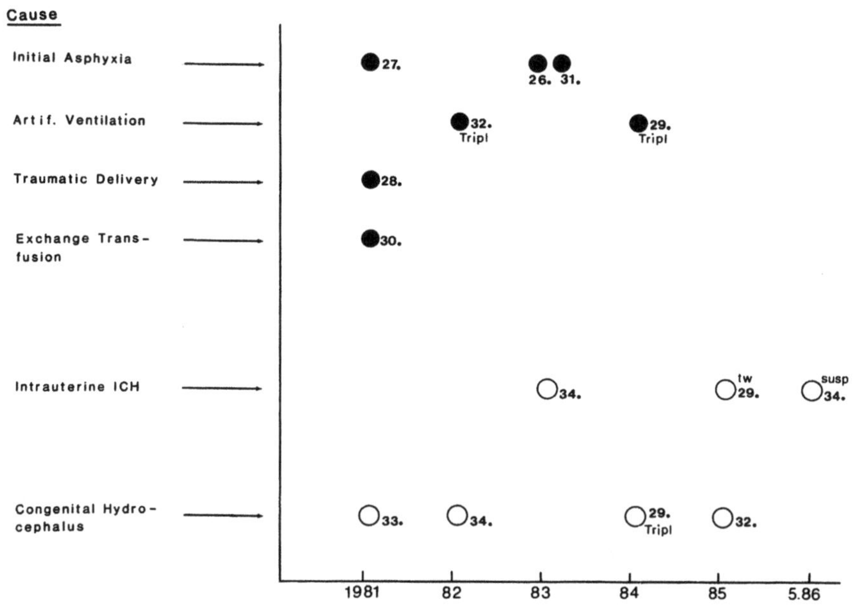

Fig. 2. Etiology of hydrocephalus in VLBW infants. Treatment-related and congenital causes, 1981–May 1986. ● Treatment related ○ congenital

Since the development of CVH in survivors may be of even greater interest, we calculated the incidence in survivors (Table 6). A CVH could be found in 24% by sonographic studies which were performed in all VLBW infants. Meaningful hemorrhages (IVH/IPH) were detected in 19%. PHH occurred in the 26th–27th week of gestation in 10%, and in the 27th week in 7% of the infants. In comparison with data in recent literature, the incidence of IVH/IPH and PHH appears low.

In order to elucidate possible mechanisms which favor or cause severe cerebral hemorrhage with development of PHH, we classified the hydrocephali observed as treatment-related or acquired in utero (Fig. 2). During the last 5½ years hydrocephalus was observed in 14 infants, born in the 26.–34. week of gestation. In seven infants full-grown hydrocephalus presented at birth. Four suffered from congenital hydrocephalus, three developed prenatal PHH after intrauterine cere-

Table 7. Reduction of intraventricular and intraparenchymous hemorrhage after improvement of fetal and neonatal care. (Modified from Leidig 1985)

Birthweight (g)	June 1981-June 1983			July 1983-June 1985		
	Total	IVH/IPH		Total	IVH/IPH	
	(n)	*(n)*	(%)	*(n)*	*(n)*	(%)
500- 750	12	6	50	15	4	27
751-1000	31	7	23	28	4	14
1001-1500	59	9	15	65	3	5

bral hemorrhage (ICH). The other seven infants presented a PHH after CVH. The assumed causes for hemorrhage were: deep initial asphyxia, severe complications caused by artificial ventilation, traumatic delivery, and complicated exchange transfusion. Most of these treatment-related cerebral hemorrhages can be prevented. With the introduction of more strict resuscitation procedures, the occurrence of PHH in VLBW infants has become a rare exception (Fig. 2). In full agreement with this are the results published by Leidig (1985) which demonstrate a statistically significant reduction of IVH and IPH in recent years in Tübingen (Table 7). Haas and Schmitten (1986) report on the long-time outcome of VLBW infants in Tübingen in the following contribution in this volume. They have observed a decreasing incidence of neurological morbidity during the last years.

A critical analysis of the results presented confirms a dramatic decrease in mortality and morbidity. In the following we will discuss some mechanisms and changes which have probably contributed to this success to a great extent. Starting in 1973, great efforts were made in Tübingen to satisfy the requirements for giving optimal neonatal intensive care to all VLBW infants. This implied building up a special team of neonatologists, close cooperation with obstetricians and transferral of all mothers with high-risk pregnancies to Tübingen. Most of the requirements for neonatal intensive care could be established from 1975 to 1977. Within a few years an improvement of transport in utero of high-risk fetuses was reached. After 10 years of excellent cooperation with the regional obstetricians, regionalization of high-risk pregnancies was complete. For infants of 1000 g or less the incidence of outborn infants decreased from 60% in 1972-1973 to 3% in 1984-1985 (Fig. 3), correspondingly the transport in utero rose from 40% to 97%. Another procedure which underwent major changes concerned resuscitation in the delivery room. During the 1970s, approximately half the resuscitations and primary care of high-risk infants at birth were performed by pediatric senior residents with short training who were supported by residents. The other half of the infants received resuscitation by an experienced staff neonatologist.

In order to elucidate the influence which is exerted by the quality of the resuscitator on mortality, we compared a group with advanced training and daily practice with a group of resuscitators with good or moderate training and only occasional practice (Table 8). As expected the difference in mortality of high-risk infants with a birthweight below 1001 g was most striking: 88.5% mortality in non-expert resuscitation versus 37% in expert resuscitation. The recognition of these findings consequently led to a change in our policy. Resuscitation and primary

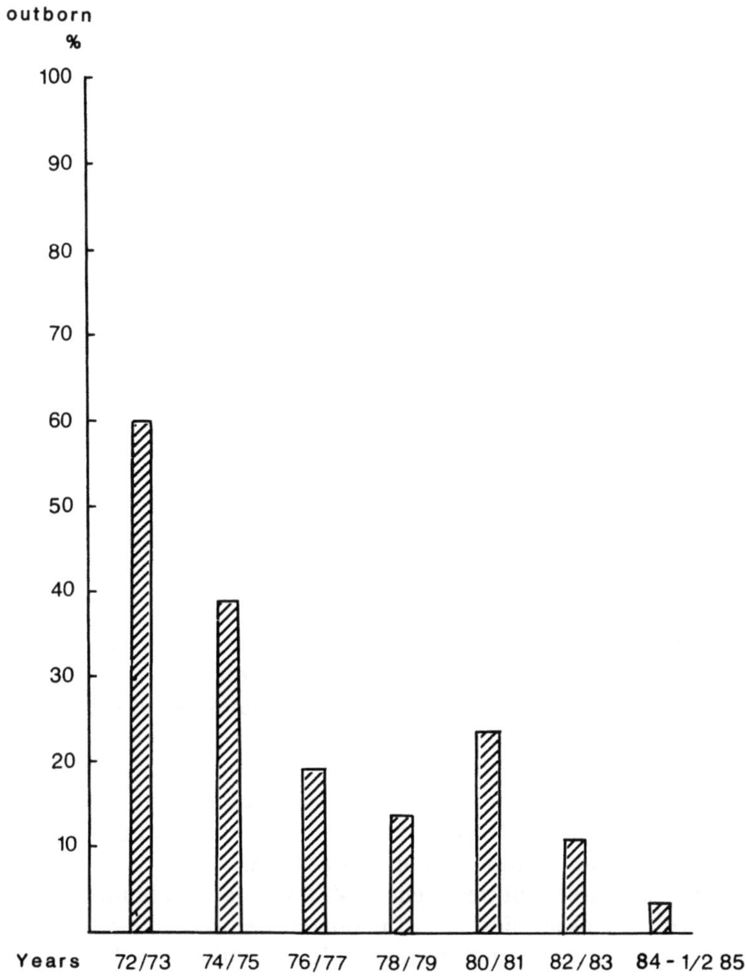

Fig. 3. Development of regionalization of high-risk pregnancies in Tübingen. Birthweight ≤1000 g

Table 8. Qualification of resuscitator at birth and mortality in VLBW infants, Tübingen 1977-1981

Birthweight (g)	Advanced training Frequent practice			Good→moderate training Occasional practice		
	Total	Deaths		Total	Deaths	
	(n)	*(n)*	(%)	*(n)*	*(n)*	(%)
500- 750	15	6	40	9	8	89
751-1000	23	8	35	17	15	88
500-1000	38	14	37	26	23	88.5

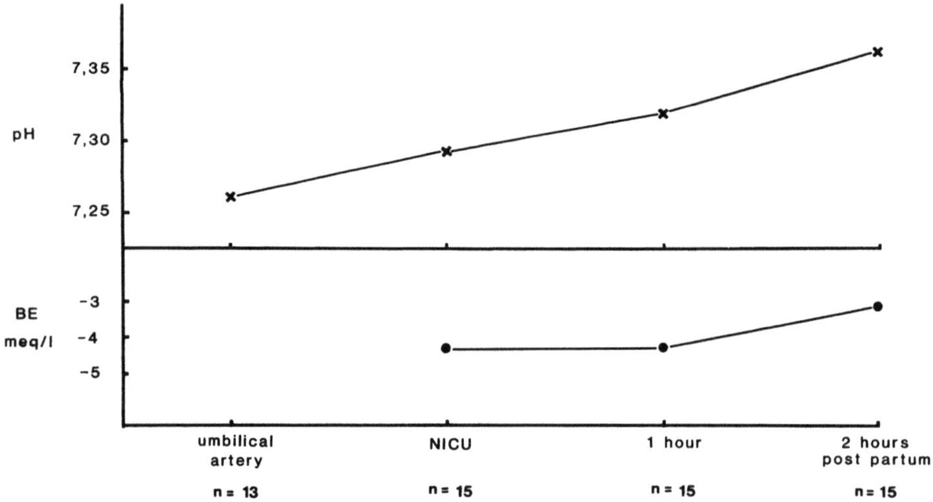

Fig. 4. pH and Base Excess (BE) in infants with a birthweight below 1000 g during the first 2 h of life under optimal fetal and neonatal care

care of high-risk infants in the delivery room is now performed exclusively by a staff neonatologist assisted by a pediatric resident and a neonatal intensive care nurse. This team will be present within minutes round the clock.

The positive effect of expert resuscitation can be shown in different ways. In Fig. 4 we present pH and base excess values of infants below 1000 g during the first 2 h of life. This proves that acidosis even in tiny infants is not an unpreventable event. Under optimal conditions, most of these infants can start extrauterine life in the same condition as infants at term.

Finally, successful treatment of VLBW infants is bound to an optimally operating NICU. This implies: a staff neonatologist available round the clock, 24-h presence of residents trained in neonatology, routine care by neonatal intensive care nurses.

In order to guarantee the absolutely necessary training and continuous practice in intubation, artificial ventilation, and other neonatal intensive care procedures, a minimum of six places for neonatal intensive care should be constantly in operation.

Conclusions

The outcome of VLBW infants in Tübingen provides all evidence that even in very tiny infants mortality and morbidity can be kept within reasonable limits which not only justify active medical care but demand it. Hopefully, the favorable results will support the establishment of Perinatal Centers where optimal neonatal intensive care in close cooperation with an obstetric team can be applied.

References

Fairweather DVI (1981) Obstetric management and follow-up of the very-low-birth-weight infant. J Reprod Med 26: 387

Goldenberg RL, Nelson KG, Davis RO, Koski J (1984) Delay in delivery: influence of gestational age and the duration of delay on perinatal outcome. Obstet Gynecol 64: 480

Haas G, aus der Schmitten I (1986) Decreasing incidence of neurological morbidity and changes of perinatal care strategies in very low birth-weight infants. International workshop on perinatal events and cerebral handicap, pathogenesis and prevention, Heidelberg June 1986. Report FIGO committee. (to be published)

Leidig E (1985) Prevention of postnatal intracerebral hemorrhage in very low birth weight infants by non-invasive monitoring. Vortrag: IV. Tübinger Symposium on newborn mortality and morbidity, Tübingen

Leidig E, Haas G, Mentzel H (1984) Prognostische Wertigkeit des Schweregrades der intra- und periventrikulären Hirnblutungen des Frühgeborenen. Monatsschr Kinderheilkd 132: 726

Stewart A (1982) Follow up bei Kindern mit sehr niedrigem Geburtsgewicht (VLBW). In: Huch A, Huch R, Duc G, Rooth G (eds) Klinisches Management des “kleinen” Frühgeborenen. Thieme, Stuttgart, pp 9-14

Decreasing Incidence of Neurological Morbidity and Changes of Perinatal Care Strategies in Very Low Birthweight Infants

G. HAAS and I. AUS DER SCHMITTEN

There is general agreement that neonatal intensive care can increase the chances of survival in very low birthweight infants (VLBW). However, there is also a controversial discussion about its efficacy in respect to the neurological morbidity in survivors. The question of whether neonatal intensive care of VLBW infants only reduces perinatal mortality at the cost of higher neurodevelopmental morbidity or whether it is able to reduce both still remains open.

In Sweden an increasing incidence of cerebral palsy was found and this unfavourable trend was considered to be due to changes in perinatal care programmes (Hagberg et al. 1984). Similarly, the incidence of surviving low birthweight infants registered in Western Australia did not indicate a beneficial effect of neonatal intensive care on the neurodevelopmental morbidity of these children (Stanley and Atkinson 1981). In these epidemiological studies, however, the perinatal care programmes applied and possible changes in perinatal care strategies have not been described or analysed. Therefore, the causal relation assumed between the increasing incidence of severe neurological sequelae in surviving low birthweight VLBW or infants and an intensification of neonatal care programmes seem not to have been fully clarified.

In our hospital, the fate and development of VLBW infants cared for in our Department of Neonatalogy has been followed since 1974. Thus, mortality and morbidity data of VLBW infants admitted to the neonatal intensive care unit (NICU) are available and changes can also be related to changes in perinatal care strategies.

In the first years of this observation period, 1974-1975, the mortality of VLBW infants to discharge was 38%, the incidence of severe neurological sequelae or "major handicaps", such as cerebral palsy, severe mental retardation, epilepsy, severe vision or hearing loss, was 12% (Michaelis et al. 1978). In the subsequent periods, a decreasing incidence of in-hospital mortality (30% in 1977-1979, 27% in 1980-1981, 23% in 1982-1983), as well as a decreasing incidence of major handicaps (9% in 1977-1979, 6% in 1980-1981, 3% in 1982-1983) of the VLBW infants admitted could be observed. The incidence of deaths after discharge from the NICU, however, was found to increase during this time period. The causes of late deaths remained partly unknown but were in some cases pulmonary hypertension due to bronchopulmonary dysplasia and therefore associated with preceding long-term artificial ventilation. The incidence of minor developmental anomalies or "minor handicaps" was approximately 5% of the VLBW infants admitted and remained unchanged in the time period observed (see Fig. 1). The decreasing inci-

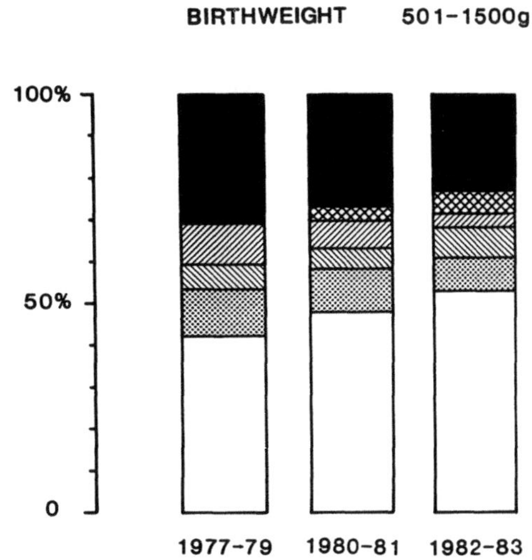

Fig. 1. Outcome of VLBW infants born in three consecutive time periods (1977-1979 $n=131$; 1980-1981 $n=113$; 1982-1983 $n=107$). ■, In-hospital deaths; ▩, deaths after discharge; ▨, major handicaps; ▧, minor handicaps; ▦, lost to follow up; □, normal development

Table 1. Neurological conditions in children with major handicaps

	1977-1979	1980-1981	1982-1983
Number of children	12	7	4[a]
Spastic diplegia	4	5	1
Spastic tetraplegia	4	2	0
Spastic hemiplegia	1	0	1
Severe mental retardation	7	3	2[a]
Epilepsy	3	2	0
Hydrocephalus	4	2	2
Severe vision loss	4	2	0
Retrolental fibroplasia	2	0	0
Atrophy of optical nerve	2	2	0
Severe hearing loss	1	0	0

[a] One child with Down's syndrome

dence of major handicaps could be seen in children with a birthweight of 1001-1500 g as well as in children with a birthweight of 501-1000 g.

Another observation made during the years 1977-1983 was a trend to fewer multiple handicaps in surviving VLBW infants with major handicaps (see Table 1). For example, severe vision loss due to retrolental fibroplasia was found only in two children born in 1977. Thereafter severe vision loss was only due to atrophy of the optical nerves caused by posthaemorrhagic hydrocephalus and increased intracranial pressure (four children born during 1978-1981). Evidently, this could be avoided in two children with posthaemorrhagic hydrocephalus born in the years 1982 and 1983.

Preliminary results of psychometric investigations of VLBW children without major handicaps born in the years 1981-1983 indicated a distribution of developmental scores or intelligence quotients which is not different from the distribution which would be expected in a standard population (see Table 2). Moreover, the

Table 2. Developmental or intelligence quotients in children with a birthweight below 1500 g and without major handicaps (1981-1983, $n=38$)

IQ	(%)
85- 90	4
91-110	70
111-115	11
>115	14

Methods applied:
Corrected age 2-3 years: Münchner Funktionelle Entwicklungs-Test (Munich functional development test)
3-4 years: McCarthy scales
3-5 years: Stanford-Binet test
4-5 years: Wechsler test for preschool age

longitudinal assessment of individual cases often showed an improvement when developmental anomalies or retardation of development were detected during the first 2 years of life.

From these results we conclude that intensive care of VLBW infants can not only increase the chance of survival, but may also improve the quality of survival, and we assume that changes in our perinatal care strategies led to an improvement in the perinatal situation of VLBW infants in our hospital.

In order to investigate this we examined records and case reports of 244 surviving VLBW infants born during 1977-1983 and treated in the NICU, and registered the occurrence of obstetrical and neonatal risk factors and complications. They were defined and categorised in a list which had to be fully completed in every case (see Table 3).

The pattern of obstetrical and neonatal risk factors and complications showed that the prenatal situation of these infants during the time periods 1977-1979, 1980-1981, 1982-1983 got even worse, indicated by a higher incidence of maternal toxaemia (16%, 14%, 26%) and intrauterine growth retardation (24%, 36%, 37%). On the other hand, the incidence of postnatal referral decreased considerably (23%, 22%, 5%), and due to an increasingly liberal use of Caesarean section if a preterm birth was inevitable, the incidence of vaginal delivery in cases with abnormal presentation decreased (16%, 4%, 3%). The postnatal situation of the VLBW infants was found to be improved in respect of low body temperature (43%, 38%, 19%) and abnormal haematocrite values at admission (50%, 45%, 17%), but obviously not in respect of low Apgar scores (50%, 51%, 47%). However, a comparison of pH values at admission in these VLBW infants after vaginal delivery and Caesarean section showed significantly higher pH values after Caesarean section (Mentzel 1984). The rate of Caesarean section in the population studied increased from 25% in 1977-1979 to 87% in 1982-1983, thus an improvement in the mean pH values of these infants at admission to the NICU may be assumed.

In total, the mean number of risk factors or adverse events per infant was found to decrease from 4.1 in 1977-1979 to 3.2 in 1982-1983 (χ^2 test, $p<0.001$). Evidently, this was mainly achieved by early intrauterine referral, consequent

Table 3. Obstetrical and neonatal risk factors and complications

1	Previous abortion or preterm delivery
2	Hyperemesis gravidarum
3	Toxaemia
4	Maternal bleeding in the first trimenon of gestation
5	Intrauterine growth retardation
6	Antepartum haemorrhage
7	Vaginal delivery if the fetus was in an abnormal presentation
8	Outborn and postnatally referred
9	Postnatal asphyxia
10	Low temperature at admission
11	Polyglobulia at admission
12	Anaemia at admission
13	Artificial ventilation longer than 7 days
14	Complications of ventilation, such as pneumothorax, severe acidosis
15	Intracranial haemorrhage
16	Exchange transfusion
17	Neonatal infection
18	Postnatal growth retardation
19	Severe postnatal disease, such as necrotising enterocolitis, sepsis, meningitis

A detailed description of the criteria applied has been published elsewhere (Haas et al. 1986).

monitoring of fetal behaviour, and early intervention if necessary in an adequately equipped perinatal centre.

Since perinatally acquired brain damage cannot be reversed and is still a frequent cause of severe handicaps in children, primary prevention is necessary and should be improved. The conclusion from our experience made during the last decade is that the improvement of perinatal care is not only a matter of improved technical means, but also the consequence of a well-organised cooperation between obstetricians and neonatologists.

References

Haas G, Asprion B, Leidig E, Buchwald-Saal M, Mentzel H (1986) Obstetrical and neonatal risk factors in very low birth-weight infants related to their neurological development. Eur J Pediatr 145: 341-346

Hagberg B, Hagberg G, Olow I (1984) The changing panorama of cerebral palsy in Sweden. IV Epidemiological trends 1959-1978. Acta Peadiatr Scand 73: 433-440

Mentzel H (1984) Sectio bei Frühgeburt aus der Sicht des Neonatologen. Indikation und Grenzen. Gynäkologe 17: 243-249

Michaelis R, Stötter M, Buchwald M, Rohr M, Mentzel H (1978) Ergebnisse der Intensivüberwachung und Intensivtherapie bei Neugeborenen mit sehr niedrigem Geburtsgewicht. Dtsch Med Wochenschr 103: 1404-1408

Stanley FJ, Atkinson S (1981) Impact of neonatal intensive care on cerebral palsy in infants of low birth-weight. Lancet II: 1162

Supported by Fonds zur Förderung der wissenschaftlichen Forschung (FWF) Wien.

Prevention of Preterm Labor – A Means of Preventing Handicaps?

E. PAPIERNIK, J. BOUYER, and J. DREYFUS

If there were a reduction in the number of preterm births which consequently lowered the number of newborn infants transferred to neonatal intensive care units, there would be immediate cost benefits and also global cost savings related to long-term disabilities, neurological disorders of perinatal origin, and mental retardation (Chapalain 1978). This assumption was the basis of one of the programs of the national perinatal care program, which was initiated in 1970 by the French Ministry of Health. The overall goal was to reduce perinatal morbidity and mortality.

This policy adopted as one of its major focuses the prevention of preterm birth since is was known that the preterm birth rate remains, despite many improvements in neonatal care, the major predictor for neonatal deaths (David and Siegel 1983), for the cost of care in neonatal intensive care units (NICU), for mental retardation, hearing and visual problems, neurological handicaps and for all their consequences. While the program for preterm birth prevention has been in effect on a national level, there have been several analyses of the program's methodology (Papiernik 1969, 1984), its social policy (Papiernik 1984), and its results (Rumeau-Rouquette et al. 1984). We feel that it is necessary to conduct a cost-benefit evaluation with regard to the program's effectiveness in terms of preterm births avoided.

We will also try to predict how many handicaps related to preterm birth could have been prevented.

Methods

Program Definition

The program for preterm birth prevention was to a large extend based upon the results of research on risk factors in relation to a woman's life style (Papiernik 1969). Specifically, the relationship between life style and uterine contractions became the keystone of the program. Furthermore, while the program was largely incentive in nature (and thus allowed for personal initiative on the part of those involved), it included the following three coordinate internventions which are described in detail elsewhere (Papiernik 1984).

- A risk factor scoring system to analyze individual preterm birth risk.
- An effort to provide the women with information regarding preterm birth, their risk status, and the relationship between life style and uterine contractions.
- A reduction in the physical workload for those women at risk of preterm delivery. In the case of physically hard work, leave of absence was proposed (this being possible with compensation owing to the nature of the French social security system).

The emphasis on life style provided a new way of modifying daily activities which may induce uterine contractions. In addition, it allowed a large degree of self-management by the individual women.

The above subsystem comprised the core of the preterm birth prevention program; however, prenatal care facilities often established additional measures to prevent preterm birth. For example, some of us thought that cervical cerclage would be an important representative measure for those women at high risk and thus we directed a lot of energy towards this procedure [which was later demonstrated as being ineffective (Lazar et al. 1984)].

We would like to evaluate, however, the core of the prevention program since that was applied on a national scale. Furthermore, since the program was introduced nationally, it was possible for us to use a district maternity hospital in Haguenau (north-eastern France) as an observation site for measuring the effects of national policy change. We developed a 12-year study, beginning in 1971, whose goal was to follow the way in which women progressively responded to the new proposals in prenatal care and to measure the effectiveness of the program. The 12-year span was divided into three 4-year periods (1971-1974, 1975-1978, 1979-1982) for which the numbers of single live births were 5763, 4957, and 5919, respectively.

The Haguenau maternity hospital serves a region defined by precise natural borders and it serves a relatively stable population (analyzed by times trends). In addition, data from census records reveal that during the study period, 90% of the births to residents of the city of Haguenau and 80% of births to residents of its surrounding area occurred in the maternity hospital. At this point, it should also be noted that another aspect of the perinatal care program was to improve the quality of delivery room care and services. No proposal for maternal transfers was established; however, a better neonatal transfer system was developed.

Effectiveness Methodology

Since the prevention program was introduced on a national level, it was impossible for us to use an experimental design in order to study exact comparisons between study and control groups. Thus, we use the Haguenau maternity hospital as our observation site.

The effect will be measured by the variation in distribution of births by gestational age (preterm birth being defined as <37 weeks since last menstrual period (LMP), using ultrasound scans for corrections since 1972) and by birthweight. The data were collected prospectively over the 12-year period by an obstetrical team which remained constant. This stability of personnel allowed for both consistency with respect to implementation of the policy and with respect to data gathering. Indirectly, the effectiveness can also be measured in terms of the number of admissions to the NICU 25 km away in the city of Strasbourg, the neonatal mortality rate, and the number of babies with abnormal neurological signs during the neonatal period. Any changes in the preterm birth rate, seen both in birthweight and gestational age distribution data, should affect the number of newborn infants at high risk (excluding malformations), and thus influence the NICU admissions, the neonatal mortality figures, and the number of newborn infants with abnormal neurological signs. The numbers for these three outcomes in each gestational age category are presented for 1000 single live births.

We can analyze the benefits which were observed after the new policy was implemented. Certain factors, such as changes in neonatal hospital days for 1000 single births and the number of NICU admissions can be measured directly. There are some benefits which are extremely difficult to quantify. It is impossible to know the actual number of handicaps avoided by the prevention program. However, we can propose a figure based upon predicted rates from literature on handicaps (Russell 1984), even if these figures have been established by birthweight more than by gestational age. Let us accept that the risk of handicap related to preterm birth is 20% for births at less than 28 weeks gestational age, 10% for births at 28-32 weeks gestational age, 5% for births at 33-34 gestational age and 0% for births at more than 34 weeks gestational age. Thus, we can apply these values to the number of single births at Haguenau and calculate the predicted numbers of handicaps for the different time periods, and test how the program could have affected this predicted number over time.

Results

Effectiveness Results

It has been shown (Papiernik et al. 1985) how the preterm (less than 37 weeks gestational age) birth rate decreased progressively at the Haguenau maternity hospital, from 5.4% to 4.1% and then to 3.7% ($p < 0.001$) over the time periods (Table 1). Specifically, the birth rate was reduced by one-third in the total preterm births and by two-thirds in the 28-32 weeks group. This reduction in the preterm birth rate is paralleled by a decreasing trend in low birthweights (Table 2): the overall low birthweight rates (for births less than 2500 g) were 4.60%, 3.95%, and 3.78% in the three successive time periods ($p < 0.001$). The largest reductions were by one-third for the 1500-1999-g group and by two-thirds for the 1000-1499-g group.

Furthermore, from Table 3 we see that the numbers of newborn infants admitted to the Strasbourg NICU per 1000 single live births decreased from 19.3 in 1971-1974 to 8.6 in 1979-1982 ($p < 0.01$). The major reduction in the number of transfers attributable to the <32 weeks category is of great importance.

Table 4 demonstrates that the rate of neonatal mortality per 1000 live births also changed over the time course of the study. This rate decreased from 8.5 per

Table 1. Preterm single live births

Gestational age (weeks)	1971-1974		1975-1978		1979-1982	
	(*n*)	(%)	(*n*)	(%)	(*n*)	(%)
26-27	11	0.2	7	0.1	4	0.06
28-32	69	1.2	44	0.9	25	0.4
33-34	60	1.1	40	0.8	40	0.7
35-36	159	2.9	106	2.2	147	2.5
less than 37	299	5.4	197	4.1	216	3.7
Total	5548	100.0	4787	100.0	5808	100.0

Preterm births (live births) were significantly reduced in successive periods ($p < 0.001$). The major reduction was observed in the gestational age group 28-32 weeks ($p < 0.001$). This table deals with pregnancies for which gestational age was known.

Table 2. Low birthweight single live births

Birthweight (g)	1971-1974		1975-1978		1979-1982	
	(*n*)	(%)	(*n*)	(%)	(*n*)	(%)
500- 999	4	0.07	5	0.10	3	0.05
1000-1499	30	0.52	21	0.42	10	0.17
1500-1999	53	0.92	44	0.89	38	0.64
2000-2499	178	3.09	126	2.54	173	2.92
less than 2500	265	4.60	196	3.95	224	3.78
Total	5760	100.00	4956	100.00	5919	100.00

This table shows the reduction in low birthweight births ($p < 0.001$), mostly in the category 1000-1499 g ($p < 0.01$).

Table 3. Number of admissions to the Strasbourg neonatal intensive care unit per 1000 single live births

	1971-1974	1975-1978	1979-1982
Live births	5760	4948	5917
Gestational age			
≤32 (per 1000)	6.6	5.4	2.0
(*n* in category)	38	27	12
33-36 (per 1000)	2.6	3.4	2.8
(*n* in category)	15	17	17
37+ (per 1000)	10.1	5.9	3.7
(*n* in category)	58	29	22
Total	19.3	14.7	8.6
	111	73	51

The number of admissions to the NICU in Strasbourg was reduced over years ($p < 0.01$) in two categories, the less than 32 weeks and the term babies

Table 4. Neonatal mortality per 1000 live births

Period	1971-1974	1975-1978	1979-1982
Neonatal deaths per 1000 live births	8.5	6.3	2.7
Actual figures	47/5548	30/4787	16/5808
Standardized rates for gestational age distribution in period 1971-1974	8.5	7.2	5.3
Confidence interval		4.8-9.6	3-7.6

Table 5. Number of abnormal neurological signs in the neonatal period by gestational age per 1000 single live births

	1971-1974	1975-1979	1979-1982
Live births	5760	4948	5917
Gestational age (weeks)			
⩽32 (per 1000)	9.2	2.6	0.3
(*n* in category)	53	13	2
33-36 (per 1000)	10.6	1.8	2.0
(*n* in category)	61	9	12
37 + (per 1000)	43.5	22.0	8.6
(*n* in category)	251	109	51
Total (per 1000)	63.3	26.4	10.9
(*n*)	365	131	65

$p < 0.001$

1000 to 6.3 per 1000 and then to 2.7 per 1000 over the successive time periods. Table 4 also presents standardized values and their confidence intervals for neonatal mortality using the same gestational age distribution for the later periods as that observed in 1971-1974. This has been done using the neonatal mortality rate for the 1979-1982 period together with the gestational age distribution for the 1971-1974 and 1975-1978 periods. These standardized values thus represent the effect of improved intrapartum and neonatal management or "better care" since the effect from "better babies" has been removed. The decreasing neonatal mortality rates for the recalculated values demonstrate that there was an improvement in the care for newborn infants apart from the preterm birth prevention program. However, since the actual neonatal mortality rates are even lower, we can hypothesize that the reduction observed resulted from both better care and from better babies. The number of abnormal neurological signs during the neonatal period per 1000 single live births attributable to each gestational age group (as indicated in Table 5) decreased over time in every gestational age group. The overall numbers for abnormal neurological signs during the neonatal period (per 1000 single live births) fell from 63.3 to 26.4 and then to 10.9 over the successive time periods ($p < 0.001$). In this case, the major improvement is seen in term babies.

Table 6. Probability of handicaps per 1000 live births

Predicted handicaps			
Gestational age (weeks)	(%)		
26-27	20		
28-32	10		
33-34	5		
Preterm births per 1000 single live births			
Gestational age (weeks)	1971-1974	1975-1978	1979-1982
26-27	2	1	0.6
28-32	12	9	4
33-34	11	8	7
Predicted handicaps per 1000 single live births			
weeks			
26-27	0.4	0.2	0.12
28-32	1.2	0.9	0.4
33-34	0.55	0.4	0.35
Total	2.15	1.5	0.87

Benefits are impossible to translate into financial terms; however, we propose to measure them in terms of "quality lives" gained. One such measure may be derived from the predicted handicap rates shown in Table 6. When examining the total predicted handicaps related to preterm births for each time period, we observe a decrease from 2.15 during 1971-1974 to 0.87 during 1979-1982, a difference of 1.28 handicaps per 1000 single live births.

Discussion

We have seen that the program for preterm birth prevention as observed in Haguenau was both effective and beneficial over the years 1971-1982. This program was also effective in France as a whole. An evaluation team performed national surveys in 1972, 1975-1976, and 1981 in order to examine the modifications in prenatal care, some of which were due to the prevention program. The 1981 survey compared its results to the other two surveys and found that the preterm (gestational age <37 weeks) birth rate decreased significantly from 8.2% to 6.8% and then to 5.6% over the three successive survey periods (Rumeau-Rouquette et al. 1984). In addition, there was a reduction in the rate of very low birthweight infants (<1500 g) from 0.8% to 0.7% and then to 0.4% over the three periods. In this way, we see that the decrease in preterm births seen at Haguenau paralleled the findings of the national evaluation team. We also know from research at a university teaching hospital, which served as an experimental site, that the prevention program was effective in reducing the preterm (<37 weeks) birth rate to 3.4% (Papiernik 1984). Another study (Papiernik et al. 1985) indicated that the prevention program targeted women across all social groups (as correlated to years of schooling) and that the preterm birth rates decreased across all categories. Furthermore, the prevention program is beginning to be applied in other countries and in very different populations.

A significant reduction in preterm births has been demonstrated in a California population, comparing an institution implementing the program to another institution not applying it (Herron et al. 1982).

The island of Martinique (with a mixed population of African and European descent) has adopted a program of preterm birth prevention similar to the one in France and this appears to be effective across all social classes (Goujon et al. 1984).

We investigated the possibility of bias which may have affected the results. It is important to remember that the French perinatal policy did not include a system for maternal transfers to tertiary perinatal centers; however, a better organized neonatal transfer system was proposed. Thus, maternal transfer could not bias the effectiveness results in Haguenau.

Ideally, we would have also liked to study both the effectiveness and cost benefit using two groups of women, one within the preterm birth prevention program and the other as a control. This was impossible as the program was introduced on a national level; we have therefore used an observation site at the Haguenau maternity hospital in order to assess the effects of the prevention program. Often, historical comparisons of prenatal practices may be misleading. Furthermore, there have been very few studies conducted justifying many of the common clinical practices (Willems et al. 1980). However, the published data on national results do not show any improvement in the preterm birth figures when specific programs have not been applied (Kessel 1984). This means that secular trends and new technologies cannot explain the reduction in preterm birth rates observed in France as a whole and at Haguenau in particular.

Why this program has not received greater acceptance in other countries is not known precisely. Often there are other factors that influence the decision to implement a program apart from cost effectiveness. We know, for example, that neonatalogists and obstetricians are often not very interested in preterm birth prevention programs. This lack of interest has begun to change and it is apparent that cost effectiveness studies may have helped. It becomes obvious for the neonatalogists that "high-tech" interventions have certain limits when the risk of handicaps and the extremely high cost per quality life saved are skyrocketing (Sinclair et al. 1981; Stewart and Reynolds 1979; Willems et al. 1980).

It seems, then, that the prevention program for preterm births as observed in Haguenau has provided both immediate and long-term benefits. For the 12-year period, the program was both effective in reducing preterm births and in reducing the number of babies at risk of handicaps. This is a new demonstration of the value of large population-based prevention programs (Russel 1984).

References

Chapalain M (1978) Perinatality: French cost-benefit studies and decisions on handicap and prevention. In: Major mental handicaps: methods and costs of prevention. no 59. Ciba Foundation Symposium. Elzevier, Amsterdam, pp 193-204

David R, Siegel E (1983) Decline in neonatal mortality, 1968 to 1977. Better babies or better care? Pediatrics 71: 531-540

Goujon H, Papiernik E, Maine D (1985) The prevention of preterm delivery through prenatal care: an intervention study in Martinique. Int J Gynaecol Obstet 23: 427-433

Herron MA, Katz M, Creasy RK (1982) Evaluation of a preterm birth prevention program: preliminary report. Obstet Gynecol 23: 427-433

Kessel SS, Villar J, Berendes HW, Nugent RP (1984) The channing pattern of low birth weight in the United States. JAMA 251: 1978-1984

Lazar P, Guegen S, Dreyfus J, Renaud R, Pontonnier G, Papiernik E (1984) Multicentered controlled trial of cervical cerclage in women at moderate risk of preterm delivery. Br J Obstet Gynaecol 91: 731-735

Papiernik E (1969) Coefficient de risque d'accouchement prématuré. Presse Med 77: 793-794

Papiernik E (1984) Proposals for a programmed prevention policy of preterm birth. Clin Obstet Gynaecol 27: 614-635

Papiernik E, Bouyer J, Dreyfus J, et al. (1985) The prevention of preterm births: the perinatal study of Haguenau. Pediatrics, 76: 154-158

Rumeau-Rouquette C, Du Mazaubrun C, Rabarison Y (1984) Naître en France: 10 ans d'évolution, vol 1. INSERM, Paris

Russell L (1984) The economics of prevention. Health Policy 4: 85-100

Sinclair J, Torrance G, Boyle M, Saigal S, Sackett D (1981) Evaluation of neonatal-intensive-care programs. N Engl J Med 305: 489-494

Stewart A, Reynolds E (1979) Intensive care and the very-low-birthweight infant. Lancet 846-847

Willems JS, Sanders CR, Riddiough MA, Belle JC (1980) Cost effectiveness of vaccination against pneumococcal pneumonia. N Engl J Med 303-553

Recent Follow-up Studies

Causes of Handicap and Impairment in a Total Population of Dundee (Scotland) Children Aged 8 Weeks to 7 Years

C. M. Drillien

Introduction

There are two main ways of carrying out folluw-up studies which try to relate perinatal events to outcome in the offspring. The first, which might be termed macroscopic, takes the broad-sweep approach, covering large populations, many data collectors and a rather limited number of specific categories of perinatal risk and childhood impairment. The United States Collaborative Project is the paradigm of this method. In the other approach, small samples of children are subjected to individual scrutiny, usually by those closely involved in their supervision. This is the method that I have chosen.

Since factors affecting child development are multiple and occur in many different combinations, there are obvious advantages in this microscopic approach. However, there is one major disadvantage: almost invariably these studies are carried out in so-called centres of excellence with high standards of perinatal care. Conclusions drawn from such centres about causes of handicap and the relation of perinatal factors to handicap could differ from those which might be deduced if the same method could be applied in areas where care and facilities are less adequate.

Dundee is an industrial city in decline. Over 20% of the population are unemployed and of the unemployed more than 40% have been unemployed for 1 year

Table 1. Perinatal mortality in Dundee

Mean perinatal mortality 1974-1983		
Dundee	12.1	
Scotland	15.6	
England and Wales	15.2	
Social class	Distribution of general population (%)	Perinatal deaths 1981-1985
I, II, III A	11.0	10.9
III B	38.0	25.0
IV, V	26.0	31.5
Unemployed	25.0	22.8

or longer. However, Dundee's perinatal record is excellent; antenatal care and special neonatal facilities are well developed. Table 1 shows that, in spite of widespread deprivation, the perinatal mortality rate in Dundee is 22% lower than that in Scotland overall or that in England and Wales. The lower half of the Table gives the distribution of perinatal deaths by social class and shows that this is approximately the same as the social class distribution within Dundee. There is no significant excess of wastage amongst the unskilled working class occupational groups nor amongst the unemployed as might be expected. This too suggests good quality of care in Dundee. Dundee also operates a comprehensive programme of total population screening for preschool developmental disorders and disabilities which facilitated the study to be presented here.

Study Sample

The study sample consisted of 5334 children born in 1974–1975 and resident in the city at any age from the first screening at 8 weeks to 5 years (I have no information about infants who moved out of Dundee before 8 weeks), and over 4000 children born in 1974–1975 who were attending city schools and institutions at age 7 years. About 85% of these samples were born in Dundee, virtually all in one National Health Service hospital, and 15% transferred in from outside.

Of the preschool group, 1.9% (that is, 104 children) were classified as handicapped - 93 came under my care, and 11 with specific conditions (such as visual defects and fatal genetically determined handicaps) were supervised elsewhere.

Categories of Handicap

Table 2 details the clinical categories to which the term 'handicap' was applied. Apart from 11 children (eight with cerebral palsy and three partially deaf and with

Table 2. Clinical conditions classified as "handicap"

Category of "handicap"	(*n*)	(%)
Mental retardation[a]	36	34
Cerebral palsy	18	17
Specific conditions with mental or physical disability[a]	10	10
Visual/hearing defects	10	10
Behavioural disorder[a]	17	16
Communication disorder[a]	8	8
Other	5	5
Total	104	100

[a] Requiring special education for ≥ 1 year

hearing aids) who entered normal school at the statutory age of 5–5½ years, all required at least 1 year of special education after that age.

Causes of Handicap

Table 3 shows what were considered to be the probable or possible prime causes of handicap after detailed examination of all suggestive causative factors in each individual case.

Postnatal Causes. There was no doubt about the cause of handicap in the six children who suffered postnatal brain damage from accident or infection.

Genetic/Familial Causes. Nor was there doubt about the 20 children who suffered from genetic and familial conditions.

Other Prenatal Causes. The presence of five or more minor congenital anomalies was considered highly suggestive of some adverse influence operating in early pregnancy. Twenty-four handicapped children presented thus. Common anomalies, such as epicanthic folds and vascular naevi, were not counted. Seven more children with no other suggestive cause for handicap had three or four minor anomalies. If these are included and added on to the 20 children with inherited defects, it can be said that in 49% of this sample handicap was certainly or probably due to prenatal causes.

Perinatal Causes. The handicaps of three children, all with cerebral palsy and normal intelligence, were attributed to very low birthweight and one more to neonatal complications. Six mildly mentally retarded children, all from poor homes, had a birthweight of less than 2200 g. Although none caused anxiety neonatally, handicap may be due in part to low birthweight in these cases. Low birthweight or trau-

Table 3. Probable or possible prime causes of handicap

Probable/possible causes of handicap	(*n*)	(%)
Genetic/familial	20	19
Prenatal MCA ≥ 5 (≥ 8)	24 (11)	23 (10)
? prenatal MCA 3–4	7	7
? pre-(MCA ≥ 5) ? perinatal	3	3
Perinatal ± social	10	10
Social/emotional	18	17
Postnatal	6	6
Not known	16	15
Total	104	100

MCA, minor congenital anomalies

matic delivery may have caused or contributed to handicap in three children who had evidence of early intrauterine insult. Thus overall, at the least, 4% of handicaps were most likely due to perinatal factors and, at the most, perinatal factors were, or may have been, involved in no more than 13%.

Social/Emotional Causes. Severe social and/or emotional deprivation was held responsible for 13% of handicaps.

Unknown Causes. In 15% of the cases no cause could be found. These children came from adequate homes with caring parents. Parents and siblings were of normal intelligence. No relevant family history was known. The children were of normal birthweight, appropriate for gestation and entirely normal neonatally. None exhibited more than two minor anomalies.

Causes by Severity of Handicap

The distribution of presumed aetiology differed with severity of handicap as shown in Table 4. Children classified as having severe handicap will need total or near-total care if they survive; some have already died. Moderately handicapped children are likely to require long-term special education and may need some supervision or assistance thereafter. Mildly handicapped children are expected to attain an independent life style and merge into the general population when adult.

Severe/Moderate Handicap. Prenatal causes predominate overwhelmingly amongst the more severely handicapped (65%). In only one child were perinatal factors probably involved and his case is worth quoting in more detail. He was the second child of a healthy, well-grown, intelligent woman. Pregnancy was uncomplicated and labour started spontaneously at 41 weeks. At 4 h the foetal heart rate dropped suddenly to less than 80 beats per minute and remained at this rate

Table 4. Causes of handicap by severity of the condition

Probable/possible causes	Handicap	
	Severe/moderate (%)	Mild (%)
Prenatal	65	23
? prenatal	–	12
? pre- ? perinatal	2	4
Perinatal ± social	–	18
Social/emotional	12	22
Postnatal	6	5
Not known	15	16
Total (%)	100	100
(*n*)	48	56

between contractions. Delivery was expedited by Ventouse extraction. The baby required external cardiac massage and prolonged ventilation. From the beginning he was grossly abnormal neurologically and the neonatal period was very stormy. He presented to me at 4 months as a severe spastic quadriplegic, profoundly retarded and epileptic. He was an odd-looking baby with microcephaly, widely spaced slanting eyes, a high arched narrow palate, abnormal palmar creases and long large first toes which were medially deviated. His obstetrician attributed his condition to injury at birth. I thought that this was a developmentally abnormal baby, possibly unable to withstand the stress of a normal labour, with superimposed anoxic brain damage. The parents were persuaded not to pursue litigation.

Mild Handicap. Amongst the mildly handicapped, prenatal and social factors head the list. Some mildly mentally retarded children had retarded parents and the prime cause of handicap could be genetic. They have been left in the social category because of the difficulty of disentangling genetic from environmental effects in these highly disorganised families. In this group of mild handicaps 7% were probably associated with perinatal factors (all of low birthweight) and these factors may have been involved in a further 15%.

Perinatal Hazards and Causes of Handicap

It is important to remember, especially when distraught parents are looking for someone to blame, that developmentally abnormal infants are prone to be of low birthweight, small for date and to have perinatal complications. Table 5 details some high-risk perinatal situations as they appeared in the birth histories of children with handicaps of probable or possible prenatal origin and those whose handicaps were due to other causes. Also given are the incidences of these complications in a randomly selected sample of infants from the general population. Neonatal complications recorded were moderate or severe. The composite additive score of four or more out of a maximum total of six indicates what would generally be accepted as severe complications of pregnancy, delivery and the neonatal

Table 5. Some high-risk perinatal factors in handicaps of prenatal and other aetiology

Perinatal complications	Cause of handicap		
	Prenatal (%)	Other (%)	Control (%)
Birthweight $\geq$ 2000 g	9	6	2
Small for date	36	10	9
Neonatal complications	18	8	3
Adverse score $\geq$ 4	14	4	3
Cases (*n*)	54	50	326

period. Table 5 illustrates the propensity of developmentally abnormal infants to be included in high-risk perinatal categories, even though these perinatal situations were very unlikely to be prime causes of handicap.

Severe Educational and Behavioural Problems in School

When children born in 1974-1975 reached the age of 7 years, a detailed questionnaire was completed by class teachers for all attending normal primary schools in the city. Amongst those experiencing the most severe schooling difficulties (all of them needing special help with lessons and most under supervision of the educational psychology department) there were 51 who had been pre-school patients of mine. Social disadvantage was the most striking feature amongst these children; 65% came from low social class families and/or from families known to have severe social difficulties. These school failures were carefully matched for sex, social class and specific social problems with an equal number of control children who had also attended my clinics pre-school but were coping reasonably well in school. The same perinatal hazards as were examined in Table 5 are detailed for these two groups of school children in Table 6. Only in the incidence of intrauterine growth retardation was there a statistically significant excess of a high-risk perinatal factor ($\chi^2=4.317$) amongst the problem children.

It was previously noted that in 36% of handicaps of prenatal origin infants were small for date. In this group of school failures the children were more than twice as likely to be small for date if they had three or more minor congenital anomalies than if they had up to two anomalies. The numbers are small and this difference is not statistically significant ($\chi^2=2.032$, applying Yates correction for small numbers). However, the 31% of problem children having multiple anomalies is significantly higher than the 14% of control children ($\chi^2=4.547$).

Table 6. Some high-risk perinatal factors in the birth histories of pupils with severe schooling problems and their controls

Perinatal complications	Problems in normal school	
	Severe (%)	Control (%)
Birthweight ≥ 2000 g	4	2
Small for date	25	10
Neonatal complications	4	6
Adverse score ≥ 4	6	8
Cases (*n*)	51	51
MCA ≥ 3 (*n*)	31	14

Impairment, Handicap, Neurology and Congenital Anomalies

There was only one other significant difference between the two groups of children in normal school and that was in the results of pre-school neurological examination as shown in Table 7. Only one-third of problem children were entirely normal neurologically pre-school compared with nine-tenths of controls. This suggests that minor cerebral damage or dysfunction is causally related to school failure.

Table 8 gives some indication of a tie-up between multiple minor congenital anomalies and early neurological abnormality, suggesting the possibility of a developmentally induced degree of cerebral dysfunction being of aetiological significance in handicap and impairment. In the top half of Table 8 are shown pre-school neurological findings and congenital anomalies in handicapped children, after excluding all with overt neurological defect, postnatal damage, specific syndromes and genetic conditions. The numbers remaining are small but, applying Yates correction to allow for this, there is still a statistically significant excess of

Table 7. Preschool neurological findings in pupils with severe schooling problems and their controls

Preschool neurology	Problems in normal school	
	Severe (%)	Control (%)
Abnormal	34	2
Doubtful	31	16
Normal	35	92
Total (%)	100	100
(*n*)	51	51

Table 8. Multiple minor congenital anomalies and neurological findings in handicapped children, and motor impairment in pupils with severe schooling problems

Handicapped	(*n*)	Preschool neurology	
		Abnormal (%)	Doubtful/normal (%)
MCA ≥ 3	30	63	37
MCA 0–2	21	29	71
School problems		**Motor impairment**	
		Marked (%)	Minor/none (%)
MCA ≥ 3	16	44	56
MCA 0–2	35	11	89

definite neurological abnormality in those having three or more minor congenital anomalies ($\chi^2 = 4.663$). The bottom half of Table 8 gives teachers' assessments of motor impairment at 7 years in children with severe schooling problems. Interestingly, marked motor impairment was recorded significantly more often for children whom I knew to have three or more minor anomalies ($\chi^2 = 5.005$).

Conclusions

In conclusion I would suggest that the concept of every child born perfect is a mirage. Unfortunately, this idea is taking hold amongst parents, possibly stimulated by the emphasis which we, in the business, put on an association between perinatal factors and handicap. If the child turns out to be less than perfect, there is an increasing tendency to find someone to blame. The most obvious scapegoat, particularly across the Atlantic, is the obstetrician. In Dundee we had (and have) handicapped children. In the great majority, no clinical expertise of obstetrician or neonatologist, or additional facilities, could have affected the outcome.

Reference

Drillien C, Drummond M (1983) Development screening and the child with special neads. Spastics International Medical, London

The Uruguayan Follow-up Study of Perinatal Events and Mental Handicaps

R. Ruggia, R. Belitzky, C. López de Cayaffa, A. Aznárez, J. L. Díaz Rossello, D. Fonseca, and R. Caldeyro-Barcia

Clinical Material

Only high-risk pregnancies were included in this study. This fact explains the high proportion of depressed and acidotic newly born infants reported here. All pregnancies were terminated by induction of labor with oxytocin infusion. Induction was made after 37 weeks since the last menstrual period. Babies weighing less than 2500 g and those born by cesarean section were not included in the study.

Methods

All labors were monitored. Uterine contractions and fetal heart rate (FHR) were recorded by internal methods (intrauterine pressure and fetal ECG) throughout the whole duration of labor. Since 1964, fetal blood samples have been obtained from the fetal scalp when FHR tracing has shown alarming signs. At birth the umbilical cord was clamped and pH, pO_2, pCO_2, and base deficit were measured in the fetal blood of the umbilical artery and vein.

Follow-up

The newly born infant was thoroughly examined and complete neurological studies were made at 1 and 24 h after birth and at discharge from the hospital (3–7 days after birth). The child was examined periodically (including EEG and psychometric tests) according to a given schedule.

All children having other diseases which may affect the central nervous system (such as severe malformations, diarrhea with dehydration, hydrocephalus, etc.) were not included in the folluw-up study.

The correlation between perinatal events and neonatal and postneonatal findings have been published elsewhere (Caldeyro-Barcia et al. 1969; Fonseca et al. 1971, 1972; Ruggia et al. 1971).

This paper concerns findings observed in children between 5 and 12 years of age.

Results

This paper studies whether there is any correlation between some perinatal events and psychomotor handicaps evaluated 5–12 years after birth.

Seizures and Abnormal EEG

Seizures

Presence of More than Three Type II Dips (Late Deceleration) in the FHR Tracing During the Last Hour Preceding Delivery

Figure 1 shows that the proportion of children with seizures is significantly higher in the group having more than three type II dips than in the control group. The difference is also significant if only the children with apiretic seizures are considered.

Seizures continued in only one child after this study finished. In the remaining children seizures were under control. Seizures appeared in children not having cerebral palsy and/or mental retardation, contrary to statements by Freeman (1985). These last two comments are also valid for seizures described in the next two sections.

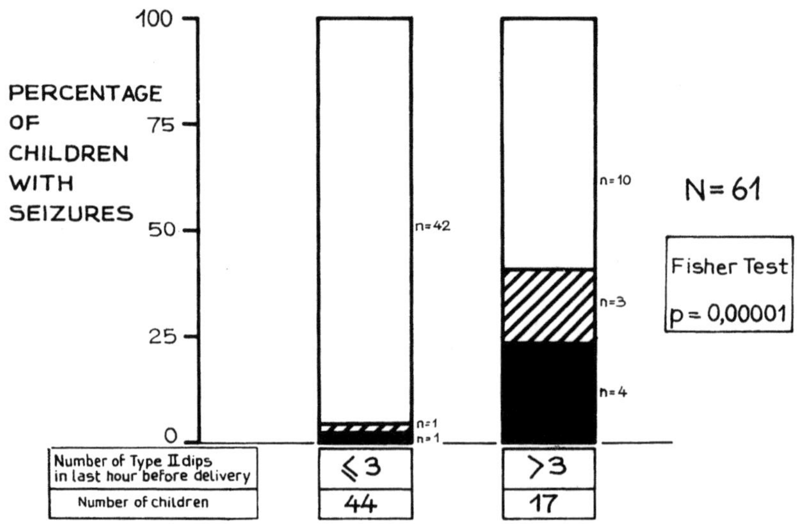

Fig. 1. Seizures – distribution according to the number of type II dips in the last hour before delivery. Age: 5 to 12 years; birthweight > 2500 g; gestational age > 37 weeks. □, Absent; ▨, febrile; ■, apiretic

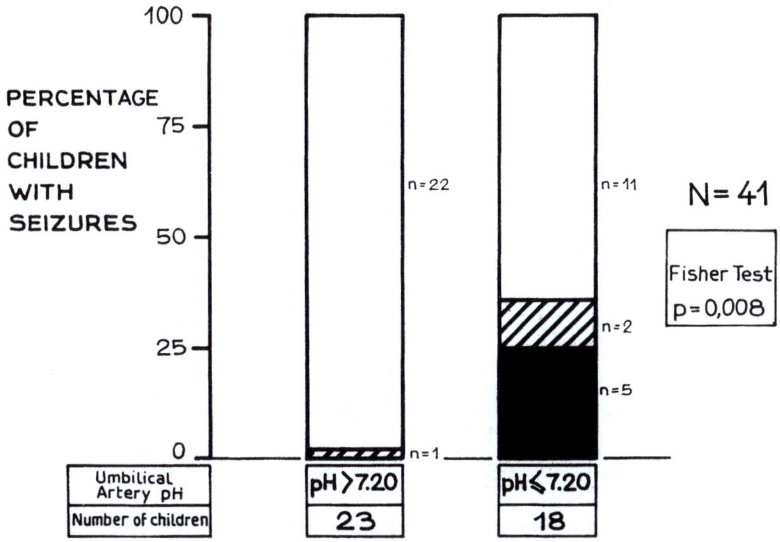

Fig. 2. Seizures - distribution according to umbilical artery pH at birth. Age: 5 to 12 years; birthweight > 2500 g; gestational age > 37 weeks. □, Absent; ▨, febrile; ■, apiretic

pH in Umbilical Artery Lower Than 7.20 at Birth

Figure 2 shows that the proportion of children with seizures is significantly higher in the group of children with actual pH of fetal blood in the umbilical artery lower than 7.20 at birth than in the control group (pH 7.20 or higher).

Very Low Apgar Score in the 1st min

Figure 3 shows that the proportion of children with apiretic seizures is significantly higher in the group which had a very low Apgar score (0–3) in the 1st min than in the other two groups with Apgar scores of 4–6 and 7–10.

The results shown suggest that a correlation might exist between some abnormal perinatal events and the presence of seizures in children between the ages of 5 and 12 years.

Abnormal Electroencephalogram

Presence of More than Three Type II Dips (Late Deceleration)
During the Hour Preceding Delivery

Figure 4 shows that the proportion of abnormal EEGs is significantly higher in the group of children who had more than three type II dips. This difference is also significant if only the "epileptic" EEGs are taken into account.

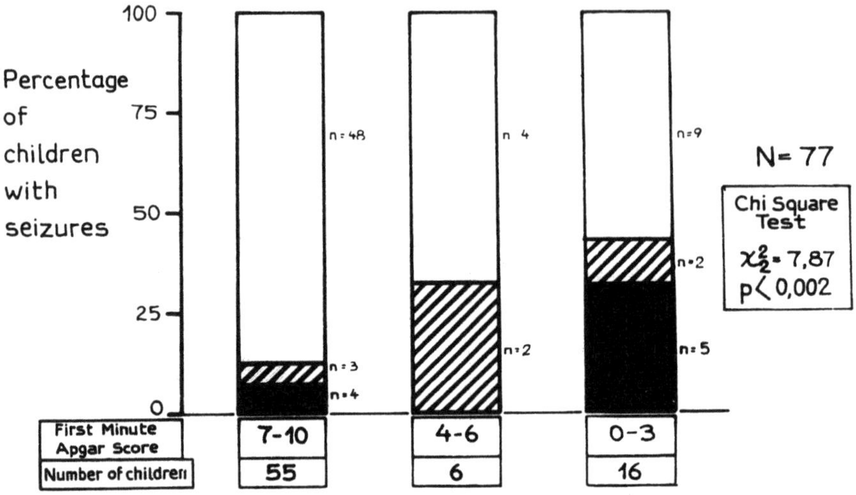

Fig. 3. Seizures - distribution according to 1st min Apgar score. Age: 5 to 12 years; birthweight > 2500 g; gestational age > 37 weeks. □, Absent; ▨, febrile; ■, apiretic

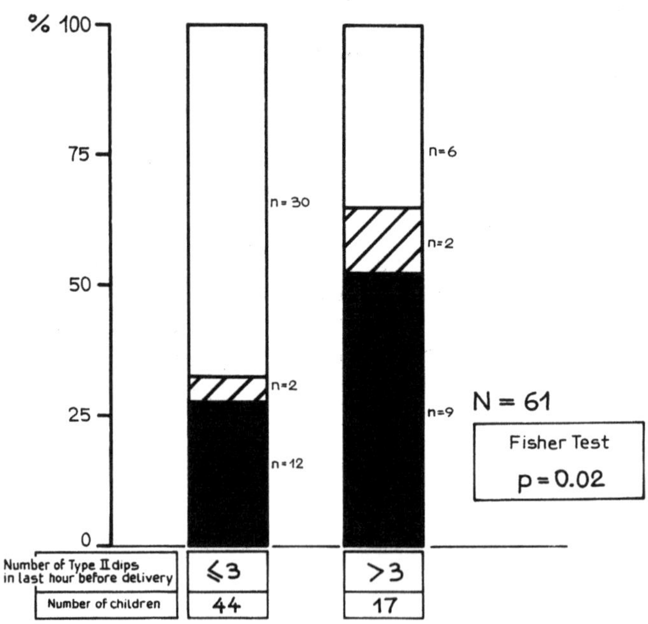

Fig. 4. EEG evolution - distribution according to the number of type II dips in the last hour before delivery. Age: 5 to 12 years; birthweight > 2500 g; gestational age > 37 weeks. □, Absent; ▨, febrile; ■, apiretic

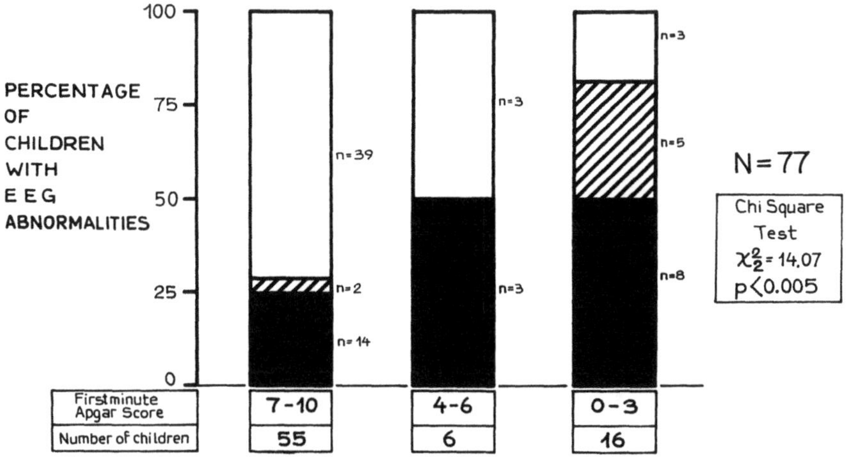

Fig. 5. Electroencephalographic evolution - distribution according to 1st min Apgar score. Age: 5 to 12 years; birthweight > 2500 g; gestational age > 37 weeks. □, Normal; ▨, nonepileptic; ■, epileptic

Table 1. Relation between perinatal events and psychologic evaluation in children aged 5-12 years

Apgar score in 1st min		Gesell test - adaptive behavior - age: 15-36 months	Terman Merril test IQ	WISC intelligence test	Bender test - differences between chronological and maturity ages at 6-10 years
0-3	*n*:	11	14	13	13
	$\bar{x}$:	98.55	94.14	89.54	7.69
	SD:	18.07	12.05	10.78	10.21
4-6	*n*:	4	6	5	5
	$\bar{x}$:	103.25	98.17	88.60	4.68
	SD:	8.46	6.43	4.93	5.94
7-10	*n*:	38	48	35	40
	$\bar{x}$:	99.11	94.75	87.46	8.33
	SD:	13.02	11.79	11.84	6.61

The differences between the different subgroups are not significant.

Low Apgar Score in the 1st min

The proportion of children with abnormal EEG (Fig. 5) is significantly higher in the group of infants who were born with very low (0-3) and low (4-6) Apgar scores than in the infants who were born with a high Apgar score (7-10) in the 1st min. The difference is also significant if only the epileptic EEGs are taken into account.

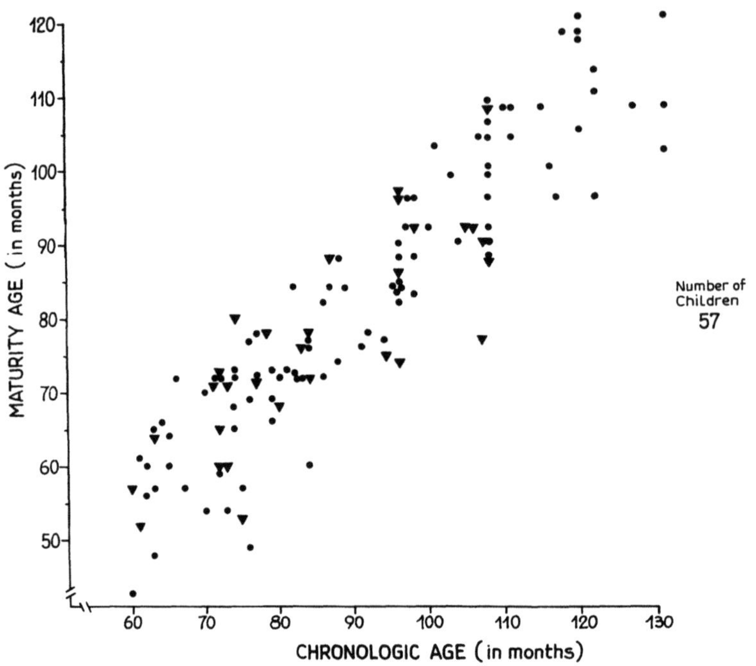

Fig. 6. Bender test motor-perceptive abilities - distribution according to 1st min Apgar score. Age: 5-12 years; birthweight > 2500 g; gestational age > 37 weeks. ●, Vigorous Apgar 7-10; ▼, depressed Apgar 0-3

Psychological Development

Very little, if any, correlation was found between ominous perinatal signs and the psychological development of children. This result agrees with the report by Freeman (1985).

Motor-Perceptive Abilities

These abilities, as measured with the Bender test (Fig. 6) between 5 and 12 years of age, showed no difference between children who had Apgar scores of 0-3 in the 1st min of life as compared with children in whom the Apgar score was 7-10.

Intelligence

Intelligence was measured with the WISC intelligence test using the difference (verbal) minus (performance IQ). There was the paradoxical result that the difference was lower (−1.95) for the group of children who had Apgar scores of 0-3 than for the group with Apgar scores of 7-10 (Fig. 7).

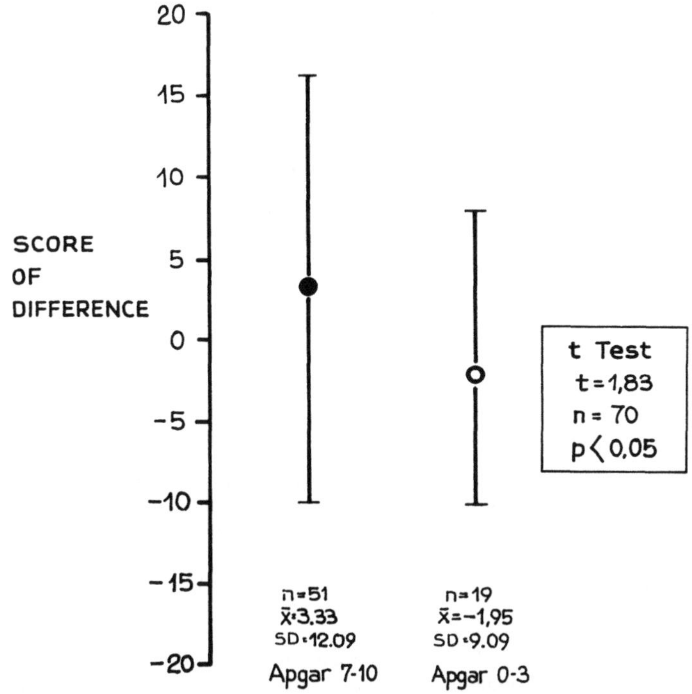

Fig. 7. WISC intelligence test difference: verbal-performance IQ - distribution according to 1st min Apgar score. Age: 5-12 years; birthweight > 2500 g; gestational age > 37 weeks

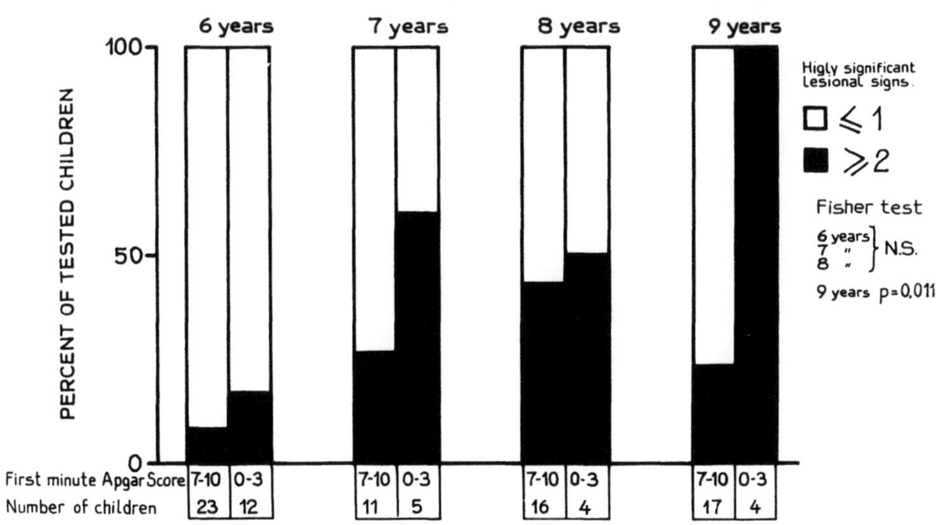

Fig. 8. Bender test (Koppitz) perceptive motor maturity - highly significant signs. Distribution according to 1st min Apgar score. Birthweight > 2500 g; gestational age > 37 weeks

Highly Significant Lesional Signs

Lesional signs were obtained using the Bender test for perceptive motor maturity using the Koppitz punctuation system. In Fig. 8, children are classified according to whether they had one or no sign or whether they had two or more signs. Comparison is made between groups of children having Apgar scores 0-3 with those with Apgar scores 7-10. No significant differences were found in children tested at 6, 7, and 8 years of age. A significant difference was found only in the children tested at 9 years of age.

References

Caldeyro-Barcia R, Casacuberta C, Bustos R, Giussi G, Gulin LO, Escarcena L, Méndez-Bauer C (1969) Correlation of intrapartum changes in fetal heart rate with fetal blood oxygen and acid-base state. In: Adamsons K (ed) Diagnosis and treatment of fetal disorders. Springer, Berlin Heidelberg New York, pp 205-225

Fonseca D, Díaz JL, Bernardi R, Bustos R, Ruggia R (1971) Alteraciones neurológicas del recién nacido con sufrimiento fetal agudo intraparto. 1er Congreso Latinoamericano de neuropediatría. Delta, Montevideo, pp 214-225

Fonseca D, Díaz JL, Bernardi R, Bustos R, Ruggia R (1972) Alteraciones neurológicas del recién nacido con sufrimiento fetal agudo intraparto. Estudios sobre el reflejo de Moro y sobre el tono muscular. Rev Argent Ginecol Obstet 3: 3

Freeman JM (1985) Prenatal and perinatal factors associated with brain disorders. National Institute of Child Health and Human Development. National Institute of Neurological and Communicative Disorders and Stroke. U.S. Department of Health and Human Services, NIH publication no 85-1149

Ruggia R, García Austt E, Fonseca D, Fasanello L, Bernardi R, Díaz JL (1971) Factores perinatales y presencia de anormalidades convulsivas y electroencefalográficas. 1er Congreso Latinoamericano de neuropediatría. Delta, Montevideo, pp 226-236

First Results of the Multicenter Finnish-Bavarian Study

K. P. RIEGEL and B. OHRT

The study we are going to describe is the third stage of an attempt to introduce quality control in regional peri- and neonatal care in Bavaria. The first step was the Munich perinatal study in 1975 (Selbmann 1980; Selbmann et al. 1977) which was succeeded by the Bavarian Perinatal survey in 1978 (Zander and Selbmann 1982) and spread to other states of the Federal Republic of Germany. Now approximately 75% of pregnancies and deliveries in the Federal Republic are followed and processed with identical questionnaires and program. Neonatal surveys of newborn infants referred to a children's hospital, based on the same principles, were adopted in Hannover and Munich in 1979. The latter started as a joint Finnish-Bavarian study (Riegel et al. 1985). From the beginning we intended to include a follow-up and this study on perinatal risks and early child development began in 1984.

Study Areas

The study population consisted of all newborn infants born during 1 year and admitted to a children's hospital in the study areas within 10 days of birth. Controls were to be recruited simultaneously from nonreferred newborn infants, matched only as far as place of residence was concerned. One study area is southern Bavaria, defined by the "catchment area" of the 19 children's hospitals in the region. These hospitals care for the sick newborn infants from approximately 65000 delivered per year in 165 obstetric units. For the comparison with Finland the region of Greater Munich (radius 30 km) was chosen. It has about 22000 deliveries per year, 24 obstetric and six children's hospitals. The Finnish study was carried out in the province of Uusimaa around Helsinki with 15000 deliveries per year, six obstetric units and five children's hospitals.

Table 1. Plan of study

	Gestation	Birth	Neonatal admission	Discharge	5 Months (corrected age)	20 Months (corrected age)
Family, socioeconomic and psychological aspects	————	————	——o	——o	——o	——o
Clinical events, course	————	——o	oooooooooooo		—o	——o
Placenta morphology	– – – –	o				
Physical state			o	o	o	o
Neurological state			o	(O)	o	o
Mental state					o	o

o, Documentation due; ——, period covered; (O), evaluation only if hospital stay exceeds 10 days

Plan of Study

Mainly financial reasons dictated the restriction of the study population to the referrals of 1 year and to having a follow-up with two tests only - one evaluation at a corrected age of 5 months (±2 weeks), the second at 20 months (±4 weeks) immediately following on the 5-month evaluation period. We shall try to continue until (at least) school-age with selected subgroups. We shall attempt to describe infants' health states and development by means of (at least) 18 different forms due at given times and investigating the environment, the obstetric and neonatal conditions, interim histories, physical, neurological, and mental (or functional) states (Table 1).

Time Course of Study

Enrollment of infants began April 1, 1985, and lasted until March 30, 1986. The 5-month evaluation started September 1, 1985. It will be finished in December 1986 with the beginning of the 20-month evaluation (until March 1988). It follows that the collection of data, even neonatal, is still going on. Completed forms have been checked for plausibility, etc., and added to our data bank for only about 65% of the expected neonatal sample and 15%-40% of the first follow-up (Table 2). For legal reasons, enrollment needed written consent of parents. Some Bavarian parents (2.5%) refused to participate, but none of the Finnish. After the newborn period, 3% of the Bavarians and 0.4% of the Finns withdrew consent or were lost. Fortunately, the majority of refusals refer to less problematic cases. Taking the deceased into account, we expect a drop-out rate of 6.6% of the Bavarian study cases and 3% of the Finnish ones in the first follow up. As can be seen in Table 2, the Finnish numbers are still too small for a meaningful evaluation.

Table 2. Cases registered by May 1 1986, in southern Bavaria (SBy) and southern Finland (SF), grouped according to birthweight

	-1000 g	-1500 g	-2000 g	-2500 g	>2499 g	Total (*n*)	Total (%)	Finally expect-ed
SBy Study group	99	208	515	1021	1739	4582	100	7249
Drop outs due to								
Hospital deaths	54	24	11	17	33	139	3.0	
Late deaths	–	–	1	2	3	6	0.1	
Withdrawals	1	2	10	26	121	150	3.3	
Control group	–	–	–	26	621	647	100	795
Withdrawals				–	10	10	1.5	
SF Study group	11	32	72	128	856	1099	100	1600
Drop outs due to								
Hospital deaths	5	6	8	3	8	30	2.7	
Withdrawals	–	–	–	1	2	3	0.3	
Control group	–	–	–	5	519	524	100	637
Withdrawals				–	3	3	0.6	

Table 3. Relative frequencies of selected items

	Southern Bavaria 1980–1981 (%)	Southern Bavaria 1985–1986 (%)	Finland 1980–1981 (%)
Perinatal survey referrals	9.5	10.3	8.9
Neonatal survey			
Pediatric transports	47.7	43.0	4.2
Gestational age < 32 weeks	6.6	6.7	6.6
Birthweight < 1500 g	6.9	6.7	6.0
Ventilated infants	17.5	13.8	8.7
Mean time on respirator (days)	7.9	5.2	5.1
Respiratory diseases	25.9	19.8	14.0
Hyaline membrane disease	16.0	10.7	7.5
Malformations	16.0	19.0	6.9
(Suspected) infections	24.4	25.2	19.0
Sepsis	6.8	8.3	2.4
Hospital mortality	6.2	3.0	3.1
Mortality < 1500 g	39.8	25.4	23.2

Profiles of Neonatal Care

Within 5 years, the perinatal landscape of Bavaria has changed considerably. Over the years the number of live born infants of less than 1000 g birthweight increased by 25%, but, more importantly, an increasing number of very low birthweight infants (< 1500 g) reach a children's hospital. Despite the former fact, mortality fell (Table 3). There are fewer pediatricly guided transports, which may reflect more referrals of high-risk women to a level 3 hospital. However, transports still exceed the Finnish figure for 1980–1981 by ten-fold. The frequency of ventilation decreased as did the mean length of stay on respirators. Not surprisingly, the incidence of respiratory diseases and, in particular, of hyaline membrane disease dropped. Whether, as compared with Finland, the relatively high frequencies of malformations and infections reflect different judgment in both countries is as yet unknown.

Health Profiles

There are many diseases a newborn infant may suffer from. Diseases can be classified according to the affected systems, to causes, and to severity (Riegel et al. 1985). An infant can be considered severely sick if one or more life-threatening diseases or events are present; negligibly or moderately sick if referral was for observation or for minor abnormalities. It is well documented that the infant's outcome is inversely related to the accumulation of risks, or, following Prechtl's concept (Prechtl 1977), to the sum of nonoptimal conditions. Among the obstetrical conditions, prematurity, malnutrition, and asphyxia play a predominant role. In a first attempt, the Bavarian study cohort was grouped into three gestational age periods, reduced obstetrical optimality (excluding prematurity), and two grades of sickness. Table 4 demonstrates that two-thirds of premature babies below 32 weeks of gestation are severely sick irrespective of the number of obstetrical risks. With increasing gestational age the percentages of severely sick newborn infants decrease in general but increase with risks, and mortality is clearly related

Table 4. Neonatal hospital morbidity as derived from diagnoses irrespective of number per infant, but graded as more or less relevant to infant's well-being (Riegel et al. 1985) and relative frequencies of a pathological neurological status at an age of 5–7 days, preliminary results

GA	<32 Weeks			32–36 Weeks			>36 Weeks		
Obst opt red	–8	>8	Total	–8	>8	Total	–8	>8	Total
(*n*)	171	125	302	908	312	1220	2385	210	2595
"Somatic" morbidity									
Negligible/moderate (%)	34	32	33	83	73	81	84	70	83
Mortality	9	7	8	0.3	0.4	0.3	0.5	1.4	0.5
Severe (%)	66	68	67	17	27	19	16	30	17
Mortality	19	36	30	5.7	11.2	7.7	4.3	7.6	4.3
Neurological status (5–7 days) pathological (%)	73	76	74	30	33	31	13	21	13

The Bavarian study cohort has been grouped according to gestational age (GA) classes with subgroups according to reduced obstetric optimality (Obst opt red, up to 8 and over 8 items out of 35, excluding GA). Figures in the table refer to percentages of frequencies of subgroups.

to risks. In terms of final outcome regarding sequelae, discrimination will be even better, because unfavorable neonatal conditions are to be added to the reduced obstetric optimality. It appears that Prechtl's concept and the grading of illness as applied are useful in describing our study population.

Neurological and Cognitive Follow up

Concept

The neurological and cognitive examinations have to evaluate the brain's maturity and integrity, and respective findings are to be correlated with all the conditions which could possibly interfere. Development is influenced by genetic determination, the course of pregnancy and delivery, health in the first years of life, socioeconomic factors and psychosocial conditions of the "environment." These influences need to be registered individually as outlined in Table 1. The concept of follow up is based on our previous experience, gained in particular from a 2-year retrospective study on the development of survivors of our intensive care unit. The following hypotheses were formed:

- The neurological assessment of the newborn infant in combination with the evaluation of pre- and perinatal risks is of high prognostic value in a postintensive care population. Additional consideration of the newborn infant's daily clinical course is of great importance.
- The prognostic value of the 5-month evaluation is increased when combined with the neonatal assessment.
- Premature infants may appear neurologically normal at about 40 weeks gestational age. This also applies to those who will later show severe neurologic impairment.
- Severe handicaps are already recognizable at 3-5 months of age, but the type of definite dysfunction is difficult to assess early in infancy.
- Some children who recover from neurological dysfunction during the first 2 years present minor neurological and learning problems again at an age of 4-5 years.

Methods

Pre- and perinatal risks are obtained from respective forms and documented on an optimal score form as suggested by Prechtl (1968). With increasing age, optimality items are added for the preceding period, thus respecting the dynamics of the developmental conditions.

The clinical course during the hospital stay is followed daily according to Casaer et al. (1982) but in a slightly modified manner. The concept of the neurological examination we use is based on suggestions of Prechtl (1977, 1982) and

Touwen (1976). The functional expression of every subsystem of the CNS has to be evaluated in a comprehensive and thorough assessment appropriate for age. The expected optimal neurological expression reflecting maturity and integrity of each system has been defined for each item, and possible deviant signs are also predefined in the forms. Our own neurological examination has developed over the years. The interscorer reliability was proven prior to the study.

Functional development is observed by means of the Griffith test (Brand 1983), as it is standard for German infants. Because of the limited value of such functional tests, the cognitive assessment at the age of 20 months will be completed by comprehensive observations of the child's play and social behavior in a free play session.

Although the 30 pediatricians participating come bimonthly for a 1-2-day seminar, confirmation of neurological examination and documentation needs long supervised training (a desirable side effect of the project). Thus, the aim of our study can only be to identify marked impairment of CNS function.

Results

The results must be regarded as very preliminary for several reasons, e.g., we report on unequally sized age groups; the sickest infants may still be hospitalized and some have not entered follow-up at the corrected age ("time lag" of very preterm babies); the cut-off points chosen for defining grades of neurological abnormality were too wide in our first data evaluation program. These restrictions need to be considered when looking at the figures of relative frequencies of a pathological neurological status at an age of 5-7 days in Table 4. It seems, though, that the figures compare favorably with those given for severe "somatic" morbidity, and that prematurity seems to outweigh other obstetric risks also with regard to neurology.

To give a short insight into the way we intend to analyze the data, two examples of selected patients in our hospital will be displayed. Figure 1 shows the changing spectrum of neurological findings within three gestational age groups during the 1 week, at discharge (which is close to 40 weeks gestational age with preterm babies), and at the (corrected) age of 5 months. As can be clearly seen, assessment at discharge can be misleading for the proposed expression of abnormal signs at this developmental stage. Two explanations may be offered (a) the infant may have recovered from the cerebral distress of the first days, and the impaired CNS system may still be in a prefunctional stage so that the neurological or cognitive disorder has not yet manifested; (b) our instruments for the neurological assessment of the preterm infant are still unsatisfactory in recognizing qualitative differences in the infants' neurological behavior. The findings are of practical relevance: the neurological status of a preterm infant must not be overemphasized at the time of discharge from hospital. Instead, frequent controls should be arranged for every child at high risk in order to recognize dysfunction early enough.

In Fig. 2, ten examples of Casaer's daily progress chart are shown. Obviously, the clinical course can be easily demonstrated from these. However, similar neona-

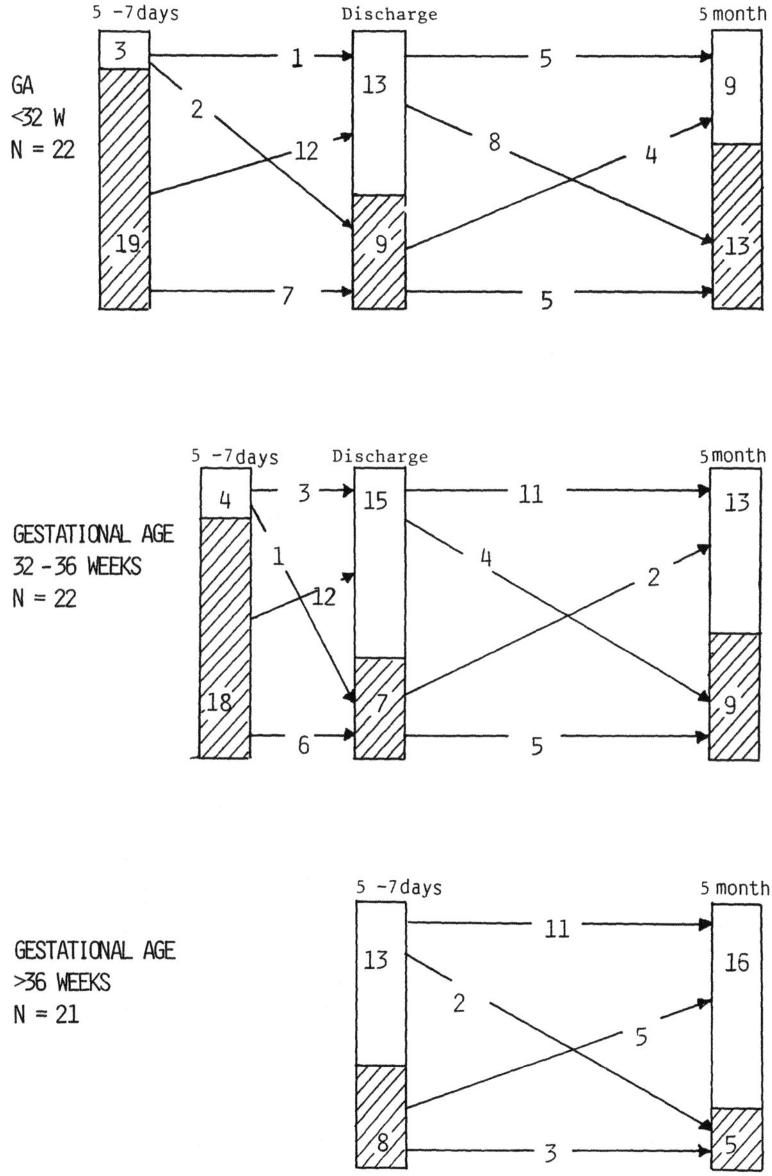

Fig. 1. Neurological findings on three gestational age *(GA)* groups of patients, aged 5–7 days, of our newborn intensive care unit at discharge (close to term), and at 5 months. The *height of columns* and the *figures* relate to number of cases. There is considerable "exchange" of normal and abnormal findings with age and rather little abnormality near term. ▨, Neurologically abnormal; □, neurologically normal

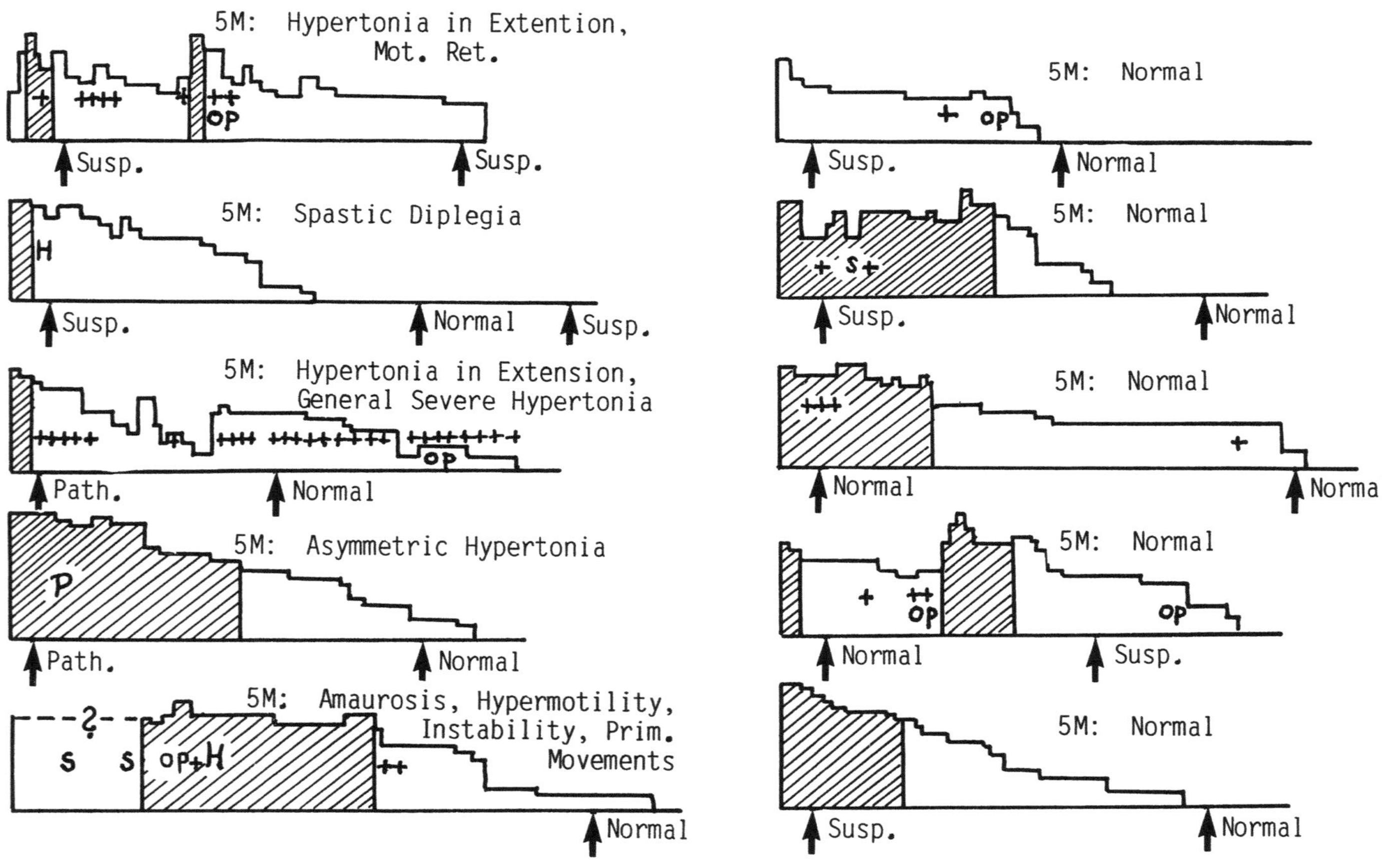

Fig. 2. Five-month outcome: neurologically abnormal *(left)* and normal *(right)* of ten premature infants (GA 26-31 weeks) related to neonatal hospital course as defined by the Casaer score. *S*, Septicemia; *op*, surgical intervention; +, apnea/bradycardia; *p*, pneumothorax; *H*, IVH; ↑, neurological examination; ▨, mechanical ventilation

tal courses with either favorable or unfavorable outcome at 5 months call for research into additional/associated factors in the preceding period.

Acknowledgement. This study was supported by the Bundesministerium für Forschung und Technologie (PKE 24), Bayerische Kommission für Perinatalogie der Bayerischen Landesärztekammer und Kassenärztliche Vereinigung Bayern.

References

Brand I (1983) Griffith Entwicklungsskalen. Beltz, Weinheim

Casear P, Eggermont E, Daniels H, Devlieger H, de Cock P, Willekens H, Jaeken J (1982) Neurological assessment in the neonatal special care unit. Pädiat Fortbildk Praxis 55: 144-166

Prechtl HFR (1968) Neurological findings in newborn infants after pre- and perinatal complications. In: Jonxis JHP, Visser HKA, Troelstra JA (eds) Aspects of prematurity and dysmaturity. Kroese, Leiden, pp 303-321

Prechtl HFR (1977) The neurological examination of the full-term newborn infant. Clin Dev Med, vol 63. Heinemann, London

Prechtl HFR (1982) Assessment methods for the newborn infant. A critical evaluation. In: Stratton P (ed) Psychobiology of the newborn. Wiley, London

Riegel K, Selbmann HK, Österlund K (1985) Perinatalrisiken und kindliche Mortalität und Morbidität. GSF, München

Selbmann HK (1980) Münchner Perinatal-Studie 1975-1977. Deutscher Ärzte-Verlag, Köln

Selbmann HK, Brach M, Höfling HJ, Jonas R, Schreiber MA, Überla K (1977) Münchner Perinatal-Studie 1975. Deutscher Ärzte-Verlag, Köln

Touwen BCL (1976) Neurological development in infancy. Lavenham, London

Zander J, Selbmann HK (eds) (1982) Wege zu einer verbesserten Perinatalversorgung. Deutscher Ärzte-Verlag, Köln

Neurological Sequelae of Infants with Very Low Birthweight in Hamburg. First Results of a Regional Study

N. VEELKEN, K. STOLLHOFF, P. WINKLER, K. HELMKE and F. J. SCHULTE

Introduction

Until 1979 the infant mortality rate in the Federal Republic of Germany used to be very high compared with most other developed countries. Since then, there has been a decrease in the mortality rate which now amounts to 9.0 per 1000 life births. This decrease is mainly due to better perinatal care and corresponds to a lowered perinatal mortality of 7.9 per 1000 births (Fig. 1). With lowered perinatal mortality, the question was raised whether a new population of handicapped children would be created by increasing perinatal survival of very low birhtweight (VLBW) infants. Research efforts have been initiated to evaluate the incidence of cerebral palsy (CP) in special risk populations in relation to mortality.

In Western Sweden, Hagberg and his co-workers were able to analyze a whole regional population of children with CP from 1954 to 1978, a period which

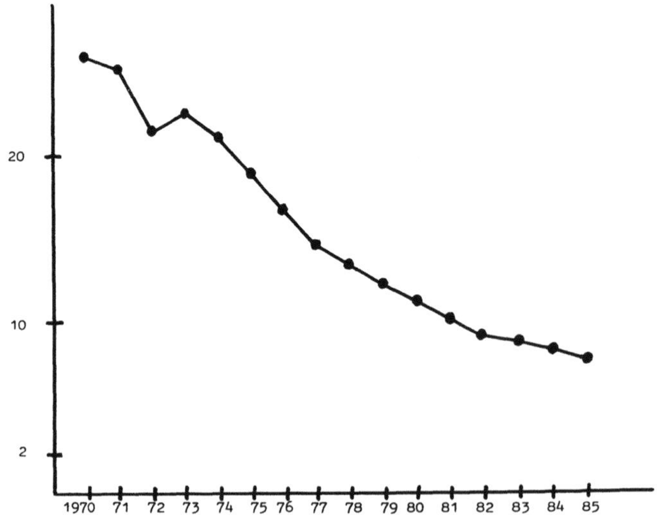

Fig. 1. Perinatal mortality rate in the Federal Republic of Germany from 1970 to 1985 per 1000 births

included the major changes in the incidence and in the panorama of CP caused by the results of modern intensive care (Hagberg and Hagberg 1984; Hagberg et al. 1975, 1984).

In the United States (Nelson and Ellenberg 1978) as well as in Australia (Dale and Stanley 1980; Stanley 1979; Stanley and English 1986) and more recently also in the Bavarian/Finnish study (see Riegel and Ohrt, this volume) a total population of newborn infants is being followed.

The third group of studies has evaluated the outcome of special risk groups, i.e., ventilated infants, severely asphyxiated infants, preterm infants with a gestational age below a certain number of weeks or infants with low or very low birthweight. With this classical approach, the study group of children was taken from one particular hospital or university. Therefore, the results are not representative for an unselected population. The overall handicap rate in a given risk group of infants is likely to be higher if patients are not selected from specially equipped neonatal intensive care units with highly motivated personnel.

We, therefore, embarked on a study to evaluate the developmental outcome of all children born in Hamburg with a birthweight of less than 1500 g. Figure 2 shows the geographical area of Hamburg with points marking the location of six neonatal intensive care units where all VLBW infants are taken care of. Five obstetric departments are in the immediate vicinity of the neonatal care units, 57% of the VLBW infants are transferred by a neonatal transport system.

The birth rate in Hamburg has remained constant over the last few years and amounts to 12000 in a population of 1.56 million. The rate of low birthweight infants (<2500 g) is 6% and the group of <1500 g is about 1% of all live births. For 1983-1986 the survival rate of VLBW infants was about 65%. The population of surviving VLBW infants has doubled since 1977.

Methods

From 1983-1986 all VLBW infants born in Hamburg were enrolled in the study; about 450 children are now being thoroughly evaluated (Table 1). The first neurological examination was done at 40 weeks conceptional age, and the infants were re-examined at 6, 12, and 18 months (corrected age). At the same time, developmental testing was performed using the Griffith developmental scale. Further evaluation of both neuro- and psychological development, as well as hearing capacity will be performed at 4 and 6 years of age. At 6 months of age, ultrasound examination was done by two experienced pediatric radiologists who were not informed about the perinatal history and the results of former examinations. The age of 6 months was chosen for practical reasons and since at this age permanent morphological brain damage due to infarcts and/or bleeding is clearly demonstrable.

Repeated ophthalmological examinations were done in all infants to detect and follow retinal changes as well as other abnormalities like myopic and hyperopic changes, astigmatism and squint. Standardized documentation of prenatal,

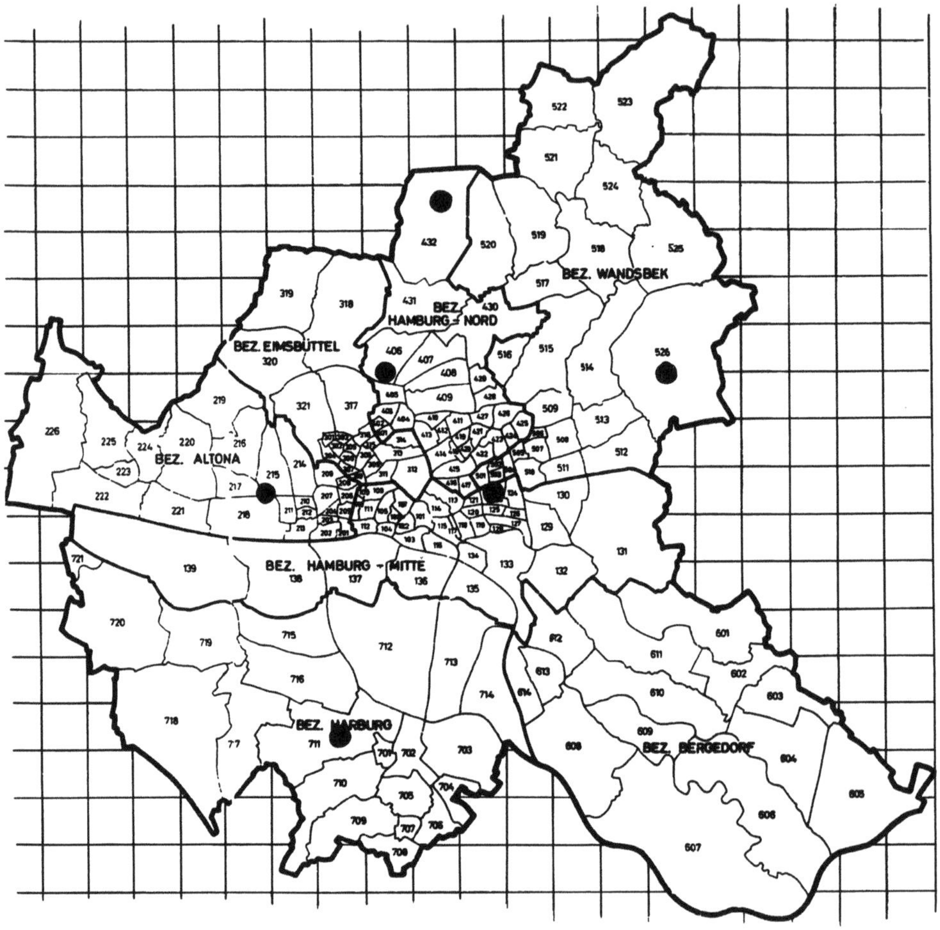

Fig. 2. Geographical area of Hamburg (FRG) marking the location of the six neonatal intensive care units

Table 1. Design of the regional follow-up study of all surviving VLBW infants in Hamburg over a 3-year period

Neurological examination	At term At 6, 12 and 18 months of age (corrected after GA) At 4 and 6 years of age
Griffith developmental scale	At 6, 12, and 18 months of age (corrected after GA)
Testing of mental capacity	At 4 and 6 years of age
Cerebral ultrasound	At 6 months of age (corrected after GA)
Repeated ophthalmological examinations	
Audiometry	At 2 and 4 years of age
Analysis of obstetric and pediatric journals	

perinatal, and neonatal events is part of our study and will be the subject of a later publication.

This study design has some advantages over previous research into the complex problem of preterm infant development: (a) Hamburg is a clearly defined region with a uniformly distributed health care system; (b) the loss to follow up rate is not only reasonably low but we were also able to get at least some information about the children who could not be examined longitudinally; (c) there is no selection of children with special risk factors from one hospital or university with particular facilities and expertise; (d) finally, we were able to have all examinations performed by two examiners only and intend to follow the study population up to school age by including one psychologist and one speech therapist.

Results

In the 1st year, 147 VLBW infants survived the neonatal period (Fig. 3), five died later during infancy. Eighteen cases were lost to follow up. According to reliable information from their private doctors, in nine of these infants motor function is quite normal. Two are still being ventilated because of severe bronchopulmonary dysplasia and there are only seven cases (4.8%) where we do not know the outcome. Thus, we were able to evaluate 124 children (Table 2): 85 (68.5%) had a birthweight appropriate for gestational age (AGA), and 39 (31.5%) were small for gestational age (SGA).

Sixteen (12.9%) of the 124 cases developed clear signs of CP (Table 3). Of these 16 children, 14 had some degree of spastic diplegia: five were able to walk inde-

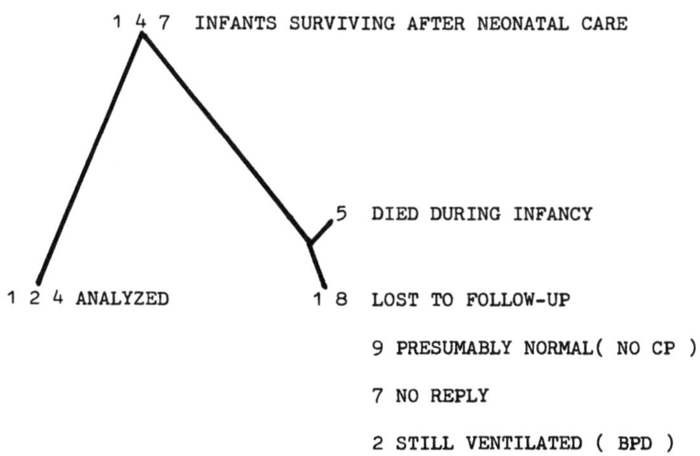

Fig. 3. Study population of the 1st year's analysis - total number and cases which were lost to follow up. *BPD*, broncho pulmonary dysplasia

Table 2. Study population of the 1st year's (July 1983-July 1984) analysis - birthweight and rate of SGA infants

Birthweight (g)	Cases	
	(*n*)	(%)
1250-1500	46	37.1
1000-1249	42	33.9
800- 999	30	24.2
<800	6	4.8
All cases	124	100.0
SGA	39	31.5

Table 3. Total number and different syndromes of CP

		Cases
Spastic diplegia		14
	Mild	5
	Moderate	4
	Severe	5
Spastic hemiplegia		1
Dystonic cerebral palsy		1

pendently (mild spasticity) at age 18 months, four had achieved at least some kind of locomotion (moderate spasticity) and five were unable to move around (severe spasticity); these five children could be classified as tetraplegic. One child seemed to have spastic hemiplegia. The ultrasound, however, showed bilateral ventricular dilatation with some accentuation of the side corresponding to the hemiplegia, better defined as hemilateral tetraplegia. The only child with aggressive hydrocephalus treated by a shunt had dystonic CP. All but two CP cases were in the AGA group (Table 4). The two SGA infants who developed CP were quite immature with a gestational age of 29 and 31 weeks, respectively. The birthweight of the children with CP did not differ significantly from the entire group. In the group with a birthweight below 800 g there was no case with CP. The rate of CP in the group < 1000 g was only slightly higher (13.9%) than in the group with a birthweight > 1000 g (12.5%). In addition to CP, there was marked developmental delay. However, these results are preliminary since the children are still too young for a final developmental diagnosis. Fourteen children had a developmental quotient (DQ) below 80, eight (57%) were SGA. Nineteen children with a DQ between 80 and 90 were classified as borderline.

Prolonged mechanical ventilation was only a weak additional risk factor for the development of CP (Table 5). Fifty percent of the children with CP, compared with 36% of the total group, were ventilated for more than 28 days. As to the ultrasound findings, there was a clear correlation between severe ventricular dilatation

Table 4. Differences in the rate of CP and developmental delay between AGA and SGA infants

	CP		DQ<80		DQ 80-90		Normal	
	(*n*)	(%)	(*n*)	(%)	(*n*)	(%)	(*n*)	(%)
AGA	14	16.5	6	7.1	11	12.9	54	63.5
SGA	2	5.1	8	20.5	8	20.5	21	53.9

Table 5. Duration of mechanical ventilation of VLBW infants in relation to intrauterine growth retardation, CP, and developmental retardation

	None		1-7 days		8-14 days		15-28 days		28 days	
	(*n*)	(%)	(*n*)	(%)	(*n*)	(%)	(*n*)	(%)	(*n*)	(%)
AGA	13	15.3	24	28.2	8	9.4	6	7.1	34	40.0
SGA	14	35.9	10	25.6	2	5.1	2	5.1	11	28.2
CP	-	-	7	43.8	-	-	1	6.2	8	50.0
DQ<80	3	21.4	-	-	1	7.1	2	14.3	8	57.1

Table 6. Ultrasound findings in VLBW infants in relation to CP and developmental retardation

Outcome		Abnormalities on ultrasound		
		None	Slight	Severe
Normal	(*n*)	62	8	1
CP	(*n*)	1	2	12
DQ<80	(*n*)	11	-	3
DQ 80-90	(*n*)	13	2	2
All	(*n*)	87	12	18
	(%)	74.3	10.3	15.4

and CP (Table 6). There was only one child with mild spastic diplegia showing no abnormalities on ultrasound. Eleven (78.5%) of the children with marked developmental delay had normal cerebral morphology on ultrasound.

Discussion

This regional study of the development of preterm infants gave slightly more pessimistic results than those which were obtained from single hospitals or universities with a high standard of knowledge, motivation, and equipment. The difference in the CP rate amounts to about 13% (regional) versus 8%-10% (single units) (Haas et al. 1983; 1986b; Stewart et al. 1981). It is quite obvious that the regional figures are more realistic for the population as a whole. Studies from Sweden have emphasized that with decreasing perinatal mortality the rate of cerebral handicap might increase again (Hagberg et al. 1984). Similar figures are not available for the Federal Republic of Germany or any other country and they are, therefore, still open to discussion and interpretation. It is at least feasable that the slight increase in CP in western Sweden during the most recent past has been the result of a methodological error, i.e., more CP children were detected because of greater sensitivity of the medical as well as paramedical profession. It is, however, also possible that intensive care management, particularly of the very small preterm infants, ascertained survival of more brain-damaged children or even included adverse factors which can cause brain damage. It is, therefore, mandatory to longitudinally examine for developmental outcome versus perinatal mortality. As in previous studies, CP in our series of VLBW infants occurred mainly in AGA infants, whereas SGA infants were prone to developmental delay. It has recently been shown by de Vries and her co-workers (De Vries et al. 1983) that periventricular leucomalacia detected by ultrasound is most likely to be indicative for CP. This assumption has been strongly confirmed by our regional results. Therefore, periventricular infarcts rather than only bleeding are a most valuable, though negative, prognostic sign.

Summary

The neurological prognosis of VLBW infants has been widely evaluated in the last few decades. However, the information has been derived from studies covering the population of single and highly equipped intensive care units. Representative figures for an entire region are still rare. This is particularly true for the Federal Republic of Germany. Therefore, in 1983 a prospective follow-up study of all VLBW infants born in Hamburg was initiated. Neurological examinations were done at term and at 6, 12, and 18 months thereafter. Re-examinations will follow at 4 and 6 years of age. Ultrasound studies were performed at 6 months corrected age. The results were based upon the evaluation of the 1st year's population at age 18 months. Mortality for this group of infants was 34%. A total of 147 infants survived the neonatal period. Five died later during infancy, 18 were lost to follow up. Sixteen (12.9%) of the 124 children thus evaluated had CP, 14 suffered from spastic diplegia, one from hemiplegia and one from dystonia. In addition, 14 (11.3%) children were severely retarded (DQ < 80). Fourteen children with CP were appropriate for gestational age. Developmental retardation without CP was mainly encountered in infants who were small for gestational age. The CP rate in the group below 1000 g was slightly higher (13.9%) than in the group with a birthweight between 1000 and 1500 g (12.5%). Prolonged artificial ventilation was only a weak additional risk factor for later CP. Twelve (80%) of the cases with CP had major ventricular dilatation in ultrasound. Fifteen (83%) with major abnormalities on ultrasound had either CP (12 or 67%) or severe developmental retardation (3 or 17%).

References

Dale A, Stanley FJ (1980) An epidemiological study of cerebral palsy in Western Australia, 1956-1975. II. Spastic cerebral palsy and perinatal factors. Dev Med Child Neurol 22: 13-25

De Vries LS, Dubowitz V, Lary S, Whitelaw A, Dubowitz LMS, Kaiser A, Silverman M, Wigglesworth JS (1985) Predictive value of cranial ultrasound in the newborn baby: a reappraisal Lancet I: 137-40

Haas G, Buchwald-Saal M, Mentzel H, Michaelis R (1983) Mortalität und neurologische Morbidität bei ehemaligen Frühgeborenen und untergewichtigen Termingeborenen. Monatsschr Kinderheilkd 131: 735-5

Haas G, Buchwald-Saal M, Leidig E, Mentzel H (1986a) Improved outcome in very low birthweight infants from 1977 to 1983. Eur J Pediatr 145: 337-40

Haas G, Asprion B, Leidig E, Buchwald-Saal M, Mentzel H (1986b) Obstetrical and neonatal risk factors in very low birthweight infants related to their neurological development. Eur J Pediatr 145: 341-6

Hagberg B, Hagberg G (1984) Prenatal and perinatal risk factors in a survey of 681 Swedish cases. In: Stanley FJ, Alberman E (eds) The epidemiology of the cerebral palsies. Clin Dev Med no 87. Spastics Int Med, Oxford

Hagberg B, Hagberg G, Olow I (1975) The changing panorama of cerebral palsy in Sweden 1954-1970. II. Analysis of the general changes. Acta Paediatr Scand 64: 187-92

Hagberg B, Hagberg G, Olow I (1984) The changing panorama of cerebral palsy in Sweden. IV. Epidemiological trends 1959-78. Acta Paediatr Scand 73: 433-40

Nelson KB, Ellenberg JH (1978) Epidemiology of cerebral palsy. Adv Neurol 19: 421-34

Stanley FJ (1979) An epidemiological study of cerebral palsy in Western Australia 1956-1975. I. Changes in total incidence of cerebral palsy and associated factors. Dev Med Child Neurol 21: 701-13

Stanley FJ, English DR (1986) Prevalence of and risk factors for cerebral palsy in a total population cohort of low-birthweight (<2000 g) infants. Dev Med Child Neurol 28: 559-68

Steward A, Reynolds EOR, Lipscomb AP (1981) Outcome for infants of very low birthweight: survey of world literature. Lancet I: 1038-40

Appendix

Perinatal Mortality Statistics of the Avon County (UK) Population, 1976–1985, Using FIGO 1982 Methodology

P. M. DUNN and C. B. VULLIAMY

The FIGO Standing Committee on Perinatal Mortality and Morbidity had its first meeting under the chairmanship of Professor Kubli in Heidelberg in 1982. The report of that workshop on Monitoring and Reporting Perinatal Mortality and Morbidity was formally approved by FIGO at its meeting in San Francisco later that year. It was then published and widely circulated in the form of a red booklet (International Federation of Gynecologists 1983). All FIGO members were requested to follow the guidelines contained in the Report and regularly make such statistics available either to FIGO headquarters or directly to P. M. Dunn, who, as Chairman of the FIGO sub-committee on perinatal epidemiology and health statistics, had been asked to collate such statistics as they became available. Not unexpectedly, progress has been slow and by the time of the World Congress of Gynaecology and Obstetrics in September 1985 only a handful of countries had provided comparable data. However, it is clear from correspondence that considerable progress is being made in many countries in persuading government departments and others to adopt the standard methodology. It is our hope that at the next World Congress in Brazil in 1988 it will be possible to achieve a much more complete account of perinatal mortality throughout the world. The 1986 workshop on Perinatal Events and Cerebral Handicap tackled the much more difficult task of long-term perinatal morbidity occurring in babies that survive this most dangerous period; however, it is not inappropriate that we should also remember those who die.

The 1982 FIGO recommendations on perinatal mortality statistics were based on, and entirely compatible with, those made by the World Health Organization in 1976 and published in the 9th edition of the International Classification of Diseases (ICD) (WHO 1979). They were that *national* perinatal mortality statistics should include all fetuses or infants weighing 500 g or more (equivalent approximately to 22 weeks' gestation) whether alive or dead. However, for *international* comparison, data should be confined to fetuses and infants weighing 1000 g or more (roughly equivalent to 28 weeks' gestation). In addition, the FIGO Working Party pointed out that as the number of preventable perinatal deaths fell with improved care, an increasing proportion of the residual deaths would be due to lethal malformation. If perinatal mortality statistics were to be used to evaluate the effectiveness of care, then it was important to be able to distinguish deaths due to lethal malformation from those due to other causes.

The question arose as to what constitutes a lethal congenital anomaly or malformation. This was defined as the death of a baby with a malformation (see ICD, chapter 14) (WHO 1979) when the malformation was considered to be responsible for the train of events leading to the fatal outcome. In order to avoid subjective decisions, it was felt best to *include* those cases when the train of events leading to death might have been interrupted by different management. Thus the following examples ought to be classified as deaths from lethal malformation: an infant with undiagnosed duodenal atresia who vomits and dies from aspiration pneumonia; an infant with a myelocele who is not operated on and dies from meningitis; an infant with a diaphragmatic hernia who dies during surgery. On the other hand, an infant with a minor malformation such a polydactyly or hare lip who dies from some unconnected cause such as infection should not be classified as a lethal malformation. One area of difficulty requires special mention. This is the case of the infant who dies as a result of respiratory problems, possibly due to pulmonary hypoplasia secondary to oligohydramnios. In this difficult area, which may not even be clarifed by necropsy, it is necessary to make an arbitrary decision: this is that in such circumstances the diagnosis of pulmonary hypoplasia as a lethal malformation is acceptable provided that the infant also shows evidence of external compression in the form of at least two congenital postural deformities (Dunn 1976).

The 1982 FIGO methodology for reporting perinatal statistics has been in use in Bristol since 1970 (Dunn 1980). In 1974 the Royal Borough of Bristol was extended to form Avon County and since 1976 population perinatal statistics have been collected for all births to Avon residents. The first 5 years 1976-1979, involving 36, 810 births have been reported elsewhere (Mutch et al. 1981). This brief report extends our results through the second quinquennium. First it may be appropriate to give some demographic details of the area.

The County of Avon is in the west of England on the south-eastern shore of the Bristol Channel which partially separates England from Wales. It has an area of 1341 km^2 and a population of approximately 900000. About half the population lives in the city of Bristol while the remainder lives in five small towns and the surrounding rural area. The social class distribution when last studied by us in 1977 was not appreciably different from the rest of England and Wales. There are approximately 10000 births to Avon residents each year. The great majority of these births, over 95% of them, take place in the two main maternity hospitals (the Bristol Maternity Hospital and Southmead Hospital) which also contain the departments of obstetrics and child health of the University of Bristol. Perhaps most important from the point of view of population study, Bristol is the main referral centre for a wide area extending far beyond the boundaries of Avon County and Avon residents are *not* referred out of the county for obstetric care or delivery.

During the whole decade 1976-1985 there were 95459 births weighing $\geqslant 500$ g to Avon residents. There were 594 stillbirths making an overall stillbirth rate of 6.2/1000. The SB rate trends over the decade may be seen in Fig. 1. It is interesting to observe how the three lines in the figure converge with the passage of time. We interpret this secular change as being due to, on the one hand, the prenatal diagnosis of babies with lethal malformation and their abortion and, on the other, to improved diagnosis of fetal distress in the second trimester, coupled with an increased use of elective delivery. As a result most stillborn fetuses now have a birthweight of > 1 kg and fewer are malformed.

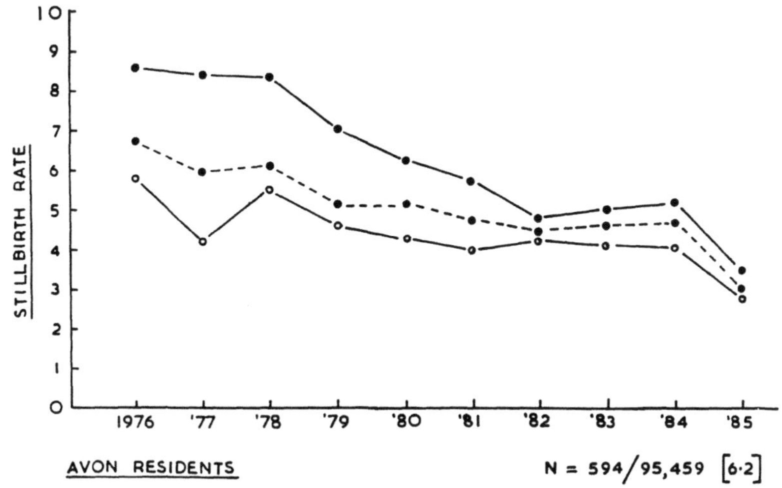

Fig. 1. Stillbirths rates for Avon residents, 1976-1985 (see text). ●——●, Total; ●----●, minus malformations; ○——○, minus malformations plus↓1 kg

Among the 94868 live births ⩾ 500 g during the decade there were 672 neonatal deaths, making an overall neonatal mortality rate of 7.1/1000. As may be seen in Fig. 2, once again the trend has been steadily downwards. The number of infants with lethal malformations has clearly diminished over the decade, once again no doubt due to improved prenatal diagnosis. The number of deaths associated with a birthweight < 1 kg at first increased but thereafter has remained fairly steady. The first of these changes was undoubtedly due to the fact that in 1977 we instituted intensive care for these tiny babies. Our success no doubt encouraged our obstetric colleagues to extend elective delivery, when appropriate, down into the second trimester, occasionally even as low as 25 weeks' gestation. Since 1977 the proportion of survivors in this extremely low birthweight group has more than doubled to 61%. The fact that the number of neonatal deaths has altered little in the last 5 years is attributable to an increasing incidence of notified live births (Dunn 1985; Dunn and Lashford 1984).

The trends for perinatal mortality may be seen in Fig. 3. Among the 95459 births there were 1132 stillbirths and early (1st week) neonatal deaths, making an overall perinatal rate for births ⩾ 500 g of 11.9/1000. Once again there is an encouraging downward trend in all three curves, though it is the lowest of the three which is the most meaningful; it excludes the very tiny babies, the reporting of whom is very variable from country to country, and also the infants with lethal malformations whose incidence again varies greatly from place to place and whose survival is only marginally affected by the standard of perinatal care.

In order to re-emphasise the way in which it is hoped that FIGO members will collect and report their perinatal statistics, we have included a Table (Table 1) showing the figures for Avon residents during the year 1985. Once again, it is the "bottom line" in which we should be most interested, as it reflects most accurately

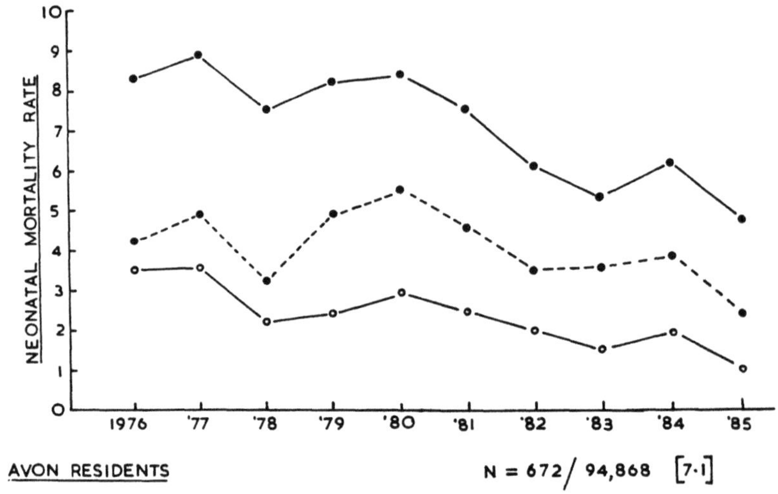

Fig. 2. Neonatal mortality rates for Avon residents, 1976–1985 (see text). ●——●, Total; ●- - - -●, minus malformations; O——O, minus malformations plus↓1 kg

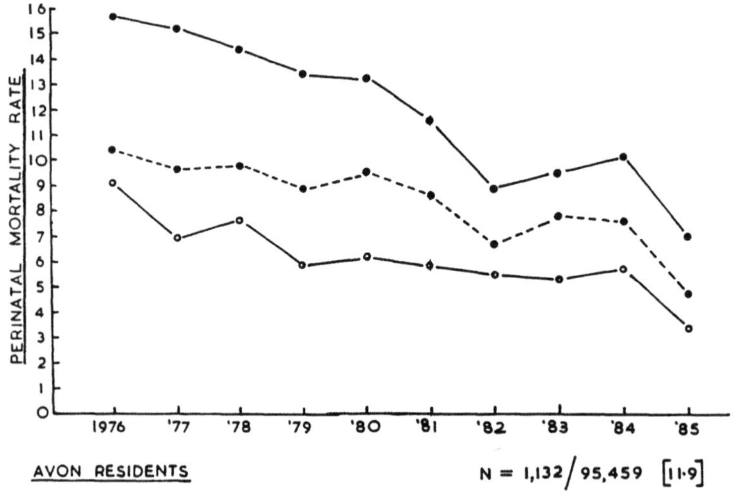

Fig. 3. Perinatal mortality rates for Avon residents, 1976–1985 (see text). ●——●, Total; ●- - - -●, minus malformations; O——O, minus malformations plus↓1 kg

the standard of obstetric and neonatal care. As may be seen, among the 10146 births ⩾ 500 g the mortality rates, after excluding lethal malformations and birthweight < 1 kg, were: stillbirth mortality rate: 2.8/1000, perinatal mortality rate: 3.5/1000 and neonatal mortality rate: 1.3/1000. In actual numbers this represents 28 stillbirths, 35 perinatal deaths and 13 neonatal deaths. With such small numbers, it is no major task to scrutinise each death individually. In respect to the

Table 1. Perinatal mortality statistics[a] for babies of Avon residents born in Avon, UK, in 1985 (excludes all births < 500 g, $n = 5$)

Number of total births ≥ 500 g	10146
Number of stillbirths ≥ 500 g	36
Number of live births ≥ 500 g	10110
Number of early (1st week) neonatal deaths	35
Number of late (2nd–4th weeks) neonatal deaths	12
Number of perinatal deaths	71
Number of births < 1 kg	39
Number of stillbirths < 1 kg	2
Number of early neonatal deaths < 1 kg	13
Number og late neonatal deaths < 1 kg	1
Number of infants with lethal malformations	28 (2 < 1 kg)
Number of stillbirths with lethal malformations	6
Number of early neonatal deaths with lethal malformations	17 (2 < 1 kg)
Number of late neonatal deaths with lethal malformations	5
Perinatal statistics	
Lethal malformation rate per 1000 total births (28/10146)	2.8
Stillbirth rate per 1000 total births (36/10146)	3.6
Neonatal mortality rate per 1000 live births (47/10110)	4.7
Perinatal mortality rate per 1000 total births (71/10146)	7.0
Excluding lethal malformations (includes < 1 kg)	
Stillbirth rate per 1000 total births (30/10118)	3.0
Neonatal mortality rate per 1000 live births (25/10088)	2.5
Perinatal mortality rate per 1000 total births (48/10118)	4.7
Excluding births < 1 kg (includes malformations)	
Stillbirth rate per 1000 total births (34/10107)	3.4
Neonatal mortality rate per 1000 live births (33/10096)	3.3
Perinatal mortality rate per 1000 total births (56/10109)	5.5
Excluding lethal malformations and births < 1 kg	
Stillbirth rate per 1000 total births (28/10091)	2.8
Neonatal mortality rate per 1000 live births (13/10045)	1.3
Perinatal mortality rate per 1000 total births (35/10091)	3.5

[a] Format according to recommendations of a report of the FIGO Committee on Perinatal Mortality and Morbidity following a workshop on Monitoring and Reporting Perinatal Mortality and Morbidity, Heidelberg, March 1982.

28 stillbirths, the most clearly defined group were eight associated with placental abruption. There was then a large group of 15 less well-defined antenatal deaths, five of which were associated with placental insufficiency and fetal growth retardation, three with suspected cord complications, two were macerated twins, one was born to a mother with diabetes and four were macerated (no cause found). There were four fresh stillbirths that appeared to be caused by intrapartum asphyxia, one following shoulder dystocia. The factors associated with the 13 neonatal deaths were easier to define: five near-stillbirths as the result of severe birth asphyxia, four due to the respiratory or intraventricular haemorrhage complications of preterm delivery, two due to infection, while one was a "cot death". The cause of the remaining death remained in doubt, though an inborn error of metabolism was suspected.

It remains for us to make one more plea. In submitting perinatal and mortality statistics, it would be helpful and illuminating to include information on the incidence of low birthweight ($\leqslant$2500 g) in each population. Throughout the world this varies form 4% to 40% or more, and clearly identifies one of the most important factors underlying perinatal death.

Acknowledgement. Dr. Vulliamy was supported by a research grant from the Van Neste Foundation.

References

Dunn PM (1976) Congenital postural deformities. Br Med Bull 32: 71-76

Dunn PM (1980) Perinatal Statistics, 1970 - 3. In: House of Commons Social Services Committee Session 1979-80 (eds). Second report: perinatal and neonatal mortality, vol 2. HMSO, London, pp 256-67

Dunn PM (1985) Fetal viability: a perinatal viewpoint. In: Beard RW, Sharp F (eds) Preterm labour and its consequences. Proc. 13th study group Royal College of Obstetricians and Gynaecologists. RCOG, London, pp 295-301

Dunn PM, Lashford AM (1984) Limit of fetal viability. Lancet I: 1079

International Federation of Gynecologists and Obstetricians' Standing Committee on Perinatal Mortality and Morbidity. In: Report following a workshop on monitoring and reporting perinatal mortality and morbidity, Heidelberg, 1982. FIGO, London

Mutch LM, Brown NJ, Speidel BD, Dunn PM (1981) Perinatal mortality and neonatal survival in Avon: 1976 - 9. Br Med J 282: 119-122

World Health Organization (1979) Definitions and recommendations. International classification of diseases, 9th edn, vol 1. WHO, Geneva, pp 763-768

MIX
Papier aus verantwortungsvollen Quellen
Paper from responsible sources
FSC® C105338

If you have any concerns about our products,
you can contact us on
ProductSafety@springernature.com

In case Publisher is established outside the EU,
the EU authorized representative is:
Springer Nature Customer Service Center GmbH
Europaplatz 3, 69115 Heidelberg, Germany

Printed by Libri Plureos GmbH
in Hamburg, Germany